ic Press is an imprint of Elsevier
eet, Suite 1800, San Diego, CA 92101-4495, USA
stown Road, London NW1 7BY, UK
man Street, Waltham, MA 02451, USA

British Library Cataloguing-in-Publication Data
A catalogue record for this book is available from the British Library

Library of Congress Cataloging-in-Publication Data
A catalog record for this book is available from the Library of Congress

ISBN: 978-0-12-411464-7

For information on all Academic Press publications
visit our website at elsevierdirect.com

Printed and bound in the United States of America

14 15 16 17 18   10 9 8 7 6 5 4 3 2 1

GLOBAL CLINICAL TRIALS FOR ALZHEIMER DISEASE

Design, Implementation, Standardization

Edited by

MENGHIS BAIRU, MD
President and Chief Executive Officer
Speranza Therapeutics Corp, Dublin, Ireland
Chief Medical Officer and Head of Global Development
Elan Pharmaceuticals
Cambridge, Massachusetts, USA

MICHAEL W. WEINER, MD
Director of the Magnetic Resonance Unit at the VA Medical Center
Professor of Radiology, Medicine, Psychiatry and Neurology
University of California at San Francisco, School of Medicine
San Francisco, California, USA

ELSEVIER

AMSTERDAM • BOSTON • HEIDELBERG • LONDON
NEW YORK • OXFORD • PARIS • SAN DIEGO
SAN FRANCISCO • SINGAPORE • SYDNEY • TOKYO

Academic Press is an imprint of Elsevier

Academ
525 B St
32 Jame
225 Wy

Copyr

No pa
in any
other

Perr
Dep
ema
wel

No
N
or
o
B

International Editorial Advisors

GLOBAL CLINICAL TRIALS FOR ALZHEIMER'S DISEASE

Edited by
Menghis Bairu & Michael W. Weiner

Praise for *Global Clinical Trials for Alzheimer's Disease: Design, Implementation, and Standardization*

Edited by Menghis Bairu, MD and Michael W. Weiner, MD

Global Editorial Board Members: Ezio Giacobini, Jean Georges, Maria Carillo, Michael Grundman, Marc Wortmann and Susan Abushakra

"Alzheimer's disease is among the most critical problems facing the world's aging populations. For this global epidemic, we need not a few national plans, but rather a well-coordinated, ambitious international plan. This book, written by outstanding experts in AD clinical trials, surveys the landscape and lays down the groundwork essential for progress."
—Paul Aisen, MD, Director, Alzheimer's Disease Cooperative Study and Professor, Department of Neurosciences, University of California, San Diego, School of Medicine, San Diego, CA

"Alzheimer's disease is quite possibly the largest worldwide medical problem of this decade. Despite a great deal of research and discussion about the disease in the U.S. and Europe, a global solution to making progress in the field is seldom discussed. *Global Clinical Trials for Alzheimer's Disease* is an excellent resource for anyone interested in solving the Alzheimer's Disease challenge as it offers real world solutions to achieving successful clinical trials globally."
—Dale Schenk, PhD, President and CEO of Prothena Corporation, San Francisco, CA

"Alzheimer's disease is rapidly becoming perhaps the most important disease in modern society. Development of new therapies for this disease is a very important yet challenging task. This book covers every aspect of the field and will doubtlessly become the seminal textbook for the development of new therapies for Alzheimer's disease."
—Richard Chin, MD, CEO, Kindred Bio, Burlingame, and Associate Professor, University of California, San Francisco School of Medicine, San Francisco, CA

Contents

I

ALZHEIMER'S DISEASE: THE TWENTY-FIRST CENTURY EPIDEMIC

II
GLOBAL ALZHEIMER'S DISEASE: CLINICAL TRIALS

III
CHALLENGES AND OPPORTUNITIES TO CONDUCT GLOBAL ALZHEIMER'S DISEASE CLINICAL TRIALS

IV

GLOBAL REGULATORY ENVIRONMENT SURROUNDING ALZHEIMER'S DISEASE TRIALS

V

STANDARDIZATION OF DIAGNOSTIC AND OUTCOME MEASURES IN GLOBAL ALZHEIMER'S DISEASE TRIALS

VI

OPERATIONALIZATION OF GLOBAL ALZHEIMER'S DISEASE TRIALS

VII

ENHANCING LOW AND MIDDLE INCOME COUNTRIES' CAPACITY AND CAPABILITY TO CONDUCT ALZHEIMER'S DISEASE TRIALS

VIII

PHARMACOGENETICS AND PHARMACOGENOMICS CONSIDERATIONS

IX

HUMAN RESOURCES PLANNING

Preface

Alzheimer's Disease (AD) is *the* 21st Century epidemic. Today, nearly 35 million individuals worldwide live with Alzheimer's-related dementia. By 2050, that number will more than triple to 115 million, a potentially catastrophic global challenge already impacting families, social service and healthcare delivery systems in every nation on earth. In 2010, Alzheimer's-related costs were estimated at $604 billion, approximately one percent of the world's GDP, and rising. AD impacts far more than the individual victim: family members, the first line of care in much of the world, suffer additional billions in lost income and life opportunities.

In 2011, President Barak Obama could have been addressing an audience far beyond the U.S. borders when he declared, "... Alzheimer's Disease burdens an increasing number of our elders and their families. It is essential that we confront the challenge it poses to our public health."

Time grows short. Of the 193 World Health Organization (WHO) member nations, fewer than 10 have implemented comprehensive national AD strategies, all of which are developed countries. Despite billions invested in research, and a clearer understanding, for example, of AD's etiology and pathology, no cure or effective treatment is in sight.

Sixty percent of Alzheimer's victims—the majority still undiagnosed—live in lesser developed countries; by 2030, that figure will top 75 percent, with the heaviest burden on Africa, Asia, and Latin America. Like the disease itself, the clinical trials vital to AD advances will take place in the developing world. Here, too, the clock is ticking, with much of the groundwork—including addressing the stigma so often associated with the disease—still to be done.

Global Clinical Trials for Alzheimer's Disease: Design, Implementation, and Standardization provides a clear blueprint for the road ahead. It is a comprehensive, yet detailed analysis—drawing on the knowledge and insight of the world's leading experts—of the benefits, challenges, costs, design, implementation, standardization, ethics, efficacy, and regulatory considerations necessary to conduct effective Alzheimer's trials in the developing world. From the field, researchers and public health officials review decades of clinical studies, as well as strategies being developed in Latin America, India, China, Korea, Turkey, and elsewhere; lessons that provide invaluable insight and hands-on experience for the next generation of AD researchers.

Global Clinical Trials for Alzheimer's Disease is also a call to action. The great challenge of the next decades will be to find the resources, financial and humanitarian, to better care for those afflicted with AD, and to refine and redouble research efforts to develop new therapies, and hopefully, the cure. As we see in these pages, this will require a collaboration of all stakeholders—academia, the pharmaceutical industry, public health organizations both domestic and international, and, foremost, the patients in the developing world who will be both subjects as well as the measurement of our success in the difficult battle ahead.

Menghis Bairu
Michael W. Weiner

About the Editors

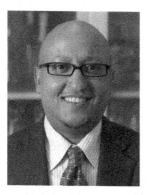

Menghis Bairu, M.D.—physician, editor, author, philanthropist and healthcare business executive—has more than two decades of international experience in the biotechnology, pharmaceutical, global health and non-profit arenas. Dr. Bairu serves as Executive Vice President, Chief Medical Officer and Head of Global Development at Elan. His responsibilities include, but are not limited to clinical development, biometrics, regulatory, CMC, QA, safety-and-risk management, clinical operations and medical affairs. Previously he served as head of Onclave Therapeutics, a wholly Elan-owned oncology biotech company.

He lectures extensively on global health and biopharmaceutical issues with particular focus on Emerging Markets (e.g. India, China, Latin America, Singapore, Middle East, South East Asia and Africa). He served as editor and co-author of *Global Clinical Trials: Effective Implementation and Management* (Elsevier, 2011), a textbook designed to help researchers develop and implement effective and ethical international clinical trials. Dr. Bairu is also editor/co-author of *Global Clinical Trials Playbook: Management and Implementation* (Elsevier, 2012).

Prior to joining Elan, Dr. Bairu worked at Genentech for more than five years in a number of managed care, medical and commercial (Oncology, Immunology, and Cardiovascular) roles. He served as managed care Medical Director for Fremont Health Corporation/II before joining Genentech. He served on the board of directors for One World Health, a nonprofit drug development company funded by the Bill and Melinda Gates Foundation and A-Cube, a privately held pharma startup.

In 2013, Dr. Bairu was named to the boards of directors of Dubai-based NewBridge Pharmaceuticals (he also serves as chairman of NewBridge's science and technology committee), and ADVentura Capital SL, a Barcelona, Spain-based venture capital firm focused on funding and mentoring promising healthcare, IT and GreenTech companies. In 2011, Dr. Bairu joined the advisory board of the China Trials 5, a global clinical trials development summit focusing on China and north Asia. He currently serves as Adjunct Faculty at the University of California San Francisco School of Medicine where he lectures on global clinical trials' design, development and conduct.

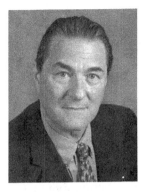

Dr. Michael W. Weiner attended Johns Hopkins University and the State University of New York, and worked at Mount Sinai Hospital in New York (Resident), and Yale University (Fellow). After service in the US Air Force, in 1971 at the University of Wisconsin he was awarded a VA Research Associate at the Madison VA. Subsequently he was awarded a VA Clinical Investigatorship and relocated to the Palo Alto VA/Stanford University, where he received the Young Investigator Award of the American College of Cardiology in 1976. In 1980 he performed the first experiment using implanted coils to obtain 31P NMR spectra from the kidney of living rats, beginning his work using NMR/MRI for research. Since 1980 he has been at the San Francisco VA/UCSF. Dr. Weiner is currently Director of the Center for Imaging of Neurodegenerative Diseases. He is Professor of Radiology, Medicine, Psychiatry, and Neurology at UCSF. He has published over 600 peer reviewed scientific papers. His grants include studies of Alzheimer's Disease, vascular dementia, frontotemporal dementia, HIV/AIDS, gulf war illness, posttraumatic stress disorder, traumatic brain injury, amyotrophic lateral sclerosis, epilepsy, and other neurodegenerative conditions. He is the Principal Investigator of: the NIA funded Alzheimer's Disease Neuroimaging Initiative (ADNI)/Grand Opportunities (GO) Grant, and the renewal of ADNI (total funding over $150 million for these 3 grants). Recently he was awarded a grant from the DOD entitled *Effects of traumatic brain injury and post traumatic stress disorder on Alzheimer's Disease in Veterans using ADNI*. In 2006, Dr. Weiner was awarded the Middleton Award, for outstanding research in the VA. He was awarded the Gold Medal of Paul Sabatier University in Toulouse France, and the Gold Medal of the city of Toulouse, France in 2010. In 2011 he accepted the Ronald and Nancy Reagan Research Award from the Alzheimer's Association on behalf of ADNI. In 2013, Dr. Weiner was awarded the Potamkin Prize for Research in Pick's, Alzheimer's, and Related Diseases from The American Academy of Neurology and The American Brain Foundation.

List of Contributors

Susan Abushakra Élan Pharmaceuticals, San Francisco, California, USA

Ricardo F. Allegri MD, PhD, FAAN Aging and Memory Center, Neurological Research Institute, Buenos Aires, Argentina

H. Michael Arrighi PhD Janssen Research and Development, South San Francisco, California, USA

Pablo M. Bagnati Aging and Memory Center, Neurological Research Institute, Buenos Aires, Argentina

Menghis Bairu MD Chief Medical Officer and Head of Global Development, Elan Pharmaceuticals, Cambridge, Massachusetts, USA and President and Chief Executive Officer, Speranza Therapeutics Corp, Dublin, Ireland

Sonia Brucki MD Department of Neurology, University of São Paulo School of Medicine, Sao Pãulo, Brazil

Tal Burt MD Duke Global Proof-of-Concept Research Network, Duke Clinical Research Unit and Duke Clinical Research Institute, Department of Psychiatry and Behavioral Sciences, Duke University, Durham, North Carolina, USA

Lorne Cheeseman Anidan Inc, Irvine, California, USA

Richard Chin MD Kindred Bio, Burlingame, San Francisco, California, USA

Debbie N. Cote Debbie Cote Associates, California, USA

Jeffrey Cummings MD Cleveland Clinic Lou Ruvo Center for Brain Health, Las Vegas, Nevada, USA

Stephanie Danandjaja MD Sanofi, Singapore

P. Murali Doraiswamy MD Departments of Psychiatry and Medicine, and the Duke Institute for Brain Sciences, Duke University, Durham, North Carolina, USA

Murat Emre MD Department of Neurology, Istanbul University Faculty of Medicine, Istanbul, Turkey

James (Dachao) Fan MD, MBS ICON Clinical Research, Singapore

Yoko Fujimoto PhD, MD Pfizer Japan Inc, Japan

Michel Grothe PhD DZNE, German Center for Neurodegenerative Diseases, Rostock, Germany

Ibrahim Hakan Gürvit MD Department of Neurology, Istanbul University Faculty of Medicine, Istanbul, Turkey

Spencer Guthrie MBA, PMP Genentech, Elan, Jansen Alzheimer's Immunotherapy and Ultragenyx Pharmaceutical, Novato, California, USA

Harald Hampel MA, MD, MSc Department of Psychiatry, University of Frankfurt, Germany

Lynne Hughes BMedSci, PhD, PMP   Quintiles, Reading, Berkshire, UK

Michael Hüll   University of Freiburg Medical School, Freiburg, Germany

Hilal İlbars PhD   Turkish Medicines and Medical Devices Agency, Ankara, Turkey

Takeshi Iwatsubo MD, PhD   Department of Neuropathology and Neuroscience, University of Tokyo, Japan

Roy W. Jones BSc, FRCP, DipPharmMed   Research Institute for the Care of Older People, Royal United Hospital, Bath, and University of Bath, Bath, UK

Nadina C. Jose MD   Anidan Group Pte Ltd, Singapore

Amir Kalali   Quntiles Inc, USA

Seong Yoon Kim MD, PhD   Department of Psychiatry, Asan Medical Center, University of Ulsan, Seoul, Korea

Miia Kivipelto MD, PhD   Karolinska Institute, Gävlegatan, Stockholm, Sweden

Amos D. Korczyn MD, MSc   Tel Aviv University, Ramat Aviv, Israel

Bernd J. Krause MD   Department of Nuclear Medicine, University of Rostock, Germany

Jens Kurth   Department of Nuclear Medicine, University of Rostock, Germany

Huafang Li MD, PhD   Shanghai Mental Health Center, Shanghai, China

Francesca Mangialasche MD, PhD   Aging Research Center, Karolinska Institutet-Stockholm University, Stockholm, Sweden

Zeev Meiner MD   Hadassah Hebrew-University Hospital, Jerusalem, Israel

Hans J. Möbius MD, PhD   EnVivo International, Brunnen, The Netherlands

Ricardo Nitrini MD   Department of Neurology, University of São Paulo School of Medicine, Sao Pãulo, Brazil

Tiia Ngandu MD   National Institute for Health and Welfare, Helsinki, Finland

Muriel O'Byrne PhD   Elan Pharma International Ltd, Dublin, Ireland

Peter Schüler MD   Global Medical and Safety Services, ICON Clinical Research, Germany

Klaudius Siegfried PhD   ICON Clinical Research, Germany

Sidney A. Spector MD   VA Medical Center, Phoenix, Arizona, USA, and Global Biopharma, Scottsdale, Arizona, USA

Stefan Teipel MD   DZNE, German Center for Neurodegenerative Diseases, Rostock, Germany and Department of Psychosomatic Medicine, University of Rostock, Rostock, Germany

Yağiz Üresin MD   Department of Pharmacology, Istanbul University Faculty of Medicine, Istanbul, Turkey

Bruno Vellas MD, PhD   University Hospital Center, Toulouse, France and Clinical Nutrition Laboratory University of New Mexico, USA

Michael Weiner MD   UCSF Professor of Medicine, Radiology, Psychiatry & Neurology, University of California, California, USA

Jing Yin   ICON Clinical Research Pte Ltd, Singapore

Xue (Kate) Zhong MD   Cleveland Clinic Lou Ruvo Center for Brain Health, Las Vegas, Nevada, USA

Dedication

This book is dedicated to Alzheimer's Disease (AD) patients, caregivers, all clinical investigators, and research and development industry colleagues that continue to work hard so that our kids, nephew and nieces don't face the devastating global impact of AD.

This book is also dedicated to all international AD expert authors that have been the source of strength and inspiration since the inception of this project. We want to thank everyone at Elsevier for their hard work and invaluable help.

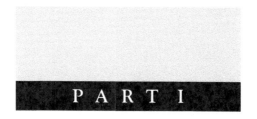

PART I

ALZHEIMER'S DISEASE: THE TWENTY-FIRST CENTURY EPIDEMIC

CHAPTER 1

The Epidemiology and Prevention of Alzheimer's Disease and Projected Burden of Disease

Tiia Ngandu[1,2], Francesca Mangialasche[3] and Miia Kivipelto[1,2,3,4]

[1]Department of Chronic Disease Prevention, National Institute for Health and Welfare, Helsinki, Finland [2]Alzheimer's Disease Research Center, Karolinska Institutet-Stockholm University, Stockholm, Sweden [3]Aging Research Center, Karolinska Institutet-Stockholm University, Stockholm, Sweden [4]Department of Neurology, University of Eastern Finland, Kuopio, Finland

1.1 OCCURRENCE OF DEMENTIA AND ALZHEIMER'S DISEASE

The occurrence of dementia, and its major subtype, Alzheimer's disease (AD), is strongly influenced by age. The prevalence of dementia nearly doubles every five years after the age of 60. The World Alzheimer Report 2009 by Alzheimer's Disease International (ADI) estimated that currently the age-standardized prevalence for those aged 60 or older is 5–7%. Among persons aged 60–64 years the prevalence is 0.7–1.8%, but among those aged over 90 years, the prevalence is 29–64% [1,2]. Several other meta-analyses have reported fairly similar prevalence estimates even if methods of individual studies have not been identical [3,4]. With the aging of populations, the prevalence of dementia and AD is increasing rapidly. It is estimated that in 2010 there were 35.6 million demented people worldwide. This number is expected to increase to 115.4 million

M. Bairu & M.W. Weiner (Eds):
Global Clinical Trials for Alzheimer's Disease.
DOI: http://dx.doi.org/10.1016/B978-0-12-411464-7.00001-8

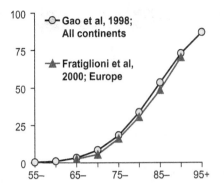

FIGURE 1.1   Incidence of dementia by age per 1000 person years [90].

by 2050 if efforts to prevent the disease fail [2]. The greatest increase is expected in less developed countries, in which the annual growth rate of older adults (aged 60+) is higher than in more developed countries. Indeed, by 2050, nearly 80% of the world's older population is expected to live in less developed countries, making dementia a global challenge [5].

The incidence of dementia and AD increases almost exponentially with age [6] (Figure 1.1). The pooled incidence from European studies among people aged 65 or above was 19.4 per 1,000 person-years [6]. The total number of new cases of dementia each year worldwide is nearly 7.7 million [7]. There are indications that the incidence rate might plateau or even decline among very old people [8]. A recent report also proposed that there may be a decline in the dementia incidence over time, but this remains to be confirmed [9].

AD is the most important cause of dementia. It accounts for between 50 to 70% of all dementia cases [6,10]. The majority of AD cases are sporadic, while the familial forms caused by autosomal dominant mutations are very rare. There is increasing evidence from population-based neuropathological and neuroimaging studies showing that mixed brain pathologies (AD, vascular) account for most dementia cases, especially among very old people [11]. This has relevant implications for the planning of preventive and therapeutic measures, since in the general population 70% of all dementia cases occur in people aged 75 or older [6].

1.2 RISK FACTORS FOR DEMENTIA AND AD

AD is a multi-factorial syndrome resulting from genetic–environmental interactions. Advanced age, familial aggregation, and the susceptibility gene apolipoprotein E (ApoE) ε4 allele have long been recognized as significant risk factors for AD. Mutations in genes APP, PSEN1, or PSEN2 have been identified behind the familial, early-onset form of AD, but the sporadic form differs from the familial type and presents considerable heterogeneity in terms of risk factor profiles, pathogenesis, and neuropathological findings. In recent years, several possibly modifiable risk and protective factors have been examined, and many vascular and lifestyle-related factors have been linked to the disease [3]. Most of the current evidence is based on observational studies. The lessons learned from the few randomized controlled trials are discussed later on in section 1.3.

The pathologic processes leading to AD probably start decades before the first symptoms are manifested [12]. The life-course approach is important: The role of different risk factors may vary in different periods of life. This stresses the importance of investigating the risk factors in long-term cohort studies with preferably both the exposure and outcome information collected several times during the lifespan. This would also enable us to find "optimal time windows" for preventive interventions.

Table 1.1 presents a summarized overview of these main putative risk or protective factors, which are discussed in this section. The accumulated evidence on risk or protective factors for dementia and AD has also been summarized in a recent report by the National Institutes of Health (NIH) [13]. The report indicated that there is still a need to refine knowledge about modifiable risk factors for dementia and AD, and in particular multidimensional intervention studies are needed.

1.2.1 Genetic, Socio-demographic, and Socio-economic Risk Factors

Age and family history were the first established risk factors for sporadic dementia and AD. Those individuals who have at least one first-degree relative with dementia are at an increased risk of developing dementia compared with persons without a family history [14]. Thus far ApoE ε4 allele has been the only established susceptibility gene for sporadic or late-onset AD. It has been estimated that it accounts for about 60% of the genetic component of late-onset AD [15]. With the era of genome-wide association studies, new candidate risk genes have been identified, but the associations are less consistent [16]. These are mainly genes involved in the metabolism and processing of the amyloid precursor protein (APP) and β-amyloid, as well as tau protein, including the GSK3β, DYRK1A, Tau, and CLU genes [17,18]. Until now, mutations in APP have not been implicated in the late-onset form of AD, with the exception of the rare variant, N660Y, which was recently identified in one case from a late-onset AD family [19]. Another recent study identified a mutation in the APP gene that can be protective against AD and age-related cognitive decline. This mutation is associated with a reduced production of amyloidogenic peptides [20].

TABLE 1.1   The Main Risk and Protective Factors for Dementia and AD

Risk Factors	Protective Factors
Genetic	**Socio-demographic**
ApoE ε4 allele	High education
Familial aggregation	High SES
Candidate genes: CR1, PICALM, CLU, TOMM40	
Vascular	**Vascular**
High blood pressure	Anti-hypertensive drugs
High cholesterol levels	Statins
Diabetes	Physical activity
High homocysteine levels	Social and mental activity
Cardiovascular disease	Mediterranean diet
Cerebrovascular disease	Vitamin B6 and B12, folate, vitamin E
Lifestyle-related	**Lifestyle-related**
Obesity	Polyunsaturated fats and fish
Smoking	Moderate alcohol use
Saturated fats	HRT?
Heavy alcohol drinking	NSAIDs?
Others	**Others**
Depression Negative stress?	
Occupational exposure (heavy metals, ELF-EMFs)?	
Head trauma	

ApoE: apolipoprotein E. CR1: complement component receptor 1. PICALM: phosphatidylinositol binding clathrin assembly protein. CLU: clusterin. TOMM40: Translocase of Outer Mitochondrial Membrane 40 homolog (www. alzgene.org). ELF-EMFs: extremely-low-frequency electromagnetic fields. HRT: hormone replacement therapy. NSAIDs: non-steroidal anti-inflammatory drugs. SES: socio-economic status.

Other genes that have been associated with increased risk of AD are TOMM40, CR1 and PICALM. The TOMM40 gene is located in a region of chromosome 19, which is in linkage disequilibrium with ApoE, and its polymorphism affects the age of onset of AD in subjects with an ApoE genotype [21]. CR1 is involved in the complement cascade, while

PICALM encodes a protein that is involved in clathrin-mediated endocytosis, an essential step in the intracellular trafficking of proteins and lipids such as nutrients, growth factors, and neurotransmitters [22].

Sex may also play a role in the risk of AD; especially among the older age groups, women have higher rates of AD compared with men [6]. Somewhat higher rates of dementia have been reported among African American and Latino populations than in Caucasians [23], but the role ethnic background plays is still controversial. Higher educational level and socio-economic status are associated with a lower risk of dementia and AD [24–26]. One of the main hypotheses behind this is that persons with higher education may have greater cognitive reserve capacity that postpones the clinical manifestation of the disease.

1.2.2 Vascular Risk Factors

Since the late 1990s, when the first prospective cohort studies became available, the research on vascular and lifestyle-related risk factors of dementia and AD has been advancing rapidly. The hope of identifying modifiable risk factors that could be used as targets for preventive efforts is the key driving force behind this line of research.

Several population-based studies have demonstrated that elevated blood pressure in midlife can increase the risk of dementia and AD in late-life [27–29]. However, a decline in blood pressure is seen in the years preceding the diagnosis of dementia [30–32]. A similar association has been detected between serum cholesterol values and dementia/AD risk, i.e., high cholesterol in midlife has been shown to increase the risk of dementia and AD [27,29,33], but a decline in cholesterol after midlife is observed in those individuals who will develop dementia/AD in late-life [34]. It has been speculated that the reductions in blood pressure and cholesterol levels may reflect the ongoing neurodegenerative disease process in the brain, and it may even represent a risk marker for late-life cognitive impairment. However, the relationships between these factors are complex and may also partly reflect phenomena related to physiological aging and also changes in lifestyle (such as diet, physical activity, or smoking). The role of these vascular risk factors seems to be different in different time points in life. Therefore it is crucial to take into account the life course perspective when investigating these risk factors and interpreting the results.

There is growing evidence that type 2 diabetes mellitus/impaired glucose tolerance is associated with an increased risk of cognitive impairment and AD, even though not all research confirms this relationship [35,36]. There are many mechanisms through which diabetes may influence the risk of dementia, including hyperinsulinemia, cerebrovascular disease, increased oxidative stress, and generation of advanced glycosylated end

(AGE) products [37]. Observational studies have also suggested that persons using antihypertensive drugs [38], or statins [39], may have a decreased risk of developing dementia and AD. Until recently, clinical vascular diseases were seldom studied in relation to AD. However, recent studies have proposed an association between various vascular disorders like myocardial infarction, atrial fibrillation, heart failure and AD [40,41].

1.2.3 Lifestyle-related Risk Factors

While earlier reports on smoking and AD showed negative results, the evidence from prospective cohorts clearly shows that smoking is associated with the increased risk of developing dementia and AD, and the risk may increase in a dose-dependent manner [42–44]. Nowadays, obesity is one of the major public health problems in Western countries [45]. Obesity, especially in midlife [46–48] but also in late-life [49], has been linked to an increased risk of dementia and AD in several studies. A diet rich in saturated fats may increase the risk of dementia and AD irrespective of the BMI value, whereas moderate intake of unsaturated fats may be protective [50,51]. A Mediterranean type of diet may, on the other hand, be protective [52]. Moderate alcohol drinking has also been shown to be protective of dementia, while frequent alcohol drinking may predispose one to the disease [53,54]. Regular physical activity [55,56] as well as a rich social network [57], being married [58], and social and mental activities [59] have all been associated with a reduction of the risk of dementia and AD.

An interaction between genetic susceptibility and lifestyles has been observed: Persons with ApoE e4 and an unhealthy lifestyle (smoking, frequent alcohol drinking, lack of physical activity, or a diet with an abundant intake of saturated fatty acids or little unsaturated fatty acids) may be especially vulnerable to developing dementia and AD [60]. Further investigation of gene–environment interactions both in epidemiologic and experimental settings are needed to increase our understanding of the disease process and for planning interventions.

Vascular and lifestyle-related risk factors and diseases often occur simultaneously, and clustering of vascular risk factors has been shown to additively increase the risk of dementia [29,46,61,62]. This has led to the development of risk scores to assess the risk of cognitive impairment or dementia on an individual level. These practical tools are used for identifying individuals who may benefit from intensive lifestyle consultations and pharmacological interventions, and for health education. The first such tool was based on data from the Cardiovascular Risk Factors, Aging and Dementia (CAIDE) study, and this dementia risk score includes easily measurable variables (age, sex, education, midlife hypertension, hypercholesterolemia, obesity, and physical inactivity) that are associated with the risk of dementia later in life [63]. The risk score instruments can be further improved as more comprehensive datasets become available (e.g., by adding new variables and age groups), but initially they are used as educational tools to demonstrate the role of modifiable vascular factors in dementia syndrome.

1.3 INTERVENTIONS TO PREVENT THE DISEASE

The multi-factorial and heterogeneous character of late-onset AD allows multiple prevention approaches (Figure 1.2). The intervention studies conducted so far have had somewhat disappointing results. There have been trials for cholinesterase inhibitors (donepezil, galantamine, rivastigmine), vitamin E supplements, vitamin B6, B12 or folic acid supplements, vitamin C, beta carotene or multivitamin supplements, omega-3 fatty acid, gingko biloba, statins, antihypertensive drugs, acetylsalicylic acid, and gonadal steroids that have shown no effect; some trials for estrogen plus progesterone and non-steroidal anti-inflammatory drugs (rofecoxib and naproxen) have even shown an increased risk of dementia/AD in the treatment group [13]. These trials have mostly used a single agent and they have been conducted on older and/or already cognitively impaired populations. Many of these trials were planned for other outcomes and cognitive outcomes were secondary. Therefore, they may have been underpowered to detect true associations.

There are, however, some positive signs that antihypertensive drug treatment, vitamin B supplementation, physical activity, and cognitive training may be beneficial, at least in certain groups of persons. The positive effect of antihypertensives has been suggested in a few clinical trials: In the Systolic Hypertension in Europe (Syst-Eur) trial, active treatment of isolated systolic hypertension with nitrendipine, a

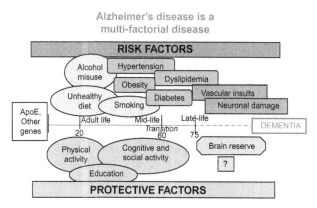

FIGURE 1.2   Risk and protective factors for Alzheimer's disease

calcium-channel blocker, was found to halve the incidence of AD [64]. The Study on Cognition and Prognosis in the Elderly (SCOPE) showed, in sub-group analyses among the subjects with lower baseline cognition, that Mini Mental State Examination (MMSE) score declined less in the candesartan than in the control group [65]. The Perindopril Protection Against Recurrent Stroke Study (PROGRESS) among subjects with a history of stroke or transient ischemic attack showed a decreased risk of decline in MMSE among persons with active treatment with perindopril [66]. Pooled analyses based on the Hypertension in the Very Elderly Trial (HYVET-COG), Systolic Hypertension in the Elderly Program (SHEP), Syst-Eur, and PROGRESS suggested that antihypertensive treatment could reduce the risk of dementia by up to 13% [67].

Single trials on other agents/interventions have also signaled possible beneficial effects, although none of them has had clinical dementia as an outcome. The VITACOG study reported that two-year supplementation with vitamin B12 plus B6 plus folic acid may slow cognitive and clinical decline in people with mild cognitive impairment (MCI) and elevated homocysteine level [68]. The Fitness for the Aging Brain Study (FABS) of adults with subjective memory impairment, proposed that a six-month home-based physical activity program provided a modest improvement in cognition measured with the cognitive section of the Alzheimer Disease Assessment Scale (ADAS-Cog) [69]. The Advanced Cognitive Training for Independent and Vital Elderly (ACTIVE) study reported that 10 sessions of cognitive training over six weeks resulted in improved cognitive abilities specific to the abilities trained that continued for five years after the initiation of the intervention [70].

Some key issues that need to be considered in all AD prevention trials are:

- *Intervention*: Given the diversity of risk and protective factors identified in observational studies, it may be more effective to have multi-domain interventions targeting several of these risk factors simultaneously, instead of just a single component intervention.
- *Timing and target group*: As the pathologic disease process takes years, even decades, the trials starting only a short time before the manifestation of clinical dementia syndrome may be too late to have results. Also, different risk factors and interventions may have their own optimal time windows, and initiating the treatment in the wrong age group may even lead to an increase in risk as was seen in trials with non-steroidal anti-inflammatory drugs or hormone replacement therapy. On the other hand, long-term interventions are challenging as they need considerable financial resources. Further, drop-out rates may increase as the duration of the intervention is prolonged. The participants that drop out may have a higher rate of cognitive decline,

and this would bias the results away from the null effect, especially if the intervention requires much more active participation than the control condition.

- *Outcome measures*: Due to a very long preclinical phase, it is difficult to determine the exact time of onset of AD. Lately, there has been a shift toward earlier diagnosis of AD [71]. When the symptoms reach the clinical threshold for dementia, the neurodegenerative processes are at a very advanced stage. Cognitive decline may be a better endpoint than conversion to dementia. The appropriate cognitive test battery should be sufficiently sensitive to detect small changes, but at the same time specific to changes that are closely related to the development of AD. The optimal test battery may also depend on the characteristics of the population.
- *Ethical issues*: Persons with high blood pressure or cholesterol levels need to be treated because of the risk of developing cardiovascular and cerebrovascular disorders, and thus true placebo-controlled trials in regards to this issue may no longer be possible to conduct. The same is true for unhealthy lifestyle factors that need to be addressed. This treatment contamination would decrease differences between groups.

Intervention studies combining several different approaches have not been conducted for AD so far, but at least three large European studies are ongoing. The Finnish Geriatric Intervention Study to Prevent Cognitive Impairment and Disability (FINGER) is a multicenter, randomized, controlled trial (RCT) with 1,260 individuals aged 60–77 who are at risk of cognitive decline [72]. The two-year multi-domain intervention consists of nutritional guidance, exercise, cognitive training, social activity, and management of metabolic and vascular risk factors. The primary outcome is cognitive performance as measured by the modified Neuropsychological Test Battery, Stroop test, and Trail Making Test. Main secondary outcomes are dementia, disability, depressive symptoms, vascular risk factors and outcomes, quality of life, and neuroimaging measures. The intervention will be completed during 2014.

The Multi-domain Alzheimer Preventive Trial (MAPT) study is a three-year randomized, controlled trial ongoing in France [73]. It has enrolled 1,200 frail elderly individuals aged 70 years or older. The participants are randomized into one of the following four groups: omega 3 alone, multi-domain intervention alone, omega 3 plus multi-domain intervention, or placebo (n = 300 each). The principal outcome measure is a change in cognitive function at three years, as determined by the Grober and Buschke Test. Final results should be available in 2013.

The Prevention of Dementia by Intensive Vascular Care (PreDIVA) study is a cluster-randomized, six-year trial ongoing in the Netherlands.

It has enrolled 3,700 elderly individuals (aged 70–78) to assess whether nurse-led intensive vascular care in primary care decreases the incidence of dementia and reduces disability. Secondary outcome parameters are mortality, incidence of vascular events, and cognitive functioning. Intensive vascular care comprises: treatment of hypertension, hypercholesterolemia, and diabetes; help with weight loss and smoking cessation; and stimulation of physical exercise [74].

Irrespective of methodological differences, all three trials target vascular and lifestyle-related risk factors for dementia and AD. In 2011, researchers leading these three studies launched the European Dementia Prevention Initiative (EDPI) (www.edpi.org). EDPI is at the forefront of international collaborative efforts to solve the clinical and public health problems of early identification of individuals at increased risk of late-life cognitive impairment, and of developing intervention strategies to prevent or delay the onset of cognitive impairment and dementia. As a first step in this direction, in 2013 EDPI members started a multinational project: the Healthy Aging Through Internet Counseling in the Elderly (HATICE) project (www.hatice.eu).

1.3.1 Pre-symptomatic AD Treatment: Anti-amyloid Drugs

Pre-symptomatic (or preclinical) AD treatments have been defined as interventions initiated before apparent cognitive decline and are intended to reduce the chance of developing AD-related symptoms [75]. The term refers to an intervention whether it is started before or after biological evidence of the underlying disease, and whether it postpones the onset, partially reduces the risk of, or completely prevents symptomatic AD [76]. Increased knowledge of the AD phenotype, particularly of the biomarkers which have been incorporated in the new diagnostic criteria for dementia and MCI due to AD, as well preclinical AD, has provided the basis for intervention studies evaluating pharmacological interventions in asymptomatic subjects who are at risk of AD, because of an established biomarker burden or a specific genetic profile.

Three RCTs are planned to start in 2013 to verify safety and efficacy of anti-amyloid drugs as a preventive measure in AD. The Alzheimer's Prevention Initiative (API) and the Dominantly Inherited Alzheimer's Network (DIAN) studies will enrol subjects who carry genetic mutations for dominantly inherited AD: mutations in the APP, presenilin-1 (PSEN1), and presenilin-2 (PSEN2) genes can cause early-onset familial AD that accounts for no more than 5% of all cases [77]. The API RCT will focus on the world's largest early-onset AD kindred in Antioquia, Columbia. Of about 5,000 individuals in this kindred, approximately 1,500 carry a mutation in the PSEN1 gene causing early-onset AD [78,79]. The trial will also include a small number of individuals in the United States, recruited in collaboration with researchers from the DIAN study [80]. The drug used in the API study is the anti-amyloid antibody crenezumab, which promotes the removal of β-amyloid from the brain [79]. The trial within the DIAN cohort will include people with mutations in any of the three genes linked to early-onset AD: PSEN1, PSEN2, and APP. Two anti-amyloid monoclonal antibodies will be tested: gantenerumab and solanezumab. A third trial, the Anti-Amyloid Treatment of Asymptomatic Alzheimer's (A4) RTC, aims to prevent sporadic AD and will evaluate the effect of solanezumab in older adults with evidence of brain amyloid accumulation at neuroimaging evaluation [79].

Overall, these studies provide the opportunity to test the efficacy of AD-modifying treatments in an earlier stage of AD compared to the pharmacological RCTs done so far. While testing these compounds in young, healthy individuals would require enormous financial resources and too long follow up, the recruitment strategies implemented in these studies allow testing the benefit of anti-amyloid drugs earlier than otherwise possible. This approach also provides the opportunity to further verify the amyloid hypothesis, which has been reconsidered many times over the past decades and criticized in light of the recent failures of RCTs testing anti-amyloid drugs in subjects with mild-to-moderate AD. A possible interpretation of these failures is that the anti-amyloid therapies have missed their "window of opportunity," since they have been provided too late. The preventive RCTs on anti-amyloid drugs are based on the assumption that an earlier interference on amyloid accumulation, before irreversible brain damage occurs, would exert a significant disease-modifying effect.

1.4 POPULATION AGING AND PROJECTED BURDEN OF DISEASE

The worldwide aging of the population will more than triple the projected number of demented persons between 2010 and 2050 [2]. This represents a huge social as well as economic burden to society. The worldwide costs of dementia were estimated to be US$ 604 billion in 2010, and this may increase by 85% by 2030 [81]. The costs for dementia include informal care (unpaid care provided by family and others), direct costs of social care (provided by community care professionals, and in residential home settings), and the direct costs of medical care (the costs of treating dementia and other conditions in primary and secondary care). The societal costs of dementia increased by 34% between 2005 and 2009. Some studies have compared estimates of the societal costs for dementia with those of other chronic diseases. A report from the United Kingdom estimated the annual societal cost of dementia at £23 billion, £12 billion for cancer, £8 billion for heart disease, and £5 billion for stroke. The societal costs of dementia almost matched those of cancer, heart disease, and stroke combined [82]. In a Swedish study the annual costs of dementia (50 billion Swedish Kronor [SEK]) was higher than for depression (32.5 billion SEK), stroke (12.5 billion SEK), alcohol abuse (21–30 billion SEK), and osteoporosis (4.6 billion SEK) [83].

The majority (70%) of costs related to dementia occur in Western Europe and North America, while nearly two-thirds of persons with dementia live in low and middle income countries. The per-capita costs of dementia have been estimated to vary from US$ 868 in countries with low incomes, to US$ 6,827 in upper middle income countries, to US$ 32,865 in countries with high incomes [84]. This difference is mainly due to the fact that in less developed countries the formal social care sector (accounting for the direct costs of care in the community by paid social care professionals, and of care homes) is almost non-existent. In these regions, informal care costs predominate, while in more developed countries the direct costs of social care account for nearly half of all costs [84]. The availability of disease-modifying treatments for AD might further increase the difference in costs between sectors, since it is reasonable to hypothesize that high income countries might be more likely to be able to pay for treatments and the preceding diagnostic procedures.

Dementia is an important cause of disability and dependence among older people. In many of the high income countries, dementia is present in a large proportion of older adults living in nursing homes or institutions. In terms of years lived with disability, AD and other dementias rank as the fourth most important disorder in high income countries (after depression, hearing loss, and alcohol abuse, for all age-groups) [85]. Among older people in countries with low and middle incomes, dementia is the most important independent contributor to disability [86].

Future projections of AD prevalence and related burden of disease may be modified in several ways. There have been important changes in risk factors during the past decades, for example cholesterol and blood pressure levels have declined, smoking has become less frequent, but on the other hand obesity and diabetes are reaching epidemic proportions. How this will be reflected in the future incidence of dementia is still unknown. There are some indications that dementia incidence might be decreasing, but current data are scarce and inconclusive [9,87].

Finding and applying effective preventive interventions would decrease disease incidence and prevalence. Based on relative risk estimates and prevalence of seven central risk factors including diabetes, midlife hypertension, midlife obesity, smoking, depression, cognitive inactivity or low educational attainment, and physical inactivity, it has been estimated that 10–25% reduction in all of these risk factors would result in the prevention of 1.1–3.0 million cases of AD worldwide [88]. Improvements in treatment may result in increased prevalence due to prolonging survival of persons with dementia. Disease-modifying treatments that would stop or slow down the progression of the disease may also increase the prevalence of the disease, but this may nevertheless reduce the individual, social, and economic burden of the disease if the time lived with severe dementia can be shortened. A two-year delay in both the onset and progression of AD has been suggested to reduce AD prevalence by more than 20% and the late-stage of the disease by more than 30% by 2050 [89].

1.5 CONCLUSION

Given the projected increase in the occurrence of dementia/AD, our societies are facing an enormous challenge in the coming years. Finding effective prevention and treatment strategies for dementia should be one of the top priorities in public health politics worldwide. AD is a multi-factorial disease resulting from an interaction between genetic and environmental factors. The evidence from observational studies shows that many modifiable, both vascular and lifestyle-related, risk factors lie behind the disease. Optimal control of vascular risk factors and maintenance of an active lifestyle are the key issues on the path to preventing AD. Detailed research is still needed on the association of these factors to identify specific targets and time frames for intervention. As the pathologic processes leading to AD may take decades to develop, starting earlier may lead to better effects. It is also becoming clear that targeting several risk factors simultaneously, as well as having a long intervention period, is needed for optimal preventive effects.

Multi-domain interventional trials are now ongoing and will provide new insights into the prevention of dementia and AD. The multi-domain intervention studies are at one end of the current spectrum of intervention trials in dementia/AD. At the other end are studies testing disease-modifying drugs (i.e., anti-amyloid therapy) in genetically at-risk groups or those with established biomarker burden. The shift towards pre-symptomatic and pre-dementia stages of AD has brought prevention and treatment trials much closer to each other than before. Since a cure for dementia is not yet available, finding effective preventive strategies is essential for a sustainable society in an aging world. As dementia, cardiovascular diseases, stroke, and diabetes mellitus—all major public health problems—share several risk factors, public health efforts promoting a healthier lifestyle have the potential to enhance health status in advanced age.

References

[1] Alzheimer's Disease International   World Alzheimer Report 2009. London: Alzheimer's Disease International; 2009.
[2] Prince M, Bryce R, Albanese E, Wimo A, Ribeiro W, Ferri CP. The global prevalence of dementia: a systematic review and meta-analysis. Alzheimers Dement. 9: 63–75 e62.

[3] Qiu C, Kivipelto M, von Strauss E. Epidemiology of Alzheimer's disease: occurrence, determinants, and strategies toward intervention. Dialogues Clin Neurosci 2009;11:111–28.

[4] Reynish E, Fratiglioni L, Prince M, Bickel H, Kiejna A, Georger J. EUROCODE: prevalence of dementia in Europe. Alzheimer Europe; 2006.

[5] United National Department of Economic and Social Affairs. Magnitude and speed of population ageing. Chapter II, World population Aging 2007; 13–16.

[6] Fratiglioni L, Launer LJ, Andersen K, Breteler MM, Copeland JR, Dartigues JF, et al. Incidence of dementia and major subtypes in Europe: a collaborative study of population-based cohorts. Neurologic Diseases in the Elderly Research Group. Neurol 2000;54:S10–15.

[7] World Health Organization Dementia: a public health priority. Geneva: World Health Organization—Alzheimer's Disease International; 2012.

[8] Miech RA, Breitner JC, Zandi PP, Khachaturian AS, Anthony JC, Mayer L. Incidence of AD may decline in the early 90s for men, later for women: the Cache County study. Neurology 2002;58:209–18.

[9] Schrijvers EM, Verhaaren BF, Koudstaal PJ, Hofman A, Ikram MA, Breteler MM. Is dementia incidence declining?: Trends in dementia incidence since 1990 in the Rotterdam Study. Neurology 78: 1456–63.

[10] Lobo A, Launer LJ, Fratiglioni L, Andersen K, Di Carlo A, Breteler MM, et al. Prevalence of dementia and major subtypes in Europe: a collaborative study of population-based cohorts. Neurologic Diseases in the Elderly Research Group. Neurology 2000;54:S4–S9.

[11] Schneider JA, Arvanitakis Z, Bang W, Bennett DA. Mixed brain pathologies account for most dementia cases in community-dwelling older persons. Neurology 2007;69:2197–204.

[12] Braak H, Thal DR, Ghebremedhin E, Del Tredici K. Stages of the pathologic process in Alzheimer's disease: age categories from 1 to 100 years. J Neuropathol Exp Neurol 70: 960–969.

[13] Williams J, Plassman B, Burke J, Holsinger T, Benjamin S. Preventing Alzheimer's Disease and Cognitive Decline. Evidence Report/Technology Assessment No. 193. (Prepared by the Duke Evidence-based Practice Center under Contract No. HHSA 290-2007-10066-I.) AHRQ Publication No. 10-E005. Agency for Healthcare Research and Quality, Rockville, MD; 2010.

[14] Devi G, Ottman R, Tang MX, Marder K, Stern Y, Mayeux R. Familial aggregation of Alzheimer's disease among whites, African Americans, and Caribbean Hispanics in northern Manhattan. Arch Neurol 2000;57:72–7.

[15] Rubinsztein DC, Easton DF. Apolipoprotein E genetic variation and Alzheimer's disease. a meta-analysis. Dement Geriatr Cogn Disord 1999;10:199–209.

[16] Bettens K, Sleegers K, Van Broeckhoven C. Genetic insights in Alzheimer's disease. The Lancet Neurol 2013;12:92–104.

[17] Qiu C, Kivipelto M, Aguero-Torres H, Winblad B, Fratiglioni L. Risk and protective effects of the APOE gene towards Alzheimer's disease in the Kungsholmen project: variation by age and sex. J Neurol Neurosurg Psychiatry 2004;75:828–33.

[18] Slooter AJ, Cruts M, Kalmijn S, Hofman A, Breteler MM, Van Broeckhoven C, et al. Risk estimates of dementia by apolipoprotein E genotypes from a population-based incidence study: the Rotterdam Study. Arch Neurol 1998;55:964–68.

[19] Ballard C, Gauthier S, Corbett A, Brayne C, Aarsland D, Jones E. Alzheimer's disease. Lancet 2011;377:1019–31.

[20] Cruchaga C, Haller G, Chakraverty S, Mayo K, Vallania FL, Mitra RD. Rare variants in APP, PSEN1 and PSEN2 increase risk for AD in late-onset alzheimer's disease families. PloS one 2012;7:e31039.

[21] Jonsson T, Atwal JK, Steinberg S, Snaedal J, Jonsson PV, Bjornsson S. A mutation in APP protects against Alzheimer's disease and age-related cognitive decline. Nature 2012;488:96–9.

[22] Roses AD, Lutz MW, Amrine-Madsen H, Saunders AM, Crenshaw DG, Sundseth SS. A TOMM40 variable-length polymorphism predicts the age of late-onset alzheimer's disease. Pharmacogenomics J 2010;10:375–84.

[23] Tang MX, Cross P, Andrews H, Jacobs DM, Small S, Bell K. Incidence of AD in African-Americans, Caribbean Hispanics, and Caucasians in northern Manhattan. Neurology 2001;56:49–56.

[24] Ngandu T, von Strauss E, Helkala EL, Winblad B, Nissinen A, Tuomilehto J. Education and dementia: what lies behind the association? Neurology 2007;69:1442–50.

[25] Karp A, Kareholt I, Qiu C, Bellander T, Winblad B, Fratiglioni L. Relation of education and occupation-based socioeconomic status to incident Alzheimer's disease. Am J Epidemiol 2004;159:175–83.

[26] Evans DA, Hebert LE, Beckett LA, Scherr PA, Albert MS, Chown MJ. Education and other measures of socioeconomic status and risk of incident of Alzheimer's disease in a defined population of older persons. Arch Neurol 1997;54:1399–405.

[27] Kivipelto M, Helkala EL, Laakso MP, Hanninen T, Hallikainen M, Alhainen K. Midlife vascular risk factors and Alzheimer's disease in later life: longitudinal, population based study. Bmj 2001;322:1447–51.

[28] Launer LJ, Ross GW, Petrovitch H, Masaki K, Foley D, White LR, et al. Midlife blood pressure and dementia: the Honolulu-Asia aging study. Neurobiol Aging 2000;21:49–55.

[29] Whitmer RA, Sidney S, Selby J, Johnston SC, Yaffe K. Midlife cardiovascular risk factors and risk of dementia in late life. Neurology 2005;64:277–81.

[30] Skoog I, Lernfelt B, Landahl S, Palmertz B, Andreasson LA, Nilsson L, et al. Fifteen-year longitudinal study of blood pressure and dementia. Lancet 1996;347:1141–45.

[31] Qiu C, von Strauss E, Winblad B, Fratiglioni L. Decline in blood pressure over time and risk of dementia: a longitudinal study from the Kungsholmen project. Stroke 2004;35:1810–15.

[32] Qiu C, Winblad B, Fratiglioni L. The age-dependent relation of blood pressure to cognitive function and dementia. Lancet Neurol 2005;4:487–99.

[33] Notkola IL, Sulkava R, Pekkanen J, Erkinjuntti T, Ehnholm C, Kivinen P, et al. Serum total cholesterol, apolipoprotein E epsilon 4 allele, and Alzheimer's disease. Neuroepidemiology 1998;17:14–20.

[34] Solomon A, Kareholt I, Ngandu T, Winblad B, Nissinen A, Tuomilehto J, et al. Serum cholesterol changes after midlife and late-life cognition: 21-year follow-up study. Neurology 2007;68:751–56.

[35] Biessels GJ, Staekenborg S, Brunner E, Brayne C, Scheltens P. Risk of dementia in diabetes mellitus: a systematic review. Lancet Neurol 2006;5:64–74.

[36] Xu W, Qiu C, Winblad B, Fratiglioni L. The effect of borderline diabetes on the risk of dementia and Alzheimer's disease. Diabetes 2007;56:211–16.

[37] Sasaki N, Fukatsu R, Tsuzuki K, Hayashi Y, Yoshida T, Fujii N, et al. Advanced glycation end products in Alzheimer's disease and other neurodegenerative diseases. Am J Pathol 1998;153:1149–55.

[38] Qiu C, Winblad B, Fastbom J, Fratiglioni L. Combined effects of APOE genotype, blood pressure, and antihypertensive drug use on incident AD. Neurology 2003;61:655–60.

[39] Solomon A, Kareholt I, Ngandu T, Wolozin B, Macdonald SW, Winblad B, et al. Serum total cholesterol, statins and cognition in non-demented elderly. Neurobiol Aging 2009;30:1006–09.

[40] Newman AB, Fitzpatrick AL, Lopez O, Jackson S, Lyketsos C, Jagust W, et al. Dementia and Alzheimer's disease incidence in relationship to cardiovascular disease in the cardiovascular health study cohort. J Am Geriatr Soc 2005;53:1101–07.

[41] Bunch TJ, Weiss JP, Crandall BG, May HT, Bair TL, Osborn JS, et al. Atrial fibrillation is independently associated with senile, vascular, and Alzheimer's dementia. Heart Rhythm 7: 433–437.

[42] Rusanen M, Rovio S, Ngandu T, Nissinen A, Tuomilehto J, Soininen H, et al. Midlife smoking, apolipoprotein E and risk of dementia and Alzheimer's disease: a population-based cardiovascular risk factors, aging and dementia study. Dement Geriatr Cogn Disord 30: 277–84.

[43] Rusanen M, Kivipelto M, Quesenberry Jr CP, Zhou J, Whitmer RA. Heavy smoking in midlife and long-term risk of Alzheimer's disease and vascular dementia. Arch Intern Med 171: 333–39.

[44] Reitz C, den Heijer T, van Duijn C, Hofman A, Breteler MM. Relation between smoking and risk of dementia and Alzheimer's disease: the Rotterdam Study. Neurology 2007;69:998–1005.

[45] Mokdad AH, Marks JS, Stroup DF, Gerberding JL. Actual causes of death in the United States, 2000. Jama 2004;291:1238–45.

[46] Kivipelto M, Ngandu T, Fratiglioni L, Viitanen M, Kareholt I, Winblad B, et al. Obesity and vascular risk factors at midlife and the risk of dementia and Alzheimer disease. Arch Neurol 2005;62:1556–60.

[47] Whitmer RA, Gunderson EP, Barrett-Connor E, Quesenberry Jr. CP, Yaffe K. Obesity in middle age and future risk of dementia: a 27-year longitudinal population-based study. Bmj 2005;330:1360.

[48] Kalmijn S, Foley D, White L, Burchfiel CM, Curb JD, Petrovitch H, et al. Metabolic cardiovascular syndrome and risk of dementia in Japanese-American elderly men. The Honolulu-Asia aging study. Arterioscler Thromb Vasc Biol 2000;20:2255–60.

[49] Gustafson D, Rothenberg E, Blennow K, Steen B, Skoog I. An 18-year follow-up of overweight and risk of Alzheimer's disease. Arch Intern Med 2003;163:1524–28.

[50] Laitinen MH, Ngandu T, Rovio S, Helkala EL, Uusitalo U, Viitanen M, et al. Fat intake at midlife and risk of dementia and Alzheimer's disease: a population-based study. Dement Geriatr Cogn Disord 2006;22:99–107.

[51] Morris MC, Evans DA, Bienias JL, Tangney CC, Bennett DA, Aggarwal N, et al. Dietary fats and the risk of incident Alzheimer's disease. Arch Neurol 2003;60:194–200.

[52] Scarmeas N, Stern Y, Tang MX, Mayeux R, Luchsinger JA. Mediterranean diet and risk for Alzheimer's disease. Ann Neurol 2006;59:912–21.

[53] Anttila T, Helkala EL, Viitanen M, Kareholt I, Fratiglioni L, Winblad B, et al. Alcohol drinking in middle age and subsequent risk of mild cognitive impairment and dementia in old age: a prospective population based study. Bmj 2004;329:539.

[54] Ruitenberg A, van Swieten JC, Witteman JC, Mehta KM, van Duijn CM, Hofman A, et al. Alcohol consumption and risk of dementia: the Rotterdam Study. Lancet 2002;359:281–86.

[55] Laurin D, Verreault R, Lindsay J, MacPherson K, Rockwood K. Physical activity and risk of cognitive impairment and dementia in elderly persons. Arch Neurol 2001;58:498–504.

[56] Rovio S, Kareholt I, Helkala EL, Viitanen M, Winblad B, Tuomilehto J, et al. Leisure-time physical activity at midlife and the risk of dementia and Alzheimer's disease. Lancet Neurol 2005;4:705–11.

[57] Fratiglioni L, Paillard-Borg S, Winblad B. An active and socially integrated lifestyle in late life might protect against dementia. Lancet Neurol 2004;3:343–53.

[58] Hakansson K, Rovio S, Helkala EL, Vilska AR, Winblad B, Soininen H, et al. Association between mid-life marital status and cognitive function in later life: population-based cohort study. BMJ 2009;339:b2462.

[59] Wang HX, Karp A, Winblad B, Fratiglioni L. Late-life engagement in social and leisure activities is associated with a decreased risk of dementia: a longitudinal study from the Kungsholmen project. Am J Epidemiol 2002;155:1081–87.

[60] Kivipelto M, Rovio S, Ngandu T, Kareholt I, Eskelinen M, Winblad B, et al. Apolipoprotein E epsilon4 magnifies lifestyle risks for dementia: a population-based study. J Cell Mol Med 2008;12:2762–71.

[61] Luchsinger JA, Reitz C, Honig LS, Tang MX, Shea S, Mayeux R. Aggregation of vascular risk factors and risk of incident Alzheimer's disease. Neurology 2005;65:545–51.

[62] Qiu C, Xu W, Winblad B, Fratiglioni L. Vascular risk profiles for dementia and Alzheimer's disease in very old people: a population-based longitudinal study. J Alzheimers Dis 20: 293–300.

[63] Kivipelto M, Ngandu T, Laatikainen T, Winblad B, Soininen H, Tuomilehto J. Risk score for the prediction of dementia risk in 20 years among middle-aged people: a longitudinal, population-based study. Lancet Neurol 2006;5:735–41.

[64] Forette F, Seux ML, Staessen JA, Thijs L, Birkenhager WH, Babarskiene MR, et al. Prevention of dementia in randomised double-blind placebo-controlled Systolic Hypertension in Europe (Syst-Eur) trial. Lancet 1998;352:1347–51.

[65] Skoog I, Lithell H, Hansson L, Elmfeldt D, Hofman A, Olofsson B, et al. Effect of baseline cognitive function and antihypertensive treatment on cognitive and cardiovascular outcomes: Study on Cognition and Prognosis in the Elderly (SCOPE). Am J Hypertens 2005;18:1052–59.

[66] Tzourio C, Anderson C, Chapman N, Woodward M, Neal B, MacMahon S, et al. Effects of blood pressure lowering with perindopril and indapamide therapy on dementia and cognitive decline in patients with cerebrovascular disease. Arch Intern Med 2003;163:1069–75.

[67] Peters R, Beckett N, Forette F, Tuomilehto J, Clarke R, Ritchie C, et al. Incident dementia and blood pressure lowering in the Hypertension in the Very Elderly Trial cognitive function assessment (HYVET-COG): a double-blind, placebo controlled trial. Lancet Neurol 2008;7:683–89.

[68] de Jager CA, Oulhaj A, Jacoby R, Refsum H, Smith AD. Cognitive and clinical outcomes of homocysteine-lowering B-vitamin treatment in mild cognitive impairment: a randomized controlled trial. Int J Geriatr Psychiatry 2012;27:592–600.

[69] Lautenschlager NT, Cox KL, Flicker L, Foster JK, van Bockxmeer FM, Xiao J, et al. Effect of physical activity on cognitive function in older adults at risk for Alzheimer's disease: a randomized trial. JAMA 2008;300:1027–37.

[70] Willis SL, Tennstedt SL, Marsiske M, Ball K, Elias J, Koepke KM, et al. Long-term effects of cognitive training on everyday functional outcomes in older adults. JAMA 2006;296:2805–14.

[71] Dubois B, Feldman HH, Jacova C, Dekosky ST, Barberger-Gateau P, Cummings J, et al. Research criteria for the diagnosis of Alzheimer's disease: revising the NINCDS-ADRDA criteria. Lancet Neurol 2007;6:734–46.

[72] Kivipelto M, Solomon A, Ahtiluoto S, Ngandu T, Lehtisalo J, Antikainen R, et al. The Finnish Geriatric Intervention Study to Prevent Cognitive Impairment and Disability (FINGER): study design and progress. Alzheimer's Dement 2013 Jan 16 [epub ahead of print].

[73] Gillette-Guyonnet S, Andrieu S, Dantoine T, Dartigues JF, Touchon J, Vellas B. Commentary on "A roadmap for the prevention of dementia II. Leon Thal Symposium 2008." The Multidomain Alzheimer Preventive Trial (MAPT): a new approach to the prevention of Alzheimer's disease. Alzheimers Dement 2009;5:114–21.

[74] Richard E, Van den Heuvel E, Moll van Charante EP, Achthoven L, Vermeulen M, Bindels PJ, et al. Prevention of dementia by intensive vascular care (PreDIVA): a cluster–randomized trial in progress. Alzheimer Dis Assoc Disord 2009;23:198–204.

[75] Reiman EM, Langbaum JB, Tariot PN. Alzheimer's prevention initiative: a proposal to evaluate pre-symptomatic treatments as quickly as possible. Biomark Med 2010;4:3–14.

[76] Reiman EM, Langbaum JB, Fleisher AS, Caselli RJ, Chen K, Ayutyanont N, et al. Alzheimer's Prevention Initiative: a plan to accelerate the evaluation of pre-symptomatic treatments. J Alzheimers Dis 2011;26(**Suppl. 3**):321–29.

[77] Blennow K, de Leon MJ, Zetterberg H. Alzheimer's disease. Lancet 2006;368:387–403.

[78] Lopera F, Ardilla A, Martinez A, Madrigal L, Arango-Viana JC, Lemere CA, et al. Clinical features of early-onset alzheimer's disease in a large kindred with an E280A presenilin-1 mutation. Jama 1997;277:793–99.

[79] Miller G. Alzheimer's research. Stopping alzheimer's before it starts. Science 2012;337:790–2.

[80] Alzheimer's Prevention Initiative. Treatment Trials 2012, available from http://endalznow.org/about-api/treatment-trials.aspx.

[81] Wimo A, Jonsson L, Bond J, Prince M, Winblad B. The worldwide economic impact of dementia. Alzheimers Dement 2010;9:1–11. e13.

[82] Luengo-Fernandez R, Leal J, Gray A. Dementia 2010. Oxford: The Health Economics Research Centre, University of Oxford; 2010.

[83] Wimo A, Johansson L, Jonsson L. Prevalence study of societal costs for dementia 2000–2005. More demented people—but somewhat reduced costs per person. Lakartidningen 2009;106:1277–82.

[84] Wimo A, Jonsson L, Bond J, Prince M, Winblad B. The worldwide economic impact of dementia 2010. Alzheimer's Dement 2013;9(1–11):e13.

[85] World Health Organization The Global Burden of Disease: 2004 Update. Geneva: World Health Organization; 2008.

[86] Sousa RM, Ferri CP, Acosta D, Albanese E, Guerra M, Huang Y, et al. Contribution of chronic diseases to disability in elderly people in countries with low and middle incomes: a 10/66 Dementia Research Group population-based survey. Lancet 2009;374:1821–30.

[87] Qiu C, von Strauss E, Backman L, Winblad B, Fratiglioni L. Twenty-year changes in dementia occurrence suggest decreasing incidence in central Stockholm, Sweden. Neurology; 2013;80:1888–94.

[88] Barnes DE, Yaffe K. The projected effect of risk factor reduction on Alzheimer's disease prevalence. Lancet Neurol 10: 819–28.

[89] Brookmeyer R, Johnson E, Ziegler-Graham K, Arrighi HM. Forecasting the global burden of Alzheimer's disease. Alzheimer's Dement 2007;3:186–91.

[90] Gao S, Hendrie HC, Hall KS, Hui S. The relationships between age, sex, and the incidence of dementia and Alzheimer disease: a meta-analysis. Arch Gen Psychiatry. 1998;55:809–815.

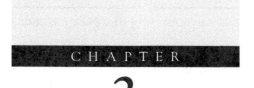

2

Developing a National Plan to Address Alzheimer's Disease

Are there lessons that emerging countries can learn from Western countries?

Menghis Bairu

Élan Pharmaceutical, California, USA

In 2050, 70 percent of all Alzheimer's cases will be in developing countries.
Source: World Alzheimer Report 2009

2.1 INTRODUCTION

More than 35 million people worldwide are living with dementia [1]. According to the Alzheimer's Association, a global advocacy group, between 50 and 80% of all dementia cases are Alzheimer's disease-related. By 2050, those afflicted with Alzheimer's disease (AD) will more than triple to 115 million [2], placing untold stress on overburdened social service and healthcare delivery systems, causing needless pain and suffering, and negatively impacting the lives of millions of family members and caregivers. Like HIV/AIDS in the early 1980s, we are seeing the leading edge of a potentially catastrophic global healthcare crisis.

Sixty percent of AD victims—the majority of them undiagnosed—now live in lesser developed countries (LDCs). In 2050, emerging countries will account for 71% of the total AD caseload, a projection driven by global population trends and the unforeseen consequences of increased life expectancy. In 2050, individuals aged 60 (the age associated with early-onset AD) will number an estimated 1.2 billion, 22% of the world's

M. Bairu & M.W. Weiner (Eds):
Global Clinical Trials for Alzheimer's Disease.
DOI: http://dx.doi.org/10.1016/B978-0-12-411464-7.00002-X

21

population. According to World Health Organization projections, four out of five of them (80%) will be living in Asia, Latin America or Africa [3].

Given the demographics, it is clear that the greatest gap in the social safety net will be in the developing world. According to projections compiled by the advocacy group, Alzheimer's Disease International (ADI), the incidence of AD-related dementia in eastern and southern Asia will more than double in the next 20 years. China already has more than 10 million people living with AD; and 75% of these have not had a timely diagnosis. According to research published by the Chinese Alzheimer's Disease Project, the number of Chinese citizens suffering from AD-related dementia will surpass the caseload of the entire developed world by 2040 [4]. In that same period, Latin America will see increases of 134–146%. North Africa and the Middle East can expect a 125% rise.

Adding to the disease burden is the widespread and unwarranted stigma associated with AD, a blame-the-victim mindset reminiscent of the early years of the HIV/AIDS epidemic: a lack of empathy and compassion triggered by scant public awareness and the exhausting, often off-putting manifestations of the disease. The end result in too many cases—isolation, abandonment, withdrawal—attempts to mask symptoms and an unwillingness to seek healthcare. All of which further diminish patients' quality of life. Nearly one in four people with AD hide or conceal their symptoms, citing social stigma or dread of being ostracized [5]. Four out of ten sufferers report being excluded from the familiar and comforting routines of everyday life [5]. "Countries are not prepared and will continue not to be prepared, unless we overcome the stigma and enhance efforts to provide better care for those who have dementia and find a cure for the future," warns ADI's Executive Director Marc Wortmann.

The future is rushing rapidly toward us and there is no cure in sight. According to the World Health Organization (WHO), AD-related dementia is accelerating at the rate of one new case every four seconds. (In the United States, the rate—one new case every 68 seconds—will accelerate to one case every 33 seconds by 2050.) Each carries an immense burden of human suffering, healthcare costs, and lost productivity, particularly among family members—the sole mechanism for caring for AD victims in much of the developing world.

In 2010, the cost of dementia was estimated at US$604 billion [5], approximately 1% of the world's gross domestic product (GDP). Cost can be visualized on a sliding scale, ranging from approximately 0.25% of GDP in lesser developed countries to 1.25% in the developed world. Eighty-four percent of the global AD cost is borne either by family members, with a resultant loss of income, livelihood, educational opportunities, etc., and community-based healthcare professionals. Direct medical costs account for the remaining 16% [5].

In the real world, statistics take on flesh and blood significance as a victim's memory, reason, judgment, and language are inevitably destroyed. Tens of millions of children and grandchildren, wives, husbands, sons, and daughters of AD patients struggle daily with the overwhelming physical and emotional burden of caring for loved ones who may not even recognize or acknowledge them.

Here again, the developing world represents the tip of the epidemiological iceberg: In 2010, LDCs accounted for 14% of AD cases, but less than 1% of total worldwide expenditures. In 2050, when developing countries will account for nearly three-quarters of all cases [6], costs of dementia care are projected to have risen by as much as 85%, with developing countries facing the greatest increase percentage-wise.

Despite the urgent need for action, only 13 of the 193 WHO member states have implemented national dementia plans, all of them in the developed world [7]. Along the Pacific Rim, only Australia, Japan, and the Republic of Korea have strategic public health initiatives in place. A number of "subnational" responses are also being developed, for example in the Canadian province of Quebec, Switzerland's Vaud Canton, and the states of New South Wales and Queensland in Australia. We're facing the specter of AD becoming yet another preventable catastrophe visited on the world's most vulnerable populations.

Time grows short. Awareness must be engendered; advocacy encouraged. If there is promising news, it is that there is a stirring of interest and concern in the international community. Models for mitigating the looming epidemic exist; research and practical recommendations are available to help blunt the worst ravages of the epidemic.

2.2 NATIONAL MODELS

2.2.1 France

2.2.1.1 Background

In 2001, when France launched Europe's first national AD campaign, there were an estimated 600,000 total cases in that country [8]: Half were diagnosed; one-third were receiving treatment; 450,000 were living at home [8]. The annual cost of nursing home care was EUR 4,600 and growing. Pressures and public concern were building (unlike cancer, for example, AD is often a very public affliction and stirs a whole spectrum of emotional responses). More than 165,000 new cases were being diagnosed annually, with a life expectancy of eight years.

The French plan is built around specific, quantifiable, cost-effective objectives (which have been continually refined over the last decade):

- identify early symptoms of AD;
- refer patients to specialists;

- create a network of "memory centers" to assist in earlier diagnosis;
- develop ethical guidelines for caregivers and nursing homes;
- provide financial support for people with dementia;
- establish day care and local information centers;
- build new residential care homes and improve existing facilities; and
- support research and clinical studies.

By 2004, France's AD caseload had grown to nearly 800,000—18% of all French citizens over the age of 75—a growing proportion of them women. Nonetheless, the impact of the national plan was evident. Among other initiatives, AD was designated a chronic disease by the *Régime Français de Sécurité Sociale*, France's social security system—a critically important step in funding caregiving.

In 2006, a second French Dementia Plan identified additional objectives: provide 100% insurance coverage for dementia; diagnose and support younger individuals with the disease; provide training and support to professional and volunteer workers; develop emergency housing facilities.

In 2008, President Sarkozy (Third Alzheimer's Plan) pledged a public investment of EUR 1.6 billion, encouraging other European Union nations to make AD a priority. In 2011, a joint government/research sector review recommended a fourth AD initiative to maintain momentum and capitalize on the advances of the prior decade. In simple terms, France's approach—summarized below—has become a 10-point user's guide for developing nations attempting to manage the AD/dementia onslaught:

1. Increase support for caregivers.
2. Strengthen coordination.
3. Enable support at home.
4. Improve access to diagnostic and care programs.
5. Improve residential care.
6. Develop training for health professionals.
7. Support new research efforts.
8. Organize epidemiological surveillance.
9. Inform the general public.
10. Promote ethical considerations.

2.2.2 India

2.2.2.1 Background

The Dementia India Report [9], published in 2010, documented the increasing magnitude of the epidemic on the Indian subcontinent. By extension, it illustrates the lack of preparedness in the developing world. More than 3.7 million Indians are living with dementia, a figure that will double in 20 years. As much as 80% of all dementia cases are AD-related. (The second leading cause of dementia is cerebrovascular (CVA) in nature.) Fewer than 10% have been diagnosed. Social costs (i.e., direct medical, community, and informal care) were estimated at US$3.4 billion in a country with a per capita income of less than US$1500. As in other lesser developed countries, the cost of caring for urban AD patients is 2.5 times greater than in rural areas.

Behind the numbers was an all-too-familiar litany of inadequacy: Extremely low awareness levels; lack of governmental policies and programs to address dementia's challenges; inadequate diagnostic facilities and tools; insufficient care facilities; limited formal training for professional caregivers and families; scarce funding for AD services and research.

India's approach is a useful model of simple but effective strategies that can be brought to bear in dealing with the AD epidemic: Mobilizing governmental and other social welfare agencies to engage in "Health Interventions," "Social Interventions," and "Policy Initiatives."

2.2.2.2 Health Interventions

1. Create national and regional centers for research, training, and treating dementia.
2. Provide periodical training of doctors and paramedical staff on the nuances of dementia, its early detection and caregiving.
3. Set up "memory clinics" at hospitals in each district to ensure early diagnosis.
4. Generate dementia/AD awareness at district and regional levels.
5. Mobilize media campaigns to extend the governmental outreach.

2.2.2.3 Social Interventions

1. Authorize the construction of assisted living facilities for AD patients (at a minimum, one for each state and in all major cities) with on-site caregiver and personnel training programs.
2. Create preliminary memory screening (MiniMental State Examination) capability.
3. Provide rehabilitative therapies including physiotherapy, occupational therapy, music, reminiscence, and yoga.

2.2.2.4 Policy Initiatives

1. Utilize the census to enumerate persons with AD.
2. Track the magnitude of the disease through epidemiological studies.
3. Provide easier access to healthcare.
4. Underwrite rehabilitative and therapeutic interventions.

2.2.3 United Kingdom

2.2.3.1 Background

Currently, there are as many as 800,000 people living with AD-related dementia in the United Kingdom; by 2040, there will be more than 1.5 million afflicted seniors. Only 45% have been diagnosed. Both Scotland and Northern Ireland have better diagnosis rates. Two-thirds now live at home (most relying on family-based caregivers, but many struggle alone with their disease); the remainder are in assisted living facilities. One in four British hospital patients suffer from AD-dementia. In 2013, AD associated costs were pegged at £23 billion annually and expected to triple by 2040.

2.2.3.2 Suffering, Isolation and Abandonment

The situation in the UK [10] mirrors the litany of suffering, isolation, and abandonment that is the hallmark of AD anywhere in the world; it underscores what must be done to alleviate the unimaginable burden of suffering, loss and stunted lives and possibilities that the world—both developed and emerging—is facing. The following is excerpted from information provided by the UK's Dementia Action Alliance and other governmental and non-governmental AD support groups:

1. Social care systems do not reflect the fact that people with dementia are now a key group using many services.
2. Only one-third of people with dementia receive a specialist diagnosis and many receive that diagnosis late.
3. General Practitioners are reluctant to diagnose dementia either because they lack the knowledge to do so, do not see the benefits of early diagnosis or because they are aware of the lack of specialist support and services.
4. Following diagnosis, many people with dementia and caregivers report receiving no information about their condition or about what support is available.
5. Many facilities are struggling to deliver quality of life for people in the later stages of the illness.
6. People with dementia struggle for too long in their own homes without the help they need.
7. People with dementia are being inappropriately prescribed or over-prescribed antipsychotic drugs which increase the risk of death and reduce quality of life.
8. Health and social care staff routinely report that they have not received training in how to treat or care for people with dementia.
9. Spending from all sources on dementia research is low compared with other disease groups and by international standards.

In 2009, the British Government unveiled the "National Dementia Strategy for England" [11]. (Note that Scotland, Northern Ireland, and Wales have developed their own strategies.) The five-year plan contained a clear message as well as actionable information for both developed and LDCs. It also signaled that despite the ravages there is hope amidst the devastation:

> People with dementia are at risk of isolation and abuse. However, if they are diagnosed early, and they and their families receive help, they can continue to live a good quality of life.

In 2010, 400 public, private and non-governmental organizations (among them pharmaceutical companies, corporations, colleges, charitable trusts, small businesses, and professional associations) formed the Dementia Action Alliance (DAA) [12]. Alliance signatories unveiled an ambitious and achievable strategy for assisting AD patients and their caregivers in the UK in living meaningful and productive lives.

A deadline (2014) was set for implementing strategic policies and recommendations. Further, the Alliance acknowledged the need for a radical change in the way societies respond to dementia, in effect, a multi-focal, cross-disciplinary approach along the lines of the "War on Cancer" begun in the USA in the early 1970s:

> The Department of Health…will set out what it intends to do to help improve the lives of people with dementia. However, radical and sustainable change will only come about through the action of individuals and organizations working together locally and nationally to challenge what is wrong and to do things better [17].

Additionally, the DAA listed goals/outcomes [13] (see Box 2.1) drawn from interviews with dementia patients and their family caregivers. These include decision-making opportunities, modes and forms of treatment, caregiving, community involvement, the right to be free of stigma and discrimination, etc. A similar set of outcomes is detailed in the UK's Department of Health's National Dementia Strategy Implementation Plan [14].

In March 2013, the National Health Service announced an initiative linking £54 million in new funding for dementia risk assessments to the quality of hospital-based dementia care. It promised to provide an additional £50 million to upgrade wards and nursing homes for people with AD, and a £300 million program to build or renovate housing for people with long-term medical conditions, including AD disease.

2.2.4 United States of America

2.2.4.1 Background

In 2012, an estimated 5.4 million Americans were living with AD disease; 200,000 were under the age of 65. According to the Alzheimer's Association [15]," nearly half of all Americans age 85 and older have AD.

BOX 2.1 GOALS/OUTCOMES

- I have control over decisions about me.
- I have control over my life and the things that matter to me.
- I have access to adequate resources to choose where and how I live.
- I can make decisions about the care I want later in my life.
- I will die free from pain, fear, and with dignity.
- My caregiver can access services that can help support them in their role.
- I can choose what support suits me best.
- I have enough information and advice to make decisions about managing, now and in the future, as my dementia progresses.
- I live in an enabling and supportive environment where I feel valued and understood.
- I am making a contribution which makes me feel valued and valuable.
- The importance of helping me to sustain relationships with others is well recognized.
- If I develop behavior that challenges others, people will take time to understand why I am acting in this way and help me to try to avoid it.
- I have a sense of belonging and of being a valued part of family, community and civic life.
- Neither I nor my family feel ashamed or discriminated against because I have dementia.
- I know there is research going on which delivers a better life for me now and hope for the future.
- I am confident that there is an increasing investment in dementia research in the UK.
- As a person living with dementia, I am asked if I want to take part in suitable clinical trials.

Women comprise almost two-thirds of all AD cases, a statistic primarily explained by the fact that women, on average, live longer than men. Proportionately, older African Americans and Hispanics are more likely than older whites to develop AD and other dementias. Health conditions (e.g., high blood pressure, diabetes) and socio-economic factors rather than genetic factors likely account for this discrepancy. By 2050, someone in the USA will develop AD every 33 seconds. Deaths from heart disease, HIV/AIDS, and strokes are declining in the USA, whereas AD deaths continue to rise—increasing 68% from 2000 to 2010.

In the USA, AD costs run to US$203 billion annually and are projected to reach US$1.2 trillion by 2050. The direct cost of AD and related dementia is greater than any other condition in the USA, including heart disease and cancer.

2.2.4.2 *The National Alzheimer's Project Act*

On January 4, 2011, President Obama signed the National Alzheimer's Project Act (NAPA) into law. With the epidemic rapidly approaching critical mass, NAPA (like the French, Indian, and British national plans described above) attempts to *coordinate* and *evaluate* AD research, clinical care, institutional, home- and community-based programs and their outcomes. The law mandates [16]:

1. A national strategic plan—updated annually and submitted to Congress—for overcoming the AD crisis.
2. Annual evaluation of all federally funded efforts in AD research, care and services—and their outcomes.
3. Annual recommendations for priority actions to lower costs of government programs; improve outcomes for AD patients; lower costs to their families.
4. The creation of an Advisory Council on Alzheimer's Research, Care and Services to assist in coordinating the work of federal agencies; to assist in developing and evaluating the national plan.

In the run-up to the NAPA legislation, the Alzheimer's Association conducted more than 130 public hearings and solicited perspectives from more than 43,000 individuals in the AD community to distill the critical challenges to containing the epidemic by 2025. Once in hand, this data became the basis for developing an appropriate governmental response. The Association's recommendations are as follows [16]:

1. Increase AD research funding to US$2 billion annually.
2. Launch a nationwide AD public awareness campaign.
3. Improve the detection and diagnosis of AD; ensure that each diagnosis is followed with care planning.
4. Establish quality care indicators for dementia; embed these measures throughout the healthcare system.
5. Include AD in the Food and Drug Administration's accelerated review processes; remove barriers to the aggressive pursuit of treatments.
6. Ensure that federal efforts to address health disparities meet the challenges that AD poses to diverse communities.
7. Create Medicare demonstration projects to expand adult day health services and home healthcare.
8. Ensure greater access to custodial care by allowing individuals to receive services without having to exhaust all of their savings first.
9. Implement evidence-based caregiver support services and interventions.
10. Ensure equal access for those with early-onset AD to all AD programs and services.

In the pharmaceutical industry, the cost of developing an AD drug could easily top US$1 billion, with no guarantees of efficacy or approval.

In fact, there have been so many negative AD trials over the past decades that there is increasing concern that publicly traded companies may be unwilling to invest in any more long and expensive trials.

In 2012, the National Institutes of Health (NIH) earmarked approximately US$450 million for AD research. An additional US$50 million was added to underwrite genetic research into the etiology of the disease, e.g., gene-sequencing of AD patients. By contrast, the agency spent about US$3.1 billion in grants for HIV/AIDS research and US$5.8 billion on cancer [17]. In the spring of 2013, President Obama asked Congress for an additional US$100 million for research and education, and in 2014 a budget supplement that would increase AD funding to US$600 million, a fraction of the US$2 billion stakeholders deem necessary in controlling the epidemic.

2.3 DEMOGRAPHICS AND DESTINY

Over the next 20 years, the number of AD cases are expected to increase by 40% in Europe, 63% in North America, 77% in South America, and 89% in Australia, New Zealand, Japan, and other developed Asia-Pacific nations. As we have seen, among LDCs the increases are much more dramatic: 117% in East Asia, 107% in South Asia, 134–146% in Latin America, and 125% in North Africa and the Middle East. As mentioned, by 2050, 70% of all AD cases will be in LDCs. It seems increasingly apparent that an international AD strategy, perhaps administered by the WHO, needs to be developed.

Awareness is key to marshaling a robust response to what is clearly "the twenty-first century epidemic." In parts of Africa and Latin America AD awareness is abysmal, with diagnoses and intervention essentially non-existent, where all too often AD is assumed to be "old age," and where vital epidemiological studies have not been undertaken. In China, 49% of individuals with AD and vascular dementia were classified as normally aging; only 20% had adequate access to diagnostic assessment, compared with 20% and more than 70% respectively, in Europe and the developed world [18].

AD is a disease that stubbornly refuses to reveal itself, either in the research lab—there is no cure in sight—or in the ill-prepared cities, villages, households, and extended families that harbor, yet all too often do not shelter, their victims.

2.4 NATIONAL DEMENTIA PLANS

The following are useful models for planning and designing workable AD responses:

Australia: http://www.alz.co.uk/plans/australia
Denmark: http://www.alz.co.uk/plans/denmark
United Kingdom: http://www.alz.co.uk/plans/england
Finland: http://www.alz.co.uk/plans/finland
France: http://www.alz.co.uk/plans/france
Republic of Korea: http://www.alz.co.uk/plans/republic-of-korea
Netherlands: http://www.alz.co.uk/plans/netherlands
Norway: http://www.alz.co.uk/plans/norway
United States: http://www.alz.co.uk/plans/usa

References

[1] World Alzheimer Report 2010: The Global Economic Impact of Dementia[Internet]. Alzheimer's Disease International; 2010 Sept. 21 [updated 2011 June; cited 2013 April]. Available from: <http://www.alz.co.uk/research/files/WorldAlzheimerReport 2010.pdf>.

[2] Dementia cases set to triple by 2050 but still largely ignored [Internet]. World Health Organization; 2012 April 11 [cited 2013 April]. Available from: <http://www.who.int/mediacentre/news/releases/2012/dementia_20120411/en/>.

[3] Dementia statistics [Internet]. Alzheimer's Disease International; 2010 [cited 2013 April]. Available from: <http://www.alz.co.uk/research/statistics>.

[4] China Alzheimer's Project[Internet]. China Contemporary TCM Institute; 2010 February [cited 2013 April].Available from: <http://www.memory360.org/en/>.

[5] World Alzheimer Report 2012: Overcoming the stigma of dementia [Internet]. London: Alzheimer's Disease International; 2012 September[cited 2013 April]. Available from: <http://www.alz.co.uk/research/WorldAlzheimerReport2012.pdf>.

[6] Ferri CP, Prince M, Brayne C, Brodaty H, Fratiglioni L, Ganguli M, et al. Global prevalence of dementia: a Delphi consensus study. Lancet 2005;366:2112–27.

[7] Government Alzheimer's Plans [Internet]. Alzheimer's Disease International; 2012 April [cited 2013 April]. Available from: <http://www.alz.co.uk/alzheimer-plans>.

[8] France–National Plans for Alzheimer and Related Diseases [Internet]. Alzheimer Europe; 2008 June [updated 2012 June; cited 2013 April]. Available from: <http://www.alzheimer-europe.org/Policy-in-Practice2/National-Dementia-Plans/France#fragment-1>.

[9] Dementia India Report 2010: Prevalence, Impact, Cost & Services for Dementia [Internet]. Alzheimer's and Related Disorders Society of India; 2010 [cited 2013 April]. Available from: <http://www.alzheimer.org.in/dementia_2010.pdf>.

[10] Who We Are [Internet]. Dementia Action Alliance 2013 [cited 2013 April]. Available from: <http://www.dementiaaction.org.uk>.

[11] United Kingdom (England) National Dementia Plans [Internet]. Alzheimer Europe; 2009 May [updated 2011 March; cited 2013 April]. Available from: <www.alzheimer-europe.org/Policy-in-Practice2/National-Dementia-Plans/United-Kingdom-England?#fragment-1>.

[12] Members Actions Plans [Internet]. Dementia Action Alliance; 2013 [cited 2013 April]. Available from: <www.dementiaaction.org.uk/members_and_action_plans>.

[13] National Dementia Declaration [Internet]. Dementia Action Alliance; 2013 [cited 2013 April].

[14] Improving care for people with dementia [Internet]. Department of Health; [updated 2013 April 23; cited 2013 April]. Available from: <http://www.gov.uk/government/policies/improving-care-for-people-with-dementia>.

[15] Alzheimer's Disease Facts and Figures 2013 [Internet]. Alzheimer's Association; 2013 [cited 2013 April]. Available from: <http://www.alz.org/alzheimers_disease_facts_ and_figures.asp>.

[16] The National Alzheimer's Project Act [Internet]. Alzheimer's Association; 2011 November [cited 2013 April]. Available from: <http://napa.alz.org/wp-content/ uploads/2011/11/2011-NAPA-Factsheet-Post-Report.pdf>.

[17] Wayne, A. US to Boost Funding for Alzheimer's Research by $50 million This Year [Internet]. Bloomberg News; 2012 February 7 [cited 2013 April]. Available from: <http://www.bloomberg.com/news/2012-02-07/u-s-to-boost-funding-for-alzheimer- s-research-by-50-million.html>.

[18] Kalaria R, Maestre G, Arizaga R, et. al. Alzheimer's disease and vascular dementia in developing countries: prevalence, management, and risk factors [print/Internet]. National Institutes of Health, National Center for Biotechnical Information; 2008 September 7 [cited 2013 April]. Available from: <http://www.ncbi.nlm.nih.gov/pmc/ articles/PMC2860610/>.

3

Preventing Alzheimer's Disease

Roy W. Jones

The Research Institute for the Care of Older People, Royal United
Hospital, Bath, and University of Bath, Bath, UK

3.1 INTRODUCTION

In 2010, there were estimated to be 35.6 million people with dementia worldwide and this number is expected to double every 20 years to an estimated 65.7 million in 2030 and 115.4 million in 2050 [1]. Currently there are more than 7.7 million new cases of dementia each year, one approximately every four seconds. The total estimated worldwide cost of dementia was US$604 billion in 2010 with 70% of these costs occurring in Western Europe and North America [1]. These costs are around 1% of the world's gross domestic product (GDP) varying from 0.24% GDP in low income countries to 0.35% in low middle income, 0.5% in high middle income, and 1.24% in high income countries. If the dementia costs were a country, it would be the world's 18th largest economy [1].

A recent US study [2] suggested that the yearly monetary cost per person that was attributable to dementia was between US$41,686 and US$56,290 depending on the method used to value informal care. This suggested that the total monetary cost of dementia in 2010 in the USA was between US$ 157 and US$ 215 billion, of which Medicare paid US$11 billion; these costs are greater than those for either cancer or heart disease [2].

Given the extreme apprehension about Alzheimer's disease (AD) in older people and their families, coupled with the enormous personal, societal, and financial costs of dementias such as AD, it is hardly surprising that there is an increasing pressure and priority to try and find effective and safe disease-modifying and preventive treatment strategies.

However, it is extremely difficult to prevent or modify a disease without a clear understanding of the aetiology and underlying pathological abnormalities and how they arise. It is not surprising therefore that the concept of developing strategies that may prevent AD is at a much

M. Bairu & M.W. Weiner (Eds):
Global Clinical Trials for Alzheimer's Disease.
DOI: http://dx.doi.org/10.1016/B978-0-12-411464-7.00003-1

33

earlier stage in comparison with strategies for preventing other conditions such as heart or lung disease. The current specific drug treatments for AD (cholinesterase inhibitors and memantine) appear to be symptomatic treatments and alternative approaches are therefore essential.

AD research has exploded over the past 25–30 years, and this has allowed the identification of a number of possible pathogenic processes and pathways and potential targets for intervention [3]. Neuropathological and neuroimaging studies have provided vital information and shown that the pathogenic process begins many years before symptoms appear. If this is the case, then—analogous to the treatment of hypercholesterolaemia to prevent heart disease—it may be necessary to commence treatments that modify the AD process many years before as well. However, the drug development process has generally remained focused on treating the disease once it is symptomatic, and regulatory authorities such as the Food and Drug Administration (FDA) and European Medicines Agency (EMEA) have difficulty in identifying a pathway for compounds that may have subtle benefits and where those benefits may not be seen for some years. Calculating the cost-effectiveness and cost–benefit of such compounds is also challenging, particularly if the cost implications are mainly considered from the point of view of health services and not the wider costs to society and the individual patient and their family.

One major initiative that has arisen as a result of concerns about the rising numbers of people with AD across the globe, and the enormous accompanying financial burden for individuals and society, is the campaign to Prevent Alzheimer's Disease by 2020 (PAD2020) that was launched in 2009 [4]. This was built from a number of think-tank meetings culminating in the specific recommendations for action based on the collective thoughts of 70 worldwide leaders in dementia research. The scientific challenge is to develop new conceptual models of dementia that will provide better explanations of the clinical underpinnings of the disease and identify new therapeutic targets. Current models fail to provide a complete account of the relationship between the clinical and biological phenotypes of the disease [4]. To prevent AD will require the development of a battery of well-validated early markers of the disease which amongst other things can identify asymptomatic people at risk of AD. Drug-discovery programs need to be expanded to identify and validate new therapeutic targets that focus on protection against synapse loss, prevention of dendritic pruning, and repair/regeneration of dying neurons [4]. Such approaches will require the appropriate infrastructure for long-term longitudinal studies and developing that infrastructure is an important part of PAD2020 [4].

3.1.1 Definitions

Primary prevention refers to strategies that alter the latent phase of AD, which will delay its development in normal people. Secondary prevention will delay the progression from the expression of the earliest symptoms, usually mild memory changes, to the stage where the individual has sufficient problems to fulfill the appropriate criteria for a diagnosis of dementia or AD to be made. Finally, tertiary prevention involves treatment that may delay, stop or reverse overt clinical disease [5].

3.2 IMPROVED UNDERSTANDING OF THE AD PROCESS

The current criteria that are most widely used to diagnose AD date back to 1984 [6] at a time when there was very little understanding about genetic factors and the underlying molecular changes that lead to AD. With these criteria, a diagnosis of definite AD is only possible after examination of brain tissue, which is rarely possible except at post-mortem. Most patients diagnosed in life as possible or probable AD [6] never come to post-mortem so an absolute pathological confirmation of the diagnosis is unusual.

More recently, new criteria have been proposed that take into account progress with the development of neuroimaging and chemical biomarkers [7,8]. The National Institute on Aging (NIA)/Alzheimer's Association (AA) proposed three different phases of the disease [7]:

1. A preclinical or pre-symptomatic phase occurring some years before symptoms become apparent.
2. A symptomatic phase characterized by mild problems in cognition, learning, and memory that are sufficient to be noticed and measured but not enough to significantly impair a person's ability to live independently or to carry out everyday activities. This phase is equivalent to the existing concept of mild cognitive impairment (MCI) [8] but includes information about biomarkers that can help to clarify the potential cause of the MCI.
3. Possible and probable AD, when the disease has progressed to a point where symptoms are more marked and a diagnosis of dementia is appropriate.

The International Working Group for New Research Criteria for the Diagnosis of AD [9] proposed a new lexicon with several similarities to the NIA/AA proposals but introduced the concept of prodromal AD, which applies to subjects with MCI and positive biomarkers that would increase the likelihood that the MCI is due to an underlying AD process.

Broadly speaking, primary prevention applies to the preclinical phase of AD, secondary prevention to the MCI/prodromal AD phase, and tertiary prevention to people with a diagnosis of AD, although in practice it remains clinically difficult to clearly delineate the three stages.

A more accurate diagnosis of AD in life is an important goal and would help to ensure that new treatments developed specifically for AD are targeted correctly and not given to people with non-AD dementia who could not benefit but might suffer harm. Earlier diagnosis in the prodromal (MCI) or the preclinical stage of AD would allow treatment to be targeted at a point where interventions are most likely to be beneficial. Finally, it would be valuable if treatment effects could be measured more objectively.

In the past few years, several major studies have begun such as the Alzheimer's Disease Imaging Initiative (ADNI) [10]. Many of these studies were designed to examine the role of chemical biomarkers and neuroimaging in assessing and predicting progression in individuals without cognitive impairment, and in individuals with MCI. These studies have given an increasingly detailed picture of the underlying events that lead to AD and dementia, including changes occurring in the pre-symptomatic phase, together with the development of biomarker and neuroimaging modalities.

A hypothetical model of dynamic markers of the AD pathological cascade has been proposed [11]. The classical lesions originally described by Alois Alzheimer are extracellular amyloid plaques and intracellular neurofibrillary tangles. The plaques are composed of the 42-amino acid β-amyloid ($A\beta_{42}$) and the tangles consist of the microtubule-associated protein tau, which becomes hyperphosphorylated. Currently available evidence suggests that the initiating event in AD is related to abnormal processing of Aβ peptide, eventually leading to the formation of Aβ plaques in the brain [11]. This process occurs while people remain cognitively unchanged. Biomarkers of brain β-amyloidosis include reductions in cerebral spinal fluid (CSF) $A\beta_{42}$ and increased amyloid positron emission tomography (PET) tracer retention (using agents such as Pittsburgh compound B (PiB) [11] and, more recently, fluorinated compounds such as florbetapir[18]F (Amyvid, Eli Lilly), which has a longer half-life of 110 minutes than PiB and is approved by the FDA and the European Commission for use in patients with cognitive impairment being investigated for AD and other causes of cognitive impairment [12]. After a variable lag period, neuronal dysfunction and neurodegeneration become the dominant pathological processes. Biomarkers of these processes are increased CSF tau and structural magnetic resonance imaging measures of cerebral atrophy. Neurodegeneration is accompanied by synaptic dysfunction, which is indicated by decreased fluorodeoxyglucose uptake on PET [11].

The hypothetical model attempts to relate the disease stage to AD biomarkers in which Aß biomarkers become abnormal first, before neurodegenerative biomarkers and cognitive symptoms, and that the neurodegenerative biomarkers correlate with clinical symptom severity [11]. Taken together, these quantifiable markers of the evolving disease process have now been replicated in numerous studies and offer an important resource for validating preventive and therapeutic agents in AD [13]. However, the situation is not straightforward if the need for complex biomarkers becomes standard practice everywhere. The availability and expense of MRI and PET scanners and amyloid imaging ligands would be an issue in many parts of the world. Reluctance and the lack of suitable facilities to do CSF testing, especially if repeat sampling were necessary, could also be a potentially limiting factor even though it has been suggested that the idea that a lumbar puncture is uncomfortable and generally unacceptable to patients is badly out of date [13]. More importantly, even in the best research centers, which have suggested that concentrations of $A\beta_{42}$, total tau, and phospho-tau in the CSF could identify with high accuracy individuals with MCI who would progress to AD [14], there are issues about the large inter-site variability in the measurements, and there have been calls for efforts to develop international standardization [14,15].

3.3 PREVIOUS PREVENTION TRIALS

A number of prevention trials have already been carried out in an attempt to delay the onset of MCI or dementia. Such trials need to recruit large numbers of participants with either no cognitive impairment or with minimal problems such as isolated memory complaints. The studies must continue for a number of years rather than a number of months as would be typical for the case of a new symptomatic treatment. As a result, the safety and tolerability of any intervention becomes critical and at least one study, the Alzheimer's Disease Anti-inflammatory Prevention Trial (ADAPT) with the non-steroidal anti-inflammatory drugs (NSAIDs) naproxen and celecoxib, has been terminated because of safety concerns [16]. The trial was initially put on hold because of concerns about increased cardiovascular risk to those taking naproxen in the trial but was then terminated permanently because of increased concerns generally about the cardiovascular and cerebrovascular risks of celecoxib [16]. The results of the study were published and neither drug improved cognition whilst there was also weak evidence of a detrimental effect of naproxen [17]. Another study that also raised safety concerns, the Women's Health Initiative Memory Study (WHI-MS), demonstrated that women on hormone replacement therapy (HRT) in the form of conjugated equine oestrogens and progesterone were more likely to develop cognitive impairment and dementia, so this approach could not be recommended for the prevention of AD [18].

Interventions evaluated to date have mainly included drugs that have already been marketed for other indications such as NSAIDs, HRT or statins, or vitamins, antioxidants and related compounds, and on the basis that inflammation, oestrogens, hypercholesterolaemia, and free radicals may be relevant factors in the AD process.

These trials have recruited from 1,000 to more than 20,000 subjects who have usually been treated for four to nine years. In some trials, like the long-term Physicians' Health Study-II (PHS-II) that examined ß-carotene, vitamins C and E, or a daily multivitamin for the prevention of cancer or cardiovascular disease, the prevention of cognitive decline was nested as a component within the main trial [19]. Some cognitive results from this study are still to be reported but the β-carotene data have been published [20]. No benefit was seen in cognitive performance after short-term (mean treatment duration of one year) β-carotene supplementation, but it was suggested that long-term supplementation might provide cognitive benefits. However, the β-carotene limb of PHS-II was halted earlier than other elements of the trial because no effects had been seen on total cardiovascular disease, total cancer cases, or total mortality [21]. The latest PHS-II results did not support multivitamin use to prevent cardiovascular disease [22].

The main outcomes in all of these prevention trials has been the onset of dementia or MCI, but so far none of the studies has demonstrated significant positive benefits and, as discussed above, some have actually shown negative effects either from a safety and/or efficacy perspective.

Three preventive trials have also been undertaken using Ginkgo biloba (as the preparation EGb 761), presumably mainly because it is considered to be a relatively safe product. One placebo-controlled trial of 118 subjects aged 85 or older without MCI or dementia, followed for 42 months, showed no benefit on an intention-to-treat analysis [23], but a secondary analysis controlling for medication adherence suggested that there might be a delay in progression to MCI and a reduction in memory decline. There were more ischaemic strokes and transient ischaemic attacks in the Ginkgo biloba group [23]. The Ginkgo Evaluation of Memory (GEM) study assessed 3,069 people with no cognitive impairment or MCI for a median duration of more than six years randomized to EGb 761 or placebo and found no benefit on cognition or the time to dementia [24]. Finally, the GuidAge study in France, which involved 2,854 people with memory complaints or MCI randomized to Ginkgo or placebo and followed for more than five years, showed that long-term use of a standardized ginkgo extract did not reduce the risk of progression to AD in comparison with placebo [25].

3.4 NEW CLINICAL TRIAL APPROACHES

Because of the urgent need to fund effective pre-symptomatic treatments that either reduce or prevent the risk of AD symptoms, new research approaches have been recommended [26]. The Alzheimer's Prevention Initiative (API) comments that it has taken too many healthy people, too much money, and too many years to evaluate the range of promising pre-symptomatic treatments using clinical endpoints [27]. Brain imaging and other measurements have already been used to track some of the earliest changes associated with the predisposition to AD. The API authors plan to evaluate investigational amyloid-modifying treatments in healthy people who are at the highest imminent risk of developing symptomatic AD using brain imaging, CSF, and cognitive endpoints [27]. One study will look at a large Columbian kindred carrying a presenilin-1 mutation close to their estimated average age at clinical onset and using crenezumab (Genentech), an experimental humanized monoclonal antibody that binds Aß peptide [28]. Another trial is proposed to study apolipoprotein E (ApoE) ε4 homozygotes (and possibly heterozygotes) close to their estimated average age at clinical onset [27].

The API's goals include: evaluating investigational AD-modifying treatments sooner than otherwise possible; determining the extent to which the treatment's brain imaging and other biomarker effects predict a clinical benefit (this information could prove useful in finding biomarker endpoints that can be used in other clinical trials); and to provide a better test of the amyloid hypothesis than is provided by clinical trials in symptomatic patients when the treatment may be being administered too late to be of significant benefit [27].

The Dominantly Inherited Alzheimer Network (DIAN) [29], started in 2008 as a network to support clinical trials for people with familial AD (FAD), is conducting a study, DIAN TU [30], with two other monoclonal antibodies that bind ß-amyloid, gantenerumab (Roche), and solanezumab (Lilly) in people with known FAD or a strong family history of AD presenting before the age of 55.

Finally, the A4 study (Anti-amyloid in Asymptomatic Alzheimer's Disease) has also selected solanezumab (Lilly) for its trial [31] of people who are amyloid biomarker positive. The therapeutic success of this study does not depend on Aβ being the cause of AD but only that it is a critical early factor in the pathogenesis of AD.

Both the DIAN and A4 studies are planned with adaptive trial design features so that ongoing information can lead to extension of the trial if it generates positive data initially or, if not, to the involvement of a new generation of drugs.

In 2012, details were presented at the Alzheimer's Association international conference about the formation of an umbrella group, the Collaboration for Alzheimer's Prevention (CAP), to look at common issues across pre-synaptic treatment trials and to harmonize the methods of the three groups, to maximize the data that will be generated, and to try and ensure that the initiatives find regulatory solutions [32]. The joint initiative has already led to one success in that regulators have indicated that it may be possible to consider preclinical treatment trials using a single cognitive composite and biomarkers for review as registration studies in these pre-symptomatic populations [32,33], although this approach has been criticized in an editorial in the *New York Times*, stating that it "lowers the bar" for AD drug development [34].

Although the term "prevention trial" is being used by the CAP group, in practice regulators such as the FDA would not grant a prevention claim without proof that the disease had effectively been prevented for the rest of the person's life and therefore the correct term should really be "preclinical AD treatment."

3.5 LIFESTYLE FACTORS, DIET, AND ALCOHOL

AD is a chronic condition presenting mainly in older adults but the onset of neuropathological changes within the brain begins some decades before clinical manifestations appear [35]. The development of the disease depends on both genetic susceptibility and other risk factors, some of which are known; such risk factors are a potential target for primary or secondary prevention. Most of the data for protective medical and lifestyle factors have emerged from retrospective case-control studies and prospective cohort studies of dementia.

Unfortunately, when people are frightened about developing a condition like AD, there is inevitabe demand for such information about possible prevention. The increasing information in the media and on websites can create the impression that there are already numerous proven preventive strategies, whereas the scientific supporting information is much more limited.

The most extensive review of risk factors came in a controversial state-of-the-science conference statement from a US National Institutes of Health panel [36]. The review included relevant studies on the relationship of multiple factors, including nutritional, medical, social, economic, behavioral, environmental, and genetic, with mild cognitive impairment or AD. The review was restricted to studies in humans from developed countries with a sample size of at least 50 for randomized, controlled trials and 300 for observational studies, and a minimum duration between exposure to preventive interventions and outcomes (in a later published report this was set at a minimum of two years [37]). The review concluded that currently there was no evidence of even moderate scientific quality to support the association of any modifiable factors (such as nutritional supplements, herbal preparations, dietary factors, prescription or non-prescription drugs, social or economic factors, medical conditions, toxins, or environmental exposures) with a reduced risk for AD [36].

Whilst a number of modifiable factors have been reported across multiple studies, the authors suggest that the overall scientific quality of the evidence is low. Conditions such as diabetes, elevated midlife blood cholesterol levels, and depression have been associated with increased risk. On the other hand, a number of lifestyle factors and medications have been linked with a reduced risk of AD, including low saturated fat consumption, an adequate intake of folic acid, high fruit and vegetable intake, use of statins, light to moderate alcohol intake, educational attainment, cognitive engagement, and participation in physical activities. Current smoking, never having been married, and having low levels of social support have all been reported to be associated with a higher risk of AD, but again, the level of the evidence was low [36]. No consistent associations for other vitamins, fatty acids, the metabolic syndrome, blood pressure, plasma homocysteine levels, obesity and body mass index, antihypertensive medications, non-steroidal anti-inflammatory drugs, gonadal steroids, or exposure to solvents, electromagnetic fields, lead or aluminum were found.

The authors also comment that there are challenges in interpreting the findings across the various studies due to the inconsistency in the definition of AD and the difficulty in separating out whether factors such as vascular disease that can itself lead to dementia are truly associated with AD and whether conditions such as depression could actually be early features of AD [36].

The primary limitation in the studies is the difficulty in recognizing causality rather than association. For example, people with higher educational levels are more likely to have greater cognitive engagement and it is hard therefore to decide whether either or both factors are important [36].

Similarly, the report suggests that for most factors, existing studies either show no association with cognitive decline or provide inconclusive evidence and where an association has been seen, the overall quality of the evidence is low.

Although the NIH report seems quite negative, it illustrates the difficulty of getting reliable information about factors that if modified might reduce the risk of AD and also the risk of dementia in general. A number of vascular risk factors have been identified that appear to be associated with dementia and cognitive decline. These factors are also usually risk factors for heart disease and have encouraged the concept that what is good for one's heart appears to be good for one's brain [38].

The Cardiovascular Risk Factors, Aging and Dementia (CAIDE) Score is a simple method for predicting the risk of late-life dementia in people of middle age, on the basis of their risk profiles [39]. The main use for such a score is to target those most at risk of the disease so that they can take preventive measures. Future dementia was significantly predicted by age ($\geq$47), low education ($\leq$10 years), hypertension, hypercholesterolaemia, and obesity. This risk score needs to be extended to other populations but highlights the relevance of midlife vascular factors.

More recently, new research has examined two Framingham vascular risk scores (for cardiovascular disease and for stroke) and compared them with the CAIDE score as predictors for 10-year cognitive decline in middle age [40]. The study participants included men and women, average age 55.6 years at baseline, from an ongoing prospective cohort study established in 1985. Cognitive tests looking at verbal fluency, vocabulary, and global cognitive scores were carried out three times over the 10-year period. Higher cardiovascular disease risk and higher stroke risk were associated with greater cognitive decline in all tests except memory; higher dementia risk was associated with greater decline in reasoning, vocabulary, and global cognitive score. The two vascular risk scores showed a slightly stronger association than the dementia risk score with 10-year cognitive decline (and this was statistically significant for semantic fluency and for global cognitive scores). The authors [40] concluded that although all three risk scores were able to predict cognitive decline in late middle age, the Framingham risk scores may have an advantage over the CAIDE score when it comes to primary prevention and targeting modifiable risk factors.

Clearly, the gold standard for showing cause and effect is to carry out a trial randomly assigning subjects either to a prevention or risk management strategy group or to a control group. However, for ethical and practical reasons it is unlikely that some strategies will ever be tested in random trials. For example, to test the impact of physical exercise on the risk of developing AD would require very large numbers of subjects and be very expensive; in addition the control group would need to go without exercise, whereas exercise already has a number of proven benefits. Like exercise, any benefit from a specific diet on the brain may relate to its effect on cardiovascular health. The best current evidence suggests that heart-healthy eating patterns, such as the Mediterranean diet, may also help protect the brain [41]. A Mediterranean diet includes relatively little red meat and emphasizes whole grains, fruit and vegetables, fish and shellfish, nuts, olive oil and other healthy fats (for example those rich in ω-3 fatty acids).

3.6 THE FUTURE

The NIH State-of-the-Science conference statement on preventing AD and cognitive decline [36] recognized the need for highly reliable consensus-based diagnostic criteria for cognitive decline, MCI, and AD, and found insufficient evidence to support the use of pharmaceutical agents or dietary supplements to prevent cognitive decline or AD. Whilst a large amount of promising research is underway, the statement called for these efforts to be increased and added to by new understandings and innovations.

For example, important ongoing trials on antihypertensive medications, ω-3 fatty acids, physical activity, and cognitive engagement might provide further insight into the prevention or delay of cognitive decline or AD [36]. This needs to be supported by further studies. Also, large-scale, population-based studies and randomized, controlled trials are needed to examine strategies for maintaining cognitive function in individuals at risk of decline, to identify factors that may delay the onset of AD among persons at risk, and to identify factors that may slow the progression of AD once a person has been diagnosed [36].

There are important conceptual differences when trying to validate the efficacy of interventions for "treatment" as opposed to "prevention" [4] and these have been well conceptualized by Meinert [42]. The basic problems and difficulties of a randomized trial for treatment or prevention are similar [42]. The differences relate to the purpose of the trial, the choice of study treatments, the choice of outcome measures, the approach to recruiting subjects and establishing inclusion and exclusion criteria such as age, and issues relating to monitoring [42]. In the context of cognitive decline and dementia, the duration of the study is also likely to be longer for preventive trials. The risk–benefit for the two types of trial also needs to be considered [42]. In a treatment trial the risks of harm occur at the same time as the potential for benefit and it is easier to assess the balance between the two. In contrast, in a prevention trial the risk begins on commencement of the intervention whereas the benefit is expected at some time in the future making the assessment of risk–benefit more difficult; strategies for prevention are usually expected to have a lower risk–benefit than interventions for "treatment."

We have entered a new era of AD and dementia research [43]. This has been driven by technological advances in imaging (MRI and PET including *in vivo* measurement of amyloid plaques) and CSF measurements that can potentially recognize risk markers for AD. Such advances will be challenging in many parts of the world where access to such facilities and the associated costs will be difficult. Nevertheless, these new technological advances are being incorporated certainly within research diagnostic criteria and can be built into primary and secondary prevention trials as well as within standard AD treatment trials.

The challenge will be to test new hypotheses and not just refine the information from imaging and chemical biomarkers further and further. Asking appropriate questions and testing new hypotheses should lead to effective preventive and therapeutic trials [43]. For example, what are the determinants of amyloid deposition and AD? What factors increase production or decrease amyloid clearance in a genetically susceptible individual? What is happening in populations that are protected against AD, such as those with the recently described Icelandic mutation [44]? Is vascular disease in the brain an important determinant of increased Aβ production? Are there unique risk factors and determinants for brain changes, such as loss of synapses, that are independent of the risk factors that determine deposition of amyloid [43]?

Successful trials could be based on a better understanding of the risk factors, whether they are lifestyle/environmental, genetic or linked to aspects of the aging process. The challenge will be to link the enhanced technological knowledge about imaging and biomarkers with relevant preventive studies that will necessarily be of long duration and expensive. The success of such an approach is vital given the predicted increase in the number of people worldwide who will develop cognitive decline or AD in the future.

References

[1] Wimo A, Prince M. World Alzheimer Report 2010: the Global Economic Impact of Dementia. Alzheimer's Disease International. 21 September 2010, cited June 2013. Available from: <http://www.alz.co.uk/research/files/WorldAlzheimerReport2010.pdf>.

[2] Hurd MD, Martorell P, Delavande A, Mullen KJ, Langa KM. Monetary costs of Dementia in the United States. N Engl J Med 2013;368:1326–34.

[3] Khachaturian ZK, Petersen RC, Gauthier S, Buckholtz N, Corey-Bloom JP, Evans W, et al. Meeting Report: A roadmap for the prevention of dementia: the inaugural Leon Thal Symposium. Alzheimer Dement 2008;4:156–63.

[4] Khachaturian ZK, Khachaturian AS. Prevent Alzheimer's disease by 2020: a national strategic goal. Alzheimer Dement 2009;5:81–4.

[5] Feldman HH, Jacova C. Primary prevention and delay of onset of AD/Dementia. Can J Neurol Sci 2007;34(**Suppl. 1**):S84–9.

[6] McKhann G, Drachman DA, Folstein M, Katzman R, Price DL, Stadlan EM. Clinical diagnosis of Alzheimer's disease – report of the NINCDS-ADRDA work group under the auspices of Department of Health and Human Services task force on Alzheimer's disease. Neurology 1984;34:939–44.

[7] Jack CR, Albert M, Knopman DS, McKhann GM, Sperling RA, Carrillo M, et al. Introduction to revised criteria for the diagnosis of Alzheimer's disease: National Institute on aging and the Alzheimer's Association workgroup. Alzheimer's Dement 2011;7:257–62.

[8] Petersen RC, Smith GE, Waring SC, Ivnik RJ, Tangalos EG, Kokmen E. Mild cognitive impairment: clinical characterization and outcome. Arch Neurol 1999;56:303–08.

[9] Dubois B, Feldman HH, Jacova C, Cummings JL, Dekosky ST, Barberger-Gateau P, et al. Lancet Neurol 2010;9:1118–27.

[10] Mueller SG, Weiner MW, Thal LJ, Petersen RC, Jack CR, Jagust W, et al. Ways toward an early diagnosis in AD: the Alzheimer's Disease Imaging Initiative (ADNI). Alzheimers Dement 2005;1:55–66.

[11] Jack CR, Knopman DS, Jagust WJ, Shaw LM, Aisen PS, Weiner MW, et al. Hypothetical model of dynamic biomarkers of the Alzheimer's pathological cascade. Lancet Neurol 2010;9:119–28.

[12] Eli Lilly and Company [press release], 2013 January 15: Available from: <http://newsroom.lilly.com/releasedetail.cfm?releaseid=733724>.

[13] Selkoe DJ. Preventing Alzheimer's disease. Science 2012;337:1488–92.

[14] Mattson N, Zetterberg H, Hansson O, Andreasen N, Parnetti L, Jonsson M, et al. CSF biomarkers and incipient Alzheimer's disease in patients with mild cognitive impairment. JAMA 2009;302:385–93.

[15] Petersen RC. Alzheimer's disease: progress in prediction. Lancet Neurol 2010;9:4–5.

[16] ADAPT Research Group Cardiovascular and cerebrovascular events in the randomized, controlled Alzheimer's disease anti-inflammatory prevention trial (ADAPT). PLoS Clin Trials 2006;1(7):e33.

[17] ADAPT Research Group Martin BK, Szekely C, Brandt J, Piantadosi S, Breitner JC, et al. Cognitive function over time in the Alzheimer's disease anti-inflammatory prevention trial (ADAPT): results of a randomized, controlled trial of naproxen and celecoxib. Arch Neurol 2008;65(7):896–905.

[18] Shumaker SA, Legault C, Rapp SR, Thal L, Wallace RB, Ockene JK, et al. Estrogen plus progestin and the incidence of dementia and mild cognitive impairment in postmenopausal women: the Women's Health Initiative Memory Study: a randomized controlled trial. JAMA 2003;289:2651–62.

[19] Christen WG, Gaziano JM, Hennekens CH. Design of physicians' health study II–a randomized trial of ß-carotene, vitamins E and C, and multivitamins, in prevention of cancer, cardiovascular disease, and eye disease, and review of results of completed trials. Ann Epidemiol 2000;10:125–34.

[20] Grodstein F, Kang JH, Glynn RJ, Cook NR, Gaziano JM. A randomized trial of ß-carotene supplementation and cognitive function in men: the Physicians' Health Study II. Arch Intern Med 2007;167(20):2184–90.

[21] Physicians' Health study: Frequently Asked Questions [Internet]. Last updated 25 June 2011, cited May 5 2013. Available at: <http://phs.bwh.harvard.edu/faqs.htm>.

[22] Sesso HD, Christen WG, Bubes V, Smith JP, MacFadyen J, Schvartz M, et al. Multivitamins in the prevention of cardiovascular disease in men: the Physicians' Health Study II randomized controlled trial. JAMA 2012;308(17):1751–60.

[23] Dodge HH, Zitzelberger T, Oken BS, Howieson D, Kaye J. A randomized placebo-controlled trial of Ginkgo biloba for the prevention of cognitive decline. Neurology 2008;70:1809–17.

[24] DeKosky ST, Williamson JD, Fitzpatrick AL, Kronmal RA, Ives DG, Saxton JA, et al. Ginkgo biloba for prevention of dementia: a randomized controlled trial. JAMA 2008;300:2253–62.

[25] Vellas B, Coley N, Ousset P-J, Berrut G, Dartigues J-F, Dubois B, et al. Long-term use of standardized ginkgobiloba extract for the prevention of Alzheimer's disease (GuidAge): a randomized placebo-controlled trial. Lancet Neurol 2012;11(10):851–59.

[26] Burton A. Preventing Alzheimer's disease: could a new kind of trial be the key? Lancet Neurol 2010;9:850–51.

[27] Reiman EM, Langbaum JB, Fleisher AS, Caselli RJ, Chen K, Ayutyanont N, et al. Alzheimer's Prevention Initiative: a plan to accelerate the evaluation of pre-symptomatic treatments. J Alzheimer's Dis 2011;26(Suppl.3):321–9.

[28] Strobel G. NIH Director announces $100m prevention trial of Genentech antibody. Alzheimer Research Forum. May 16, 2012 (updated May 21, 2012, cited June 2013). Available from: <http://www.alzforum.org/new/detail.asp?id=3155>.

[29] DIAN (the Dominantly Inherited Alzheimer Network). Cited June 2013. Available from: <http://dian-info.org>.

[30] National Institute on Aging. Dominantly inherited Alzheimer Network trial: an opportunity to prevent dementia (DIAN TU). Cited June 2013. Available from: <http://www.nia.nih.gov/alzheimers/clinical-trials/dominantly-inherited-alzheimer-network-trial-opportunity-prevent-dementia>.

[31] Strobel G, Zakaib GD. Solanezumab selected for Alzheimer's A4 prevention trial. Alzheimer Research Forum. January 18, 2013. Cited June 2013. Available from: <http://www.alzforum.org/new/detail.asp?id=3379>.

[32] Strobel G. Collaborative umbrella CAPs three prevention trial initiatives. Alzheimer Research Forum, August 7, 2012. Cited June 2013. Available from: <http://www.alzforum.org/new/detail.asp?id=3232>.

[33] FDA. Guidance for Industry – Alzheimer's disease: Developing drugs for the treatment of early stage disease. Cited May 2013. Available at: <http://www.fda.gov/downloads/Drugs/GuidanceComplianceRegulatoryInformation/Guidances/UCM338287.pdf>.

[34] The Editorial Board, New York Times Drugs for early-stage Alzheimer's. New York Times [Internet] 2013 Mar. 13. Cited June 2013. Available from: <http://www.nytimes.com/2013/03/18/opinion/drugs-for-early-stage-alzheimers.html?_r=0>.

[35] Braak H, Braak E. Neuropathological staging of Alzheimer-related changes. Acta Neuropathol Berl 1991;82:239–59.

[36] Daviglus ML, Bell CC, Berrettini W, Bowen PE, Connolly ES, Cox NJ, et al. National Institutes of Health State-of-the-Science Conference statement: preventing Alzheimer's disease and cognitive decline. Ann Intern Med 2010;153(3):176–81.

[37] Daviglus ML, Plassman BL, Pirzada A, Bell CC, Bowen PE, Burke JR, et al. Risk factors and preventive interventions for Alzheimer's disease: state of the science. Arch Neurol 2011;68(9):1185–90.

[38] Jones RW. Primary prevention of dementia. Psychiatry 2007;6(12):511–13.

[39] Kivipelto M, Ngandu T, Laatikainen T, Winblad B, Soininen H, Tuomilehto J. Risk score for the prediction of dementia risk in 20 years among middle aged people: a longitudinal, population-based study. Lancet Neurol 2006;5:735–41.

[40] Kaffashian S, Dugravot A, Elbaz A, Shipley MJ, Sabia S, Kivimaki M, et al. Predicting cognitive decline: a dementia risk score vs. the Framingham vascular risk scores. Neurology 2013;80(14):1300–6.

[41] Alzheimer's Association. Prevention and risk of Alzheimer's and Dementia [Internet]. 2013. Cited April 2013. Available from: <http://www.alz.org/research/science/alzheimers_prevention_and_risk.asp>.

[42] Meinert C. Long-term drug prevention trials. Clin Trials 2008;5:168–76.

[43] Kuller LH, Lopez OL. Dementia and Alzheimer's disease: a new direction. The 2010 Jay L. foster memorial lecture. Alzheimer Dement 2011;7:540–50.

[44] Jonsson T, Atwal JK, Steinberg S, Snaedal J, Jonsson PV, Bjornsson S, et al. Nature 2012;488:96–9.

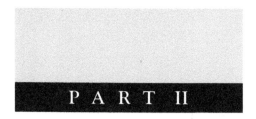

PART II

GLOBAL ALZHEIMER'S DISEASE: CLINICAL TRIALS

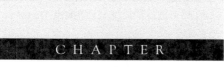

4

Overview of Global Clinical Trials: Drivers/Issues/ Opportunities of Globalization

Menghis Bairu[1], Sidney A. Spector[2] and Richard Chin[3]

[1]Elan Pharmaceutical, Cambridge, Massachusetts, USA, and Speranza Therapeutics Corp, Dublin, Ireland [2]Department of Neurology, VA Medical Center, Phoenix, Arizona, USA, and Global Biopharma, Scottsdale, Arizona, USA [3]Kindred Bio, Burlingame, California, USA

4.1 INTRODUCTION

There has been a rapid increase in the globalization of clinical trials. The proportion of clinical studies being conducted across the world, especially in developing countries, has been driven by the need for lower cost, greater speed, and higher quality. This book is a comprehensive survey of the state of global clinical trials.

Not since almost a century and a half ago, when the modern economy was created by a confluence of new inventions—telegraph, railroad, refined oil, and Bessemer steel—have we seen the wholesale transformation of entire industries that we are seeing today. Propelled by the Internet, microprocessors, mobile phones, and standardized shipping containers, the world has over the last decade or so been fast-forwarding into globalization with a rapidity and scale that is hardly imaginable.

As with other industries, such as information technology and traditional manufacturing, drug development has become highly globalized. Globalization brings both significant benefits and potential difficulties. Done correctly, global clinical trials lower the cost of drugs for everyone, distribute modern science and medicine broadly, and enhance the health of patients around the world. However, the endeavor of drug development is complicated and risky, and it is extremely important to conduct trials correctly. The goal of this book is to help physicians and clinical trial professionals everywhere to achieve that objective.

M. Bairu & M.W. Weiner (Eds):
Global Clinical Trials for Alzheimer's Disease.
DOI: http://dx.doi.org/10.1016/B978-0-12-411464-7.00004-3

49

4.2 GROWTH OF GLOBAL CLINICAL TRIALS

The number of international trials has been growing rapidly. According to a report from the Office of the Inspector General (OIG), as of 2008, 80% of marketing applications for drugs and biologicals approved by the US Food and Drug Administration (FDA) contained data from US clinical trials conducted outside the USA [1]. Table 4.1 shows the breakdown from the report [1]. According to the same source, over half of the sites and subjects in these applications were from non-US sources.

As can be seen in Table 4.2, 57% of patients in new drug applications (NDAs) and 87% of patients in biologicals license applications (BLAs) were from non-US sites. The largest proportion of non-US patients came from Western Europe, as of 2008 approvals (Figure 4.1) [1]. Figure 4.1 is based on patients in approved applications, and therefore reflects the proportion of patients enrolled into trials over the past 10 years or so.

TABLE 4.1   FDA Marketing Approval for Drugs and Biologicals Containing Clinical Data approved In Fiscal Year 2008

Marketing Applications	Drugs	Biologicals	Drugs and Biologicals
Applications with only US data	15	9	24
Applications with non-US and US data	82	5	87
Applications with only non-US data	9	1	10
Totals	106	15	121

Source: OIG analysis of FDA marketing applications approved in fiscal year 2008.

TABLE 4.2   Number and Percentage of Non-US Subjects and Sites from Clinical Trials Supporting Drug and Biological Marketing Applications Approved in Fiscal Year 2008

	Drugs	Biologicals	Drugs and Biologicals
No. of non-US and US subjects	92.859	206,842	299,701
No. of non-US subjects	52.820	179,712	232,532
Percentage of non-US subjects	56.9%	86.9%	77.6%
No. of non-US and US trial sites	11,227	717	11,944
No. of non-US trial sites	6,129	356	6,485
Percentage of non-US trial sites	54.6%	49.7%	54.3%

Source: OIG analysis of FDA marketing applications approved in fiscal year 2008.

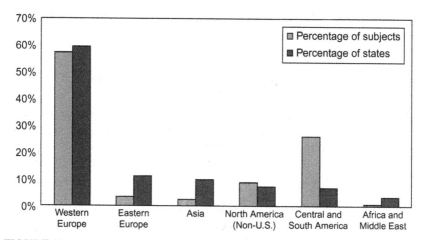

FIGURE 4.1 Percentage of non-US clinical trial subjects and sites by region for FDA marketing applications approved in fiscal year 2008. These numbers are based on data from 193 clinical trials with complete subject and site information. *Source: OIG analysis of FDA marketing applications approved in fiscal year 2008.*

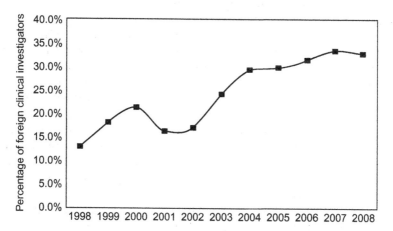

FIGURE 4.2 Trend in non-US clinical investigators as a percentage of all clinical investigators identified in investigational new drug (IND) applications from 1998 to 2008.

The proportion of non-US clinical investigators is growing rapidly (Figure 4.2) [1]. This trend is not confined to lower quality or less prominent clinical trials. An analysis by Glickman and colleagues recently found that between 1995 and 2005, the number of countries represented in a sample of studies published in the *New England Journal of Medicine* doubled from 33/150 to 70/150 [2].

These figures are largely consistent with the numbers calculated by Tufts Center for Drug Development, which estimates that in 2007, 57%

of the patients in clinical trials came from the USA, 14% from Western Europe, and 29% from the rest of the world.

4.3 DRIVERS OF GLOBALIZATION

The trend toward globalization has been fueled by several factors. The rapidly increasing cost of clinical trials—increasing at 20% per year—has been driving much of the effort. Conducting clinical trials in developing countries can easily reduce costs by 50% or more, and in some cases can reduce costs by up to 90%.

More importantly, recruitment of patients tends to be much faster in developing countries. In many cases, recruitment can be increased by 100%, and in some cases by 500% or more. In an industry such as pharmaceutical development, speed of enrollment can be a very strong driver for globalization.

In addition, in some diseases, such as in the areas of oncology and rheumatology, it can be difficult to recruit patients who are naïve to therapy into clinical trials in developed countries. In the USA and Europe, for example, most patients with severe rheumatoid arthritis may already have been exposed to biologicals such as tumor necrosis factor (TNF) inhibitors. It can be almost impossible to enroll patients who are TNF inhibitor naïve into clinical trials in those countries. Developing countries can offer a larger pool of treatment-naïve patients, when ethically permitted.

In other cases, the diseases of interest only exist in those countries, or the prevalence is much higher in those countries. Certain forms of hepatitis are one example. Global health has become an important area of drug development, largely owing to the investment by the Bill and Melinda Gates Foundation. For diseases such as malaria and visceral leishmaniasis, trials must be conducted in developing countries because that is where the diseases exist.

More recently, quality has also become a driver in some instances. Many countries that were previously being used in clinical trials because of cost advantages have now evolved. Rather than being lower cost, lower quality regions, they have become more expensive and also higher quality. In many Eastern European countries, for example, the clinical trial data from top clinical trial sites are often more reliable than in the USA.

4.4 ISSUES OF GLOBALIZATION

Of course, with globalization can come a variety of potential issues. One of the first issues, which will be discussed in Chapter 21, is potential ethical issues. An ethical problem may arise if a drug is being tested in a population where people may never stand to benefit from their voluntary acts of charity, namely in enrolling in clinical trials. For example, because of this issue, the government of Thailand insisted that human immunodeficiency virus (HIV) vaccine studies in Thailand could only proceed if the vaccine were to be made available to Thai patients upon successful development. Another ethical issue is the difficulty in obtaining true informed consent in some countries and populations. This will be discussed further in this chapter.

A second issue is regulatory harmonization, or lack thereof. Prior to the International Conference on Harmonisation (ICH), which brought the Global Cooperation Group (GCP) regulations in line across the USA, Europe, and Japan, the varied regulatory requirements for each country made international trials very onerous. The ICH was convened to harmonize regulations in those three regions, and involved the European Commission, European Federation of Pharmaceutical Industries Associations, Japanese Ministry of Health and Welfare, Japanese Pharmaceutical Manufacturers' Association, Centers for Drug Evaluation and Research, Biological Evaluations and Research, and Pharmaceutical Research and Manufacturers of America. After ICH, the developed countries largely harmonized their regulatory requirements and international trials became a lot more practicable. Today, most countries' implementation of ICH is reasonably similar and the vast majority of regulations are the same. For example, reporting requirements for suspected unexpected serious adverse reactions (SUSARs) are fairly standard.

However, even in the USA and European Union (EU), some regulations have started to diverge. For example, the USA no longer follows the Declaration of Helsinki, because the declaration considers placebo-controlled trials to be unethical in cases where an active drug is available, and the USA disagrees. New privacy regulations, especially in the EU, financial disclosure requirements in the USA, and various other non-ICH requirements are also making the clinical trial landscape more complicated than before.

In developing countries, implementation of ICH guidelines may be varied, and there may be additional requirements. In many countries, for example, Phase I studies are much more difficult to perform than in developed countries.

A third potential issue is logistics. Getting a drug in and out of the countries, through customs, can sometimes be difficult. Getting blood and tissue samples across customs can be even harder.

4.5 CONTROL AND INSPECTIONS OF FOREIGN SITES

In general, most regulatory authorities do not extend jurisdiction over conduct of studies in other countries; for example, the Spanish regulatory agency will not care that patients are being dosed in a clinical trial in Japan. However, almost all regulatory authorities will require sponsors to keep them updated of new safety events that occur anywhere in the world. A few agencies, such as the FDA, will require investigators to follow US laws if they are conducting studies under US investigational new drug (IND) applications. Of course, it is up to the sponsor to decide whether to place foreign studies under the US IND or keep them separate.

Historically, the FDA has inspected very few sites. The FDA had inspected only 1% of non-US sites as of 2008 [1]. Other countries have had a varied record with respect to audits of foreign sites. With the recent heparin contamination issue, however, inspections of foreign sites are likely to increase. The FDA recently set up an office in China, for example. It is also engaged in working more with other countries' regulatory agencies to coordinate inspections.

4.6 ETHNIC AND GENETIC ISSUES

Apart from the issues outlined above, international trials in general can raise the issue of ethnic, genetic, and other differences, as variability in these factors may make extrapolation of results from one geographical region to another problematic.

As a general rule, these differences have not historically resulted in changes to the risk/benefit ratio. There are very few drugs that have a favorable risk/benefit in one patient's population and not in another. There are, however, some drugs where the dosing needs to be adjusted in different populations; for example, tissue plasminogen activator has a substantially lower dose in Japan than in the USA.

The differences between populations and geographies can be divided into intrinsic and extrinsic differences [3]. Extrinsic differences include: environmental differences, such as climate and weather; cultural differences, such as languages and diet; medical treatment differences, such as treatment patterns and diagnosis; and population differences, such as prevalence of smoking. Intrinsic factors include: genetic factors, such as polymorphisms in drug metabolism and genetic diseases; and physiological differences, such as size and cardiovascular function. While E5 (ethnic factors in the acceptability of foreign clinical data) classifies diseases as an intrinsic factor, in many cases it can be an extrinsic factor, such as prevalence of tuberculosis in the general population.

Whenever international trials are conducted, and even when an within-nation trial is conducted, differences in these factors can play a role in the interpretability of the clinical trial. With a broader array of countries now being involved in clinical trials, these factors can sometimes be magnified.

4.7 USABILITY OF INTERNATIONAL CLINICAL DATA IN REGULATORY FILINGS

In global clinical trials, the goal is usually to file the data in another country for registration, typically in the USA and EU. Fortunately, ICH E5 has been adopted by many countries, and helps significantly in standardizing the expectations of the regulators [3].

In the USA, 21 CFR 314.106 (the acceptance of foreign data in a new drug application) is the overarching regulation that governs what foreign data are acceptable. The code makes it clear that data from US patients are not needed if three criteria are met. First, the foreign data must be relevant and applicable to the US population. Second, competent investigators must have performed the studies. Third, the FDA must have confidence in or have the ability to validate the verity of the data [4].

In the rest of the regulations, the FDA makes it clear that studies that are solely conducted outside the USA do not need to be performed under an IND. However, they must be conducted under all local regulations and ICH. (In the EU, the rules are largely similar, and foreign data are usually acceptable.) However, although regulations allow the approval of drugs with 100% data from patients outside the country, in many cases, regulatory authorities strongly prefer at least some of the data to be based on patients from within the country.

The principles outlined in ICH E5 are clear. Where possible, it is desirable to reduce duplication of data and it is beneficial to use foreign data where possible. The approval requirements for the drug remain the same, but the goal is to fit the foreign data into the framework of existing regulatory requirements.

To that end, the types of study and data required by the local registration requirements must be fulfilled. For example, if an early phase cardiac (QTc) study is required, that must be performed. Once a clinical package is assembled that meets the normal regulatory requirements, that package can be considered to be complete. A complete package would contain [3]:

- clinical efficacy and safety data, and dose response, performed under GCP and utilizing approvable endpoints and appropriate controls; the medical diagnosis and definitions must be applicable in the new region
- pharmacokinetics/pharmacodynamics/dose response/safety/efficacy in the population studied
- pharmacokinetics and where possible pharmacodynamics/dose response in the new region.

Once a "complete" package has been assembled, there may or may not be a question as to whether the population in the studies is similar enough to the target population that the data can be extrapolated. If there is doubt, bridging studies should be done to demonstrate the appropriate extrapolation.

In order to decide whether the data can be extrapolated, the drug's sensitivity to ethnic factors needs to be determined. With some drugs in some populations, there will be little ethnic impact on safety and efficacy, while in others, there may be substantial effects. The degree of potential concern depends on both the drug and the population.

Drugs that are metabolized by enzymes that are heterogeneous across populations, such as G6PD, are likely to be more problematic. Drugs that are passively excreted without undergoing metabolism are less likely to be ethnically sensitive, as are drugs with a wide therapeutic margin or a flat dose–response curve. In some cases, it is known how ethnically sensitive drugs in the same class have been, and that can help to determine the likelihood that the new drugs will be ethnically sensitive.

The lists in the following boxes summarize some of the factors that may make a drug more or less likely to be ethnically sensitive.

PROPERTIES OF A COMPOUND MAKING IT LESS LIKELY TO BE SENSITIVE TO ETHNIC FACTORS [3]

- linear pharmacokinetics (pharmacokinetics)
- a flat pharmacodynamic (effect–concentration) curve for both efficacy and safety in the range of the recommended dosage and dose regimen (this may mean that the medicine is well tolerated)
- a wide therapeutic dose range (again, possibly an indicator of good tolerability)
- minimal metabolism or metabolism distributed among multiple pathways
- high bioavailability, thus less susceptibility to dietary absorption effects
- low potential for protein binding
- little potential for drug–drug, drug–diet, and drug–disease interactions
- non-systemic mode of action
- little potential for inappropriate use.

PROPERTIES OF A COMPOUND MAKING IT MORE LIKELY TO BE SENSITIVE TO ETHNIC FACTORS [3]

- non-linear pharmacokinetics
- a steep pharmacodynamic curve for both efficacy and safety in the range of the recommended dosage and dose regimen (a small change in dose results in a large change in effect)
- a narrow therapeutic dose range
- highly metabolized, especially through a single pathway, thereby increasing the potential for drug–drug interaction
- metabolism by enzymes known to show genetic polymorphism
- administration as a prodrug, with the potential for ethnically variable enzymatic conversion
- high intersubject variation in bioavailability
- low bioavailability, thus more susceptible to dietary absorption effects
- high likelihood of use in a setting of multiple comedications
- high likelihood for inappropriate use, e.g., analgesics and tranquilizers.

Depending on the likelihood of ethnic sensitivity, more or fewer data may be required on the comparative pharmacokinetics, pharmacodynamics, and clinical relationship to dose. At a minimum, however, basic absorption, distribution, metabolism, and excretion data are required. Some drug–drug interaction and food–drug interaction data may be required as well, particularly if certain drugs and food differ significantly between two populations.

In many cases, there is sufficient evidence about the pharmacokinetics or pharmacodynamics endpoints, and their relationships to clinical data, that demonstrating equivalence at the pharmacokinetics or pharmacodynamics level may be sufficient. Occasionally, there may be a need for additional clinical data.

References

[1] Levinson DR. Challenges to FDA's Ability to Monitor and Inspect Foreign Clinical Trials. Department of Health and Human Services 2010; Office of Inspector General.
[2] Glickman SW, McHutchinson JG, Peterson ED, Cairns CB, Harrington RA, Califf RM, et al. Ethical and scientific implications of the globalization of clinical research. N Engl J Med 2009;360(8):816–23.

[3] International Conference on Harmonisation of Technical Requirements for Registration of Pharmaceuticals for Human Use (1998). Ethnic factors in the acceptability of foreign clinical data, E5(R1). Available from: <http://www.ich.org/fileadmin/Public_Web_Site/ICH_Products/Guidelines/Efficacy/E5_R1/Step4/E5_R1__Guideline.pdf>.

[4] US 21 CFR 314.106. The acceptance of foreign data in a new drug application. Available from: <http://www.fda.gov/downloads/RegulatoryInformation/Guidances/UCM294729.pdf>.

[5] World Health Organization. The WHO Prequalification Project; updated January 2013 (cited July 15, 2010). Available from: <http://www.who.int/mediacentre/factsheets/fs278/en/index.html>.

[6] World Health Organization. Procedure for prequalification of pharmaceutical products; (cited January 2013). Available from: <http://www.who.int/vaccines-documents/DocsPDF06/812.pdf>.

[7] World Health Organization. Procedure for assessing the acceptability, in principle, of vaccines for purchase by United Nations agencies, 2010. <http://who.int/vaccines-documents/DocsPDF06/812.pdf>.

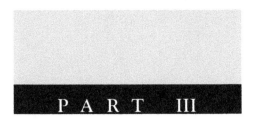

PART III

CHALLENGES AND OPPORTUNITIES TO CONDUCT GLOBAL ALZHEIMER'S DISEASE CLINICAL TRIALS

CHAPTER 5

Challenges and Opportunities to Conduct Global Alzheimer's Disease Clinical Trials

Jeffrey Cummings and
Kate Zhong

Cleveland Clinic Lou Ruvo Center for Brain Health, Las Vegas, Nevada, Cleveland, Ohio, and Weston, Florida, USA

5.1 INTRODUCTION

Alzheimer's disease (AD) is a progressive neurodegenerative disease of the brain that causes increasing cognitive and functional disability leading to death. AD is a worldwide disorder producing substantial disability for citizens—especially elderly individuals—in all countries [1]. Current treatments of AD produce modest improvement and temporary delay in deterioration [2]. It is imperative that new and more powerful drug treatments are developed to prevent, delay the onset, slow the progression, or improve the symptoms of AD. There are currently approximately 80 medications in development for AD and being assessed in clinical trials [3]. Each trial requires from 60 (small Phase I trials) to 1,200 individuals (large Phase III trials) to participate. The United States is the most common site for clinical trials [4,5] allowing companies more direct access to the Food and Drug Administration (FDA) and the world's largest pharmaceutical market, but the US cannot provide a sufficient number of patients in a timely way to test all the agents in the drug development pipeline. Trials must be "globalized" to include non-US sites to provide an adequate number of subjects for clinical trials. This chapter examines the challenges and opportunities for globalization of trials for AD treatments. We will examine the nature of globalization, the reasons for globalization, the extent of globalization, and the issues raised by globalization on clinical trial conduct.

M. Bairu & M.W. Weiner (Eds):
Global Clinical Trials for Alzheimer's Disease.
DOI: http://dx.doi.org/10.1016/B978-0-12-411464-7.00005-5

5.2 WHAT IS GLOBALIZATION?

There is no consensus definition of globalization of clinical trials. When the clinical trials enterprise began, most clinical trials were done in the US as a result of FDA policy requiring extensive data on safety and efficacy for products presented for marketing approval. Globalization has been defined with regard to the inclusion of non-US sites and is traditionally considered as the inclusion of multiple non-US sites in a trial. Globalized trials can include multicenter trials with US and non-US sites or multicenter trials that include multiple non-US sites without US participation. A more unbiased way of describing globalization might be any trial that includes trial sites from three or more international regions (US, Western Europe, Eastern Europe/Russia, Canada, South America, Southeast Asia, Central America, Australia/New Zealand, Japan, India, Middle East, Africa, China [5]).

5.3 WHY GLOBALIZATION?

Globalization has many advantages. The principal driver of globalization is the need to recruit many patients in a short period of time—more than can usually be recruited within a single nation even with multiple sites within the country. Anticipated and desirable study timelines are nearly doubled for many trials to allow the trials to meet recruitment goals [6]. Faster recruitment translates into accelerated development of desperately needed new medications, reduced costs for drug development, and longer periods of exclusivity.

There are often more patients available at international sites than at individual sites in the US. In China, for example, trial sites are located in large hospitals that provide care to thousands of patients, facilitating recruitment and patient flow into trials.

The per-patient cost of trials is typically less in developing countries where salaries, laboratory costs, imaging expenses, hospitalization costs, and administrative charges are less than in the US or Europe [5]. For some trials, costs in India are one-tenth the cost of conducting the same trial in the US [5,7]. This cost disparity is declining but remains an important reason for including international trial sites in trials.

In addition to enhancing the total number of patients available for trials, globalization also increases access to treatment-naïve patients. In many countries, the standard of care of patients with AD does not include cholinesterase inhibitors or memantine, widely used in economically advanced countries. Treatment-naïve patients allow construction of true placebo groups with no concomitant therapy and to compare disease progression in patients on test therapies compared to no treatment.

Some studies have found that retention of patients in trials is higher in trials conducted in China and India than in other countries [8]. Trial completion is critical to data quality and unbiased trial interpretation. Retention can be an important motivation to include sites with success in retaining patients in trials.

Patients and patient advocacy groups may support globalization efforts since performance of trials in low and middle income countries provides access to experimental and, in some cases, standard therapies for trial participants.

The developing world is aging rapidly. In 2010, 58% of all people with dementia lived in low or middle income countries; this will grow to 63% in 2030, and to 71% in 2050 [9]. The growth in the number of individuals with dementia translates into the growth of the market for dementia-related products including pharmaceuticals. Conducting trials in nations with growing aging populations to facilitate approval of the agent for sale in that country is an important aspect of pharmaceutical company strategy.

Patients from international sites differ ethnically and in many other ways (discussed below) from those in the US. These differences may influence AD pathophysiology and progression or response to treatment. Testing new therapies in diverse populations provides insight into these variations in disease and drug response and promotes understanding of the generalizability of clinical trial outcomes.

Cognitive impairment makes an important contribution to the disability observed in the elderly in low and middle income countries [10]. Local and national governments in these countries are motivated to find treatments. The large number of patients with these disorders in low and middle income countries means that they may benefit disproportionately from advances in therapy [7].

Physicians and physician-scientists from the international community are also motivated to participate in global trials. An increasing number of international investigators have experience and motivation to be part of the global scientific community. Participating in global trials allows them to contribute to the growth of scientific knowledge, increase their expertise, collaborate with international colleagues, and build local resources to provide infrastructure for scientific activities.

Many pharmaceutical companies are expanding their basic science and manufacturing facilities to international sites, especially Asia. Conducting drug development in these countries may conserve resources and facilitate translation of basic drug understanding to the development program. The internationalization of pharmaceutical companies is another contributor to the globalization of trials.

Taken together, there are commercial, scientific, patient-based, and investigator-based reasons for globalization of trials including those for AD.

5.4 HOW COMMON ARE GLOBALIZED TRIALS?

Globalization is progressing at a rapid rate. Glickman and colleagues [5] noted that since 2002, the number of active FDA-regulated investigators based outside the US has grown by 15% annually, whereas the number of US investigators has grown by 5% annually. Glickman et al. [5] noted that although the US conducted more trials in 2007 than any other country, the cumulative number of trials conducted outside the US exceeded the number conducted in the US.

Cummings and colleagues [4] analyzed AD trials from a global perspective. The US sites were included in 76 of 269 trials meeting study criteria and listed on clinicaltrials.gov. Thus, most AD trials are being conducted at non-US sites. The US has more trials than any other national region but the total number non-US sites is larger. Eighteen percent of trials were being conducted in the US only, the rest were multinational globalized trials. Relatively few AD trials are dependent exclusively on the US.

Given the many reasons to conduct trials with multinational locations, the trend toward globalization of trials is predicted to continue to increase.

5.5 GLOBALIZATION AND CLINICAL TRIAL INSTRUMENTATION

A concern in the globalization of trials is the comparability of data collected in different populations. Clinical trial tools must be rigorously translated to ensure the validity of the instrumentation and acculturated to ensure that the intent of the assessment is preserved. There have been few attempts to assess the validity of instruments in validation studies in cross-national comparison research but not all countries have been included, and there is no central repository of tools that have been studied.

Globalized trials may include sites in 30 or more countries and include populations speaking as many as 20 languages. This highlights the importance of valid translation of instruments to ensure that the data captured across linguistic groups are equally valid and have similar psychometric characteristics. The optimal methodology of translation, back translation, and reconciliation is often not pursued rigorously. Means of insuring best clinical practices for translation and making the best translations widely available are needed [11].

The principal tools used in AD clinical trials include the Alzheimer's Disease Assessment Scale-cognitive portion (ADAS-Cog), the Clinical Dementia Rating (CDR), the Neuropsychiatric Inventory (NPI), and some measure of activities of daily living. Pharmacoeconomic data are collected in some trials, usually with the Resource Utilization in Dementia (RUD) instrument, and quality of life (QoL) data are integrated in some trials using a variety of QoL scales. The effects of translation, culture, education, literacy, age, gender, ethnicity, and socio-economic status on data collected with these instruments have received limited study.

A frequent approach is to compare a translated version of a trial instrument with the original in a single-site study. For example, Mavioglu and coworkers [12] showed that the Turkish version of the ADAS-Cog was affected by subject age; both the Chinese version of the ADAS-Cog [13] and the Turkish version [12] were independent of education effects. This is a valuable first step but does not provide a comprehensive understanding of how instruments perform across multiple populations.

Efforts to harmonize the ADAS-Cog across European countries have been reported [14]. Among versions identified at the time of the study, there were differences in object drawings to be named, items for verbal memory, number of learning trials allowed, imagery value of the words used for memory, and number of parallel versions. These differences affect administration, performance, and scoring, creating heterogeneity in ADAS-Cog results. Harmonization of versions used across countries resulted in an ADAS-Cog that performed similarly across countries and had similar correlations with other commonly used tools. Such studies of other instruments, and including more languages and cultures, have not been reported.

The CDR collects data on memory, orientation, judgment and problem solving, community affairs, home and hobbies, and personal care. It is used in its original form to assign scores of 0.5, 1, 2, or 3, or in its amended scoring approach to total the individual item scores to produce the "Sum of Boxes" score (CDR-sb). Application of the CDR in Asia has drawn attention to the challenges of assessing judgment, community affairs, and home and hobbies in individuals who have low education, restricted roles in the family, and limited resources [15,16]. Cross-cultural implementation of the CDR requires substantial involvement of the interviewer, will be influenced by the experience and vigilance of the examiner, and may have limited reliability in some studies.

Activities of daily living (ADL) differ markedly among countries. A Thai ADL scale, for example, includes taking a taxi-boat and bicycling as means of transportation, conveyances rarely used by the elderly in the US [17]. Developing an instrument to capture ADL data across Western countries has been pursued [18] but the tool has not been widely used. Means of developing equivalent measures across multiple cultures with uniform scoring criteria have not emerged.

Behavioral changes are a major aspect of AD and the NPI is the instrument most commonly used to measure behavioral changes in patients with cognitive impairment. The NPI has been used in many cultures and nations and has been shown to have good reliability across cultural settings [19–21]. There have been few studies of the transcultural validity of the NPI compared with tools or interviews based on intra-cultural experience. Differences in NPI profiles have been reported for Chinese and American patients, with more anxiety and delusions among Chinese patients and more apathy and appetite changes observed in US patients [22]. This suggests that there may be culture-specific profiles that might respond differentially to therapeutic interventions and affect trial outcomes.

The RUD is the instrument used most often to capture pharmacoeconomic data in clinical trials. A recent review of the literature and consensus discussion advanced a revised version of the instrument more appropriate than the original for international application [23]. This revised "globalized" instrument has not been included in reported studies.

Preliminary studies of QoL have been conducted and show decline in QoL in caregivers and patients with strong correlations between depressed mood and impaired ADL [24]. The QoL-AD is the most commonly used dementia-specific tool and a few cross-cultural correlations with the original tool developed in the US have been published [25]. There has been little work in comparing the elements and assumptions of QoL scales across disparate cultures.

This review of the literature indicates that the same instruments are used in global clinical trials as in US trials where most of the original instruments were developed. The trial instruments have typically been subject to few studies of reliability or to investigation of concurrent validity. There are few studies where the applications of the tools across multiple countries in the same trial are investigated. The country-specific translation, acculturation, and adjustment of instruments may create differences that are difficult to accommodate in data analysis strategies. For example, in the Hindi version of the Mini Mental Status Examination (MMSE), 16 of the items were changed to make it more culturally appropriate [26]. Even within the US, substantial trial-to-trial differences have been observed in the scoring of the ADAS-Cog and the NPI [27,28]. The variance created by differences in instruments, administration and scoring of clinical trial instruments amplifies the "noise" of data from trials and makes it more difficult to establish drug–placebo differences. There is a need to advance studies of the cross-cultural application of tools in globalized trials and to establish a library of the best studied instruments available for use in trials.

5.6 GLOBAL EFFECTS ON DIAGNOSIS OF ALZHEIMER'S DISEASE

AD can be difficult to diagnose accurately. An autopsy confirmation study of cases observed longitudinally in US expert centers showed that sensitivity of the diagnosis ranged from 70.9% to 87.3% and specificity from 44.3% to 70.8% [29]. This indicates that diagnosis has only modest sensitivity and specificity even when patients are optimally assessed and followed until death. Diagnosis in trial centers where patients are recruited only for trials and application of diagnostic criteria in international settings are expected to be often erroneous. In recent trials of bapineuzumab, nearly 40% of apolipoprotein e4 non-carriers had no amyloid burden when scanned with amyloid brain imaging, indicating that they did not have AD. Cultural and educational differences across cultures make diagnosis challenging. A study of instrument-based diagnosis in specific international sites showed modest diagnostic accuracy that was substantially improved by the sequential use of several instruments [30]. Such quality improvement approaches are not routinely incorporated into trial methodologies.

Use of more rigorous clinical methods or introduction of biomarkers supportive of the diagnosis of AD is necessary to improve diagnostic accuracy and ensure that patients included in AD trials have the intended underlying pathology relevant to the treatment mechanism of action (MOA). These strategies will be more important as trials move to earlier stage patients where diagnostic accuracy is more difficult.

5.7 PATIENT-RELATED FACTORS TO BE CONSIDERED IN GLOBALIZED TRIALS

Subjects in international studies differ by socio-economic status, standard of care, general health, co-morbid medications, nutrition history, dietary habits, vaccination and immune history, and exercise levels. These factors create diversity among trial populations and some of these may affect trial outcomes.

Educational level may have an important impact in trials. Persons with AD and low educational levels progress more slowly than those with high education levels [31]. Subjects with high educational levels have proportionately more brain pathology, more abnormal brain metabolism, and more rapid progression than patients with lower levels of educational attainment [32–34]. Slower progression in a trial implies that there will be less decline in the placebo group and less power to identify a drug–placebo difference. US trial participants tend to have high educational levels whereas patients in many other parts of the world, especially Asia, often have lower levels. For example, a study of galantamine in Korea included patients in the four treatment arms with 5.6, 5.2, 5.6 and 1.8 years of formal education [35]. This compares with 14 years of education in most US trials [36]. Such differences may translate into impacts on predictions of progression, power calculations, and sample size estimates.

Patients in low and middle income countries are less likely to be on background antidementia therapies, may have different co-morbidity profiles (e.g., more concomitant cerebrovascular disease), and may have different concomitant medications such as statins, antihypertensives, or pulmonary drugs that may have effects on AD [37].

Diets also differ across nations. For example, flavonoid extracts may affect dementia prevalence [38]. Similarly, curcumin is used extensively in the diet in some countries (i.e., India, Thailand) and has been shown to affect multiple aspects of AD pathophysiology [39]. These dietary choices may affect rate of cognitive and functional decline and trial outcomes.

The pattern of caregiving may also differ among countries with concomitant effects on trial performance. Studies in the US show that more patients in clinical trials had spouse caregivers than caregivers of other types (adult children, others). Patients with spouse caregivers had lower rates of attrition and were more likely to complete the trial [40]. The percentage of spouse caregivers may vary among nations and cultures and affect trial participation characteristics.

There are many factors affecting patients that may translate into differences in disease progression as observed in clinical trials in different national groups. There is limited insight into the magnitude of these effects, and their impact on recruitment, stratification, analysis or interpretation of trial data is uncertain.

5.8 DISEASE-RELATED FACTORS TO BE CONSIDERED IN GLOBALIZED TRIALS

In addition to the host-related factors described above (education, diet, concomitant medications, etc.), international populations may have biological differences that affect AD progression. ApoE genotype has been shown to affect AD risk, age of onset, and rate of progression during the early phases of the disease. ApoE e4 carriers have earlier age of onset and progress more rapidly in the early/prodromal phases of the illness [41]. ApoE genotypes are not equally distributed in the world's population [42], and differences in the proportion of e4 carriers might affect trial outcomes, especially in trials of mildly affected individuals.

Small head size reduces cognitive reserve and increases vulnerability to AD [43]. Head size is related to body size; US and European populations are the tallest of the world's populations and have the largest head sizes. Asian, Indian and African populations have the smallest head size, and this may contribute to an increased risk of AD. If disease progression is similarly affected, head size may affect disease progression and trial outcomes.

5.9 PHARMACOKINETIC- AND PHARMACODYNAMIC-RELATED FACTORS TO BE CONSIDERED IN GLOBALIZED TRIALS

Ethnic factors that may affect pharmacokinetics and pharmacodynamics differ among sites in international trials and may impact trial result interpretation. Box 5.1 lists the features of compounds that are less sensitive to ethnic influences and are better candidates for global trials [4]. Agents that vary from this profile in important ways might best be studied in single-nation trials.

As noted above, height differs in the world populations with Northern Europeans being the tallest and Asians the shortest on average. Height will affect body size, volume of distribution of drugs, and brain exposure of the test compound.

Ethnic differences in the distribution of polymorphisms affecting the cytochrome P450 enzyme system are well known and affect the levels of drugs metabolized by the hepatic cytochrome system [44,45]. Knowledge of the effect of these enzymes on the metabolism of the test agent and of the distribution of the enzyme polymorphisms in the trial populations is important in the interpretation of trial results.

BOX 5.1 CHARACTERISTICS OF DRUGS THAT ARE LESS SENSITIVE TO ETHNIC INFLUENCES AND ARE BETTER CANDIDATES FOR GLOBAL TRIALS [4]

- Linear pharmacokinetics
- Wide therapeutic dose range
- Minimal or no metabolism by enzymes subject to genetic influences (e.g., cytochrome P450 enzymes)
- High bioavailability
- Little inter-subject variability in bioavailability
- Low protein binding
- Limited potential for drug–diet interactions
- Limited potential for drug–drug interactions
- Limited potential for abuse or inappropriate use
- Not a prodrug

Differences in pharmacodynamics mediated by receptor subtypes or enzymes involved in the pathophysiology affected by the drug's MOA are possible and have not been adequately studied.

5.10 SITE-RELATED FACTORS TO BE CONSIDERED IN GLOBALIZED TRIALS

Site factors have profound effects on the quality of data generated in a trial. Site variability increases with the number of sites required and globalized trials will have more variability than trials conducted in one country or a single geographic region.

As noted above, diagnosis of AD is not straightforward and accuracy is dependent on the experience of the diagnostician. The training of the clinician, time available for interviewing the patient, diligence in reviewing the history and recording the clinical and functional decline, care in reviewing the past medical history and concomitant medications, assessment of comorbid disease, review of the patient's mood state and any history of substance use all contribute to the accuracy of diagnosis. Central review of diagnostic approaches offers one means of reducing the inevitable variability associated with having multiple clinicians with varying qualifications and motivations perform diagnosis and rating of patients. The technology for recording interviews and reviewing them centrally is currently available.

International sites are not all familiar with instrumentation used in clinical trials. In a review of European centers, for example, 40–50% of sites used the CDR and an ADL measure and 20% used the NPI [46]. Sites not routinely using the trial instruments require more training and supervision to ensure quality data collection. In one review of trial sites, 27% of ADAS-Cog raters had less than one year of experience with the instrument; 40% of raters in a trial conducted in China had administered the ADAS-Cog less than five times [47]. Rater surveillance programs instituted in one trial involving 658 raters from 31 countries found that 50% of ADAS-Cog raters and 30% of MMSE raters required remediation because of evidence of erroneous performance or rater drift [47].

Review of adverse event reporting in international trials (not limited to AD trials) shows that there is excessive site-to-site variation in adverse event recording and reporting [48]. This may contribute to undesirable challenges in understanding toxicity of test compounds.

Institutional review boards (IRBs) have variable experience and not all may offer adequate protection to patients with informed consent and the necessary scrupulous attention to patient rights and safety [49]. Sites from countries that have conducted fewer trials require more instruction and supervision of the IRB process.

Some laboratory measures may also have low inter-site and intra-site measurement reliability. Serial measurements of cerebrospinal fluid (CSF) levels of beta-amyloid protein and tau protein show substantial variability between and within laboratories [50]. Standardization efforts are underway and are critical to improving the interpretation of CSF measurements in trials.

The Alzheimer's Disease Neuroimaging Initiative (ADNI) is developing methods of neuroimaging and patient assessment that standardize the approach and is building a comprehensive, publically accessible database useful for planning trials [51]. The expansion of ADNI to similar research programs in Europe, China, Korea, Japan, and Australia will provide similar comprehensive data on international populations and will help guide globalized trials. Inclusion and standardization of biomarkers will help reduce variability in international trials.

5.11 OTHER CONSIDERATIONS IN GLOBALIZED TRIALS

A variety of other influences must be considered when implementing globalized trials. Regulatory expectations differ across countries and are not completely harmonized. In addition, marketing of a compound shown to be successful in a globalized trial requires different levels of data for approval within individual countries. Bridging studies may be required to extend the results of the global trial to a specific nation [4]. In some cases, the focus of the bridging study is on patient safety and adverse events; in others, evidence of efficacy is required.

Supply line maintenance must be carefully planned in globalized trials. Export and import laws, manufacturing, and border regulations can all affect the availability of drug product for the trial sites.

Drug pricing after trial completion will be an important consideration. Countries with sites and patients that contributed to a successful trial may feel that pricing to make the drug widely accessible to disease victims is warranted.

Fairness to investigators is also an important consideration. Advancing the careers of trialists is an important goal and contributors from countries participating in trials should be included in the authorship of trial-related papers. Reviews suggest that scientists from countries that have traditionally done fewer trials are under-represented in authorship [52].

5.12 RECOMMENDATIONS

This review of globalization identifies both the benefits of international trials and the challenges associated with them. Box 5.2 lists

BOX 5.2 RECOMMENDATIONS TO IMPROVE QUALITY OF INTERNATIONAL MULTISITE CLINICAL TRIALS

- Ensure adequate training of clinicians and site personnel involved in trials
- Perform regular monitoring of site performance
- Consider central review of all or part of the trial data
- Ensure adequate training of IRBs and rigorous application of informed consent and patient protection procedures
- Develop a library of well-studied clinical trial tools whose features in international trials are known
- Create access to trial data after trial completion to enhance continuous learning from globalized trials
- Encourage harmonization of international drug development guidelines from regulatory agencies
- Study the effects of education, diet, exercise, comorbidity and concomitant medication on international trial outcomes
- Increase use of biomarkers to reduce diagnostic heterogeneity in globalized trials

recommendations for improving globalized trials suggested by this review and the available data.

Increased use of technology (e.g., central review of assessment and diagnostic procedures) and biomarkers, enhancing training, and increased regulatory harmonization all promise to promote quality of globalized trials. Creation of libraries of well-characterized trial instruments and of relevant data are important goals.

This review and similar examinations of the global clinical trial enterprise demonstrate that there has been little detailed scientific study of the effects of globalization on trials. This is an area in urgent need of research. Reducing measurement noise and improving our ability to detect drug–placebo differences is critical to advancing drug development programs and finding new treatments for AD. Globalization will increase and developing methods for improved international trials is necessary to create new drugs for patients with AD.

References

[1] Wortmann M. Dementia: a global health priority–highlights from an ADI and World Health Organization report. Alzheimers Res Ther 2012;4:40.

[2] Aisen PS, Cummings J, Schneider LS. Symptomatic and nonamyloid/tau based pharmacologic treatment for Alzheimer disease. Cold Spring Harb Perspect Med 2012;2:a006395.

[3] PhRMA. Medicines in development for Alzheimer's disease. Cited June 2013. Available from: <www.phrma.org>; 2012.

[4] Cummings J, Reynders R, Zhong K. Globalization of Alzheimer's disease clinical trials. Alzheimers Res Ther 2011;3:24.

[5] Glickman SW, McHutchison JG, Peterson ED, Cairns CB, Harrington RA, Califf RM, et al. Ethical and scientific implications of the globalization of clinical research. N Engl J Med 2009;360:816–23.

[6] Getz K, Lamberti MJ. 89% of trials meet enrollment, but timelines slip, half of sites under-enroll. Tufts Cent Study Drug Dev 2013;15:1–4. Impact Report.

[7] Lang T, Siribaddana S. Clinical trials have gone global: is this a good thing? PLoS Med 2012;9:e1001228.

[8] Perkovic V, Patil V, Wei L, Lv J, Petersen M, Patel A. Global randomized trials: the promise of India and China. J Bone Joint Surg Am 2012;94:92–6.

[9] Prince M, Bryce R, Albanese E, Wimo A, Ribeiro W, Ferri CP. The global prevalence of dementia: A systematic review and metaanalysis. Alzheimers Dement 2013;9:63–75.

[10] Sousa RM, Ferri CP, Acosta D, Guerra M, Huang Y, Jacob K, et al. The contribution of chronic diseases to the prevalence of dependence among older people in Latin America, China and India: a 10/66 Dementia Research Group population-based survey. BMC Geriatr 2010;10:53.

[11] Feldman J, Anand R, Blesa R, Dubois B, Gray J, Homma A, et al. Translation issues in clinical trials of dementia drugs. Alzheimer Dis Assoc Disord 1997;11:61–4.

[12] Mavioglu H, Gedizlioglu M, Akyel S, Aslaner T, Eser E. The validity and reliability of the Turkish version of Alzheimer's Disease Assessment Scale-Cognitive Subscale (ADAS-Cog) in patients with mild and moderate Alzheimer's disease and normal subjects. Int J Geriatr Psychiatry 2006;21:259–65.

[13] Liu HC, Teng EL, Chuang YY, Lin KN, Fuh JL, Wang PN. The Alzheimer's disease assessment scale: findings from a low-education population. Dement Geriatr Cogn Disord 2002;13:21–6.

[14] Verhey FR, Houx P, Van Lang N, Huppert F, Stoppe G, Saerens J, et al. Cross-national comparison and validation of the Alzheimer's disease assessment scale: results from the European Harmonization Project for Instruments in Dementia (EURO-HARPID). Int J Geriatr Psychiatry 2004;19:41–50.

[15] Homma A, Meguro K, Dominguez J, Sahadevan S, Wang YH, Morris JC. Clinical dementia rating workshop: the Asian experience. Alzheimer Dis Assoc Disord 2006;20:318–21.

[16] Lim WS, Chong MS, Sahadevan S. Utility of the clinical dementia rating in Asian populations. Clin Med Res 2007;5:61–70.

[17] Senanarong V, Harnphadungkit K, Prayoonwiwat N, Poungvarin N, Sivasariyanonds N, Printarakul T, et al. A new measurement of activities of daily living for Thai elderly with dementia. Int Psychogeriatr 2003;15:135–48.

[18] Reisberg B, Finkel S, Overall J, Schmidt-Gollas N, Kanowski S, Lehfeld H, et al. The Alzheimer's disease activities of daily living international scale (ADL-IS). Int Psychogeriatr 2001;13:163–81.

[19] Cheng ST, Lam LC, Kwok T. Neuropsychiatric symptom clusters of Alzheimer disease in Hong Kong Chinese: correlates with caregiver burden and depression. Am J Geriatr Psychiatry Aug 2012:29. [Epub ahead of print].

[20] Leung VP, Lam LC, Chiu HF, Cummings JL, Chen QL. Validation study of the Chinese version of the neuropsychiatric inventory (CNPI). Int J Geriatr Psychiatry 2001;16:789–93.

[21] Vellas B, Hausner L, Frölich L, Cantet C, Gardette V, Reynish E, et al. Progression of Alzheimer disease in Europe: data from the European ICTUS study. Curr Alzheimer Res 2012;9:902–12.

[22] Chow TW, Liu CK, Fuh JL, Leung VP, Tai CT, Chen LW, et al. Neuropsychiatric symptoms of Alzheimer's disease differ in Chinese and American patients. Int J Geriatr Psychiatry 2002;17:22–8.

[23] Wimo A, Gustavsson A, Jönsson L, Winblad B, Hsu MA, Gannon B. Application of Resource Utilization in Dementia (RUD) instrument in a global setting. Alzheimers Dement 2012 Nov 8. doi:pii: S1552-5260(12)02387-4.

[24] Bruvik FK, Ulstein ID, Ranhoff AH, Engedal K. The quality of life of people with dementia and their family carers. Dement Geriatr Cogn Disord 2012;34:7–14.

[25] Wolak A, Novella JL, Drame M, Guillemin F, Di Pollina L, Ankri J, et al. Transcultural adaptation and psychometric validation of a French-language version of the QoL-AD. Aging Ment Health 2009;13:593–600.

[26] Chiu HF, Lam LC. Relevance of outcome measures in different cultural groups–does one size fit all? Int Psychogeriatr 2007;19:457–66.

[27] Connor DJ, Sabbagh MN. Administration and scoring variance on the ADAS-Cog. J Alzheimers Dis 2008;15:461–64.

[28] Connor DJ, Sabbagh MN, Cummings JL. Comment on administration and scoring of the neuropsychiatric inventory in clinical trials. Alzheimers Dement 2008;4:390–94.

[29] Beach TG, Monsell SE, Phillips LE, Kukull W. Accuracy of the clinical diagnosis of Alzheimer disease at National Institute on aging Alzheimer Disease Centers, 2005–2010. J Neuropathol Exp Neurol 2012;71:266–73.

[30] Prince M, Acosta D, Chiu H, Scazufca M, Varghese M, 10/66 Dementia Research Group Dementia diagnosis in developing countries: a cross-cultural validation study. Lancet 2003;361:909–17.

[31] Stern Y, Albert S, Tang MX, Tsai WY. Rate of memory decline in AD is related to education and occupation: cognitive reserve? Neurology 1999;53:1942–47.

[32] Bennett DA, Wilson RS, Schneider JA, Evans DA, Mendes de Leon CF, Arnold SE, et al. Education modifies the relation of AD pathology to level of cognitive function in older persons. Neurology 2003;60:1909–15.

[33] Roe CM, Mintun MA, D'Angelo G, Xiong C, Grant EA, Morris JC. Alzheimer disease and cognitive reserve: variation of education effect with carbon 11-labeled Pittsburgh Compound B uptake. Arch Neurol 2008;65:1467–71.

[34] Kemppainen NM, Aalto S, Karrasch M, Någren K, Savisto N, Oikonen V, et al. Cognitive reserve hypothesis: Pittsburgh Compound B and fluorodeoxyglucose positron emission tomography in relation to education in mild Alzheimer's disease. Ann Neurol 2008;63:112–18.

[35] Suh GH, Yeon Jung H, Uk Lee C, Hoon Oh B, Nam Bae J, Jung HY, Korean Galantamine Study Group A prospective, double-blind, community-controlled comparison of three doses of galantamine in the treatment of mild to moderate Alzheimer's disease in a Korean population. Clin Ther 2004;26:1608–18.

[36] Petersen RC, Aisen PS, Beckett LA, Donohue MC, Gamst AC, Harvey DJ, et al. Alzheimer's Disease Neuroimaging Initiative (ADNI): clinical characterization. Neurology 2010;74:201–09.

[37] Appleby BS, Nacopoulos D, Milano N, Zhong K, Cummings JL. A review: treatment of Alzheimer's disease discovered in repurposed agents. Dement Geriatr Cogn Disord 2013;35:1–22.

[38] Beking K, Vieira A. Flavonoid intake and disability-adjusted life years due to Alzheimer's and related dementias: a population-based study involving 23 developed countries. Public Health Nutr 2010;13:1403–09.

[39] Candore G, Bulati M, Caruso C, Castiglia L, Colonna-Romano G, Di Bona D, et al. Inflammation, cytokines, immune response, apolipoprotein E, cholesterol, and oxidative stress in Alzheimer disease: therapeutic implications. Rejuvenation Res 2010;13:301–13.

[40] Grill JD, Raman R, Ernstrom K, Aisen P, Karlawish J. Effect of study partner on the conduct of Alzheimer disease clinical trials. Neurology 2013;80:282–88.

[41] Samaranch L, Cervantes S, Barabash A, Alonso A, Cabranes JA, Lamet I, et al. The effect of MAPT H1 and APOE ε4 on transition from mild cognitive impairment to dementia. J Alzheimers Dis 2010;22:1065–71.

[42] Singh PP, Singh M, Mastana SS. APOE distribution in world populations with new data from India and the UK. Ann Hum Biol 2006;33:279–308.

[43] Perneczky R, Wagenpfeil S, Lunetta KL, Cupples LA, Green RC, Decarli C, MIRAGE Study Group Head circumference, atrophy, and cognition: implications for brain reserve in Alzheimer disease. Neurology 2010;75:137–42.

[44] Bjornsson TD, Wagner JA, Donahue SR, Harper D, Karim A, Khouri MS, et al. A review and assessment of potential sources of ethnic differences in drug responsiveness. J Clin Pharmacol 2003;43:943–67.

[45] Faison WE, Schultz SK, Aerssens J, Alvidrez J, Anand R, Farrer LA, et al. Potential ethnic modifiers in the assessment and treatment of Alzheimer's disease: challenges for the future. Int Psychogeriatr 2007;19:539–58.

[46] Paulino Ramirez Diaz S, Gil Gregório P, Manuel Ribera Casado J, Reynish E, Jean Ousset P, Vellas B, et al. The need for a consensus in the use of assessment tools for Alzheimer's disease: the Feasibility Study (assessment tools for dementia in Alzheimer Centres across Europe), a European Alzheimer's Disease Consortium's (EADC) survey. Int J Geriatr Psychiatry 2005;20:744–48.

[47] Doody RS, Cole PE, Miller DS, Siemers E, Black R, Feldman H, et al. Global issues in drug development for Alzheimer's disease. Alzheimers Dement 2011;7:197–207.

[48] Muehlhans S, Richard G, Ali M, Codarini G, Elemuwa C, Khamesipour A, et al. Safety reporting in developing country vaccine clinical trials–a systematic review. Vaccine 2012;30:3255–65.

[49] Izadi M, Fazel M, Nasiri-Vanashi T, Saadat SH, Taheri S. Informed consent for inclusion into clinical trials: a serious subject to note in the developing world. Arab J Nephrol Transplant 2012;5:97–100.

[50] Verwey NA, van der Flier WM, Blennow K, Clark C, Sokolow S, De Deyn PP, et al. A worldwide multicentre comparison of assays for cerebrospinal fluid biomarkers in Alzheimer's disease. Ann Clin Biochem 2009;46:235–40.

[51] Weiner MW, Aisen PS, Jack Jr CR, Jagust WJ, Trojanowski JQ, Shaw L, Alzheimer's Disease Neuroimaging Initiative. The Alzheimer's disease neuroimaging initiative: progress report and future plans. Alzheimers Dement 2010;6:202–11.

[52] Hoekman J, Frenken K, de Zeeuw D, Heerspink HL. The geographical distribution of leadership in globalized clinical trials. PLoS One 2012;7:e45984.

6

Lessons Learned from Major Clinical Trials Conducted Over the Past Decades

Peter Schüler[1], Klaudius Siegfried[2] and Michael Hüll[3]

[1]Global Medical and Safety Services, ICON Clinical Research, Germany
[2]Drug Development Services, ICON Clinical Research, Germany
[3]University of Freiburg Medical School, Freiburg, Germany

6.1 INTRODUCTION

In 2007 we celebrated 100 years of publications in Alzheimer's disease (AD) research [1]. Alois Alzheimer, working in clinical psychiatry and neuropathology, linked cognitive decline with amyloid plaques and neurofibrillary tangles. Over this past century, extensive knowledge about the disease and its underlying pathophysiology has been accumulated [2]. A major therapeutic breakthrough was triggered by the findings of Drachman and Leavitt [3]. They observed that scopolamine-induced cognitive decline was similar to cognitive decline associated with aging. Together with the observation that AD is characterized by the degeneration and loss of cholinergic neurons in the nucleus basalis Meynert, located within the substantia innominata at the ventral surface of the basal forebrain [4], this ultimately led to the development of the symptomatic cholinergic drugs, with the first one being tacrine, marketed in 1991, and other better-tolerated ones to follow.

Improved biochemical analysis led to the determination of the molecular nature of amyloid plaques and neurofibrillary tangles and established the role of A-beta peptides and tau proteins [5]. In the mid 1990s, an additional major breakthrough was related to the linkage between decreased A-beta 42 levels and increased tau levels in cerebrospinal fluid (CSF) and clinical diagnosis of AD [6]. A small number of patients

M. Bairu & M.W. Weiner (Eds):
Global Clinical Trials for Alzheimer's Disease.
DOI: http://dx.doi.org/10.1016/B978-0-12-411464-7.00006-7

suffer from inherited AD, based on meanwhile well-defined mutations in one of three genes: APP (amyloid precursor protein), PSEN1 or PSEN 2 (presenelin 1 and 2). All these mutations directly affect the generation of A-beta 42, by either altering the substrate (APP) or the protease that cleaves this substrate (PSEN, the catalytic component of gamma-secretase) [5].

Over the years, based on these findings, a valuable biomarker tool for early diagnosis was developed [7]. This biomarker was based on observations that the calculated ratio of phospho-tau to A-beta 42 was significantly increased in patients with AD. Tests provided high diagnostic accuracy in distinguishing patients with AD from healthy control subjects (sensitivity, 86%; specificity, 97%), subjects with non-AD dementias (sensitivity, 80%; specificity, 73%), and subjects with other neurological disorders (sensitivity, 80%; specificity, 89%).

After this relevant step forward, the scientific field felt it would only be a matter of a few more years to find even more effective and probably also disease-modifying compounds to treat AD. In addition, from 1990 to the end of 1999, the Library of Congress and the National Institute of Mental Health of the National Institutes of Health sponsored a unique interagency initiative to advance the goals set forth in a proclamation by President George Bush designating the 1990s as the "Decade of the Brain."

After the publication of the pioneering work of Braak and Braak in 1991 [8], in coincidence with improved imaging techniques [9], the overall impression was that the pathophysiology of AD was unlikely to reveal any major secrets.

In contrast to this impression, since the introduction of the cholinesterase-inhibitors and memantine targeting NMDA receptors, incredibly, no new classes of drugs have made it to the market for the treatment of AD. According to a recent report by Pharmaceutical Research and Manufacturers of America (PhRMA) released in 2012 [10], between 1998 and 2011, 101 treatments were investigated but failed to ultimately reach patients, of which 17 projects with final clinical data that targeted A-beta [11]. The overall ratio of failure to success was 31 to 1 (Figure 6.1).

The negative projects include a wide variety of mechanisms of action:

1. Inhibition of A-beta aggregation by tramiprosate (Phase III with over 1,000 pts) and scyllo-inositole (Phase II with 353 pts).
2. A-beta antibodies: bapineuzumab (Phase III with over 2,000 pts) and solanezumab (Phase III with over 2,000 pts).
3. Inhibition of gamma-secretase by semagacestat (Phase III with over 3,000 pts) and avagacestat (Phase II with over 600 pts).
4. Modulation of gamma-secretase by (R)-flurbiprofen/tarenflurbil (Phase III with over 2,400 pts).

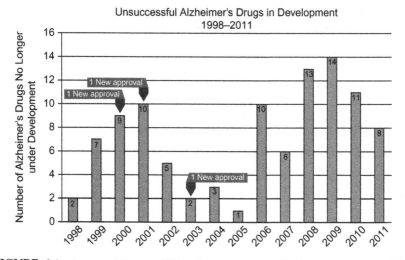

FIGURE 6.1 Between 1998 and 2011, only three new medications were approved for AD. All drugs in development since 2004 failed [10].

5. Inhibition of tau-pathology via GSK3b-inhibition; tideglusib in Phase II with over 300 pts.

Some of these programs and their potential reason for failure are described in more detail below.

According to the PhRMA report, the following potential reasons were identified:

1. Scientists still do not fully understand the underlying causes and mechanisms of the disease, particularly when trying to separate potential causes from effects of the disease.
2. The limited utility of current animal models of the disease is a huge barrier in preclinical testing of drug candidates and limits their predictive validity.
3. The absence of validated non-invasive biomarkers of disease activity and progression.

Additional reasons could be the following: [12]

1. Poor methodology of animal studies.
2. Use of models that do not accurately reflect human pathogenesis.
3. Neutral or non-significant animal studies are less likely to be published.
4. Treatment comes too late, when damage is irreparable.
5. In line with PhRMA explanation No. 1 above, D. Smith [13] sees the focus on a wrong target, i.e. we need to challenge the underlying hypothesis that the formation of amyloid-beta (A-beta) drives the

pathophysiology of AD—instead of just being a result of underlying disease progression, as a key reason for consistent failure.

Other reasons could be seen in the need to use doses that enter the central nervous system (CNS) or have relevant biological activity in CNS.

The potentially good news comes in a second 2012 PhRMA report [14]. America's biopharmaceutical companies currently have 93 medicines in development for AD and dementias—either in human clinical trials or awaiting US Food and Drug Administration (FDA) review. However, about one-third of these ongoing projects are either directly targeting A-beta or doing this indirectly through the gamma-secretase pathway. The majority of the remaining therapies represent a symptomatic approach, only. In view of the so far fairly disappointing results, the question is whether A-beta in fact is (still) a valid target for disease-modifying treatment approaches.

6.2 THE AMYLOID APPROACH

There were several approaches to reduce beta-amyloid in the brain:

1. Reduce hypercholesterolemia.
2. Limit the creation of beta-amyloid and plaques.
3. Induce anti-body response to A-beta 42 via vaccination with subsequent clearance of amyloid plaques.

There are some good arguments why A-beta is the correct target, e.g. the genetic forms of A-beta overproduction leading to AD pathology and dementia.

None of these approaches has yet survived clinical testing, mainly because of a lack of demonstrable efficacy. Thus, the question arises of whether clinical study protocol features such as subject selection criteria, the selected study design, outcome measures, or treatment duration account for this failure—or whether the underlying pathogenetic concepts are fundamentally wrong.

6.2.1 Reduce Hypercholesterolemia

The reduction of hypercholesterolemia was considered an applicable approach to address the underlying A-beta hypothesis because high total cholesterol blood levels are positively correlated with A-beta plaques in the brain. However, there is only limited evidence that cholesterol is connected to A-beta cerebrospinal fluid (CSF) levels. The study by Simons et al. [15] is the only one to find simvastatin significantly decreased A-beta-40 levels in the CSF of patients with mild AD. The Rotterdam epidemiologic study indicated that the use of statins was associated with a reduced risk of AD [16].

Lesser et al. [17] found that nursing home residents with AD pathology (Consortium to Establish a Registry for Alzheimer's Disease, CERAD) had significantly higher total serum cholesterol (TC) and low-density cholesterol (LDL) than residents without AD pathology. This was later confirmed in larger population studies, additionally showing that increasing certainty of AD (CERAD-based) [18] and increasing counts of neuritic plaques (NP), but no significant lipid neurofibrillary tangles (NF) correlations, were significantly associated with higher levels of TC and LDL.

This was confirmed recently in a series of 147 autopsies performed between 1998 and 2003 on residents in Hisayama town, Japan (76 men and 71 women), who underwent clinical examinations in 1988. Lipid profiles, such as TC, triglycerides, and high-density lipoprotein cholesterol (HDLC), were measured in 1988. Adjusted means of TC, LDLC, TC/HDLC, LDLC/HDLC, and non-HDLC (defined as TC–HDLC) were significantly higher in subjects with neuritic plaques (NPs), even in sparse to moderate stages (CERAD = 1 or 2), compared with subjects without NPs in multivariate models including ApoE4 carrier and other confounding factors [19].

In two rather small studies with 400–600 subjects, simvastatin and atorvastatin were assessed over an average of 18 months [20,21]. None of the primary and secondary endpoints showed significant improvements, though one cannot rule out that this was also due to the low statistical power of the study.

This model was also tested in the larger PROSPER (Prospective Study of Pravastatin in the Elderly at Risk) study; 5,804 patients aged 70 to 82 years without pre-existing dementia, but with a vascular risk factor such as vascular disease, nicotine-abuse, hypertonus or diabetes, were enrolled [22]. They were followed up over an average of 42 months with interim cognitive assessments at six different time points. No difference in cognitive decline at any of the cognitive domains was found in subjects treated with pravastatin compared with placebo (all $p > 0.05$). Pravastatin treatment in old age did not affect cognitive decline during a three-year follow-up period. However, pravastatin is passing the blood–brain barrier only to a very limited extent, which may also have contributed to this result [23]. Thus, what about the more targeted efforts to reduce the formation of A-beta?

An ongoing study with simvastatin, supported by the German ministry of research, now examines the potential to postpone conversion from mild cognitive impairment (MCI) to AD. However, the lack of efficacy of statins in modifying the course of AD casts a shadow on their ability to modify the course in MCI. Although cognitive data from studies with statins in vascular disease suggest a primary preventive effect of statins on cognitive decline, the effects are uncertain due to the rather small degree of cognitive decline observed and a lack of operationalized AD diagnosis.

6.2.2 Limit or Prevent Plaque Formation

Tarenflurbil is a selective A-beta-lowering agent that demonstrated encouraging results on cognitive and functional outcomes among mildly affected patients in an earlier Phase II trial. It was tested in a multi-center, randomized, double-blind, placebo-controlled trial enrolling 1,684 patients with only mild AD [24]. Co-primary efficacy endpoints were changed from baseline to month 18 in total score of the Alzheimer's Disease Assessment Scale-cognitive subscale (ADAS-Cog, 80-point version) and the Alzheimer's Disease Cooperative Studies-Activities of Daily Living (ADCS-ADL) scale. Tarenflurbil had no significant beneficial effect on the co-primary measures (difference tarenflurbil vs. placebo in change from baseline to endpoint), according to an intent-to-treat analysis. There were also no significant differences in the secondary outcome measures. The ADAS-Cog score decreased approximately by 7.1 points over 18 months in all groups (see Table 6.1). This could be interpreted as a failure of the underlying treatment approach. But, as in the previous example, the alternative explanation for this failure could be that only insufficient levels of tarenflurbil were able to cross the blood–brain barrier: Tarenflurbil only passes the blood–brain barrier at levels of 05–1.0% [25]. Tarenflurbil, however, had weak effects on amyloid levels in the brain and spinal fluid of patients with AD. But what if these biomarkers are a marker for an invalid target?

A related approach is based on the inhibition of beta or gamma-secretase—enzymes relevant to the formation of beta-amyloid in the brain; beta-secretase BACE is also under evaluation. Initial compounds had trouble reaching the brain or they got in but couldn't stay, ousted in short order by P-glycoprotein. These early problems seem to be addressed. Lilly presented Phase I data on their BACE inhibitor LY2886721 in development for AD at the annual meeting of the American Academy of Neurology on March 18, 2013, but announced termination of Phase II in June 2013, due to liver toxicity of the drug. In December 2012 Merck initiated a Phase II/III clinical trial of its AD drug MK-8931 (Merck company communication).

Cleavage of APP, first by beta-secretase and then by gamma-secretase, fuels production of several brain A-beta peptides, including the highly amyloidgenic isoform A-beta 42. Gamma-secretase inhibitors may

TABLE 6.1 Typical Example of the Summary of Primary Endpoint Results in Recent Studies with a Disease-Modifying Agent Targeting A-beta: Mean (SD) Change from Baseline in the Co-primary Endpoints in the Intention-to-Treat Population [24]

	12 Months	18 Months	Slope (SD)
ADAS-Cog			
Tarenflurbil (n = 786)	4.24 (7.99)	7.27 (10.52)	5.22 (0.272)
Placebo (n = 746)	4.28 (7.50)	7.08 (9.24)	5.06 (.274)
Pvalue	.74	.86	
ADCS-ADL			
Tarenflurbil (n = 751)	−5.36 (10.18)	−10.20 (13.31)	−7.12 (0.394)
Placebo (n = 725)	−6.05 (10.72)	−9.74 (14.01)	−7.08 (0.395)
Pvalue	.19	.48	

decrease production of amyloid and potentially modify the progression of AD.

In one such study with Lilly's gamma-secretase inhibitor, semagacestat, the clinical outcome was even worse under active treatment, compared with placebo. Development was stopped in 2010, after a pre-planned interim analysis of two Phase III trials for patients with mild to moderate AD showed that cognition and activities of daily living worsened in patients treated with semagacestat compared with those on placebo. That gave rise to the idea that beta-amyloid formation may be a result of AD progression or potentially even an attempted repair mechanism [26].

A comparable finding was seen for another investigational gamma-secretase inhibitor, avagacestat. In a Phase II dose-finding trial, trends for cognitive worsening were observed for patients on the two higher doses (100 mg and 125 mg daily) on the ADAS-Cog. Bristol-Myers Squibb planned for a new study to enroll patients in stages where clinical signs and symptoms of dementia are not yet evident, with patients identified based on biomarker evidence of AD. This pre-dementia study was planned to examine avagacesat dosed at 50 mg/day for two years but was terminated in December 2012, due to lack of biologic effect at the lower dose (BMS company communication). This project could have helped to answer the question of whether A-beta is the right target, provided treatment is initiated at the right time, in early pre-symptomatic stages, or whether the timing is irrelevant because the treatment target is wrong.

6.2.3 Vaccination/Immunotherapy

Immunotherapy covers passive (antibody application) and active immunotherapy (vaccination strategies). Vaccination refers to giving a peptide fragment to induce active antibody production by the body (active immunoterhapy).

Passive concepts: In the pivotal Phase III EXPEDITION studies in over 2,000 patients with Lilly's lead compound, solanezumab (a monoclonal antibody that binds to soluble forms of beta amyloid), only a pre-specified sub-group analysis of patients with mild/early disease revealed a statistically significant benefit over placebo [27], with a 42% reduction in cognitive decline at 18 months.

The original analysis did not indicate any significant effects on both pre-defined primary endpoints, and this was confirmed in a second trial that involved patients with mild to moderate AD. A statistically significant difference between active drug and placebo was found neither on the ADAS-Cog nor on the ADCS-ADL scale.

A possible interpretation of these findings would be that a disease-modifying therapy that targets A-beta has to start very early in the disease progression, before any major brain damage occurs.

Bapineuzumab, a monoclonal antibody that targets beta-amyloid, comes with a very similar story: Results of biomarker sub-studies, included in the bapineuzumab trials, showed significant differences in the amount of amyloid in the brain and phospho-tau in CSF between patients with AD carrying the apolipoprotein E4 (ApoE4) genotype who received bapineuzumab and those taking placebo [28]. The results of two large Phase III randomized, double-blind trials of bapineuzumab (Johnson & Johnson and Pfizer Inc.) in patients with mild to moderate AD nonetheless showed that the treatment failed to meet co-primary clinical endpoints of change in cognitive and functional performance compared with placebo in ApoE4 carriers and non-carriers, respectively.

The new biomarker results can be interpreted in different ways, depending on one's preconceived notions about the amyloid cascade hypothesis: The findings demonstrate that the antibodies reach and remove amyloid in the brain, as shown on the Amyloid-PET scans [29], and that there was less of a downstream effect from amyloid deposition, as seen from measures of phospho-tau in the CSF.

For a believer in the A-beta hypothesis, the lack of clinical effects could still be explained by a start that comes too late to have a significant impact of pathophysiological cascade of events.

With gantenerumab, a monoclonal antibody that binds to all forms of aggregated beta amyloid, Roche is also targeting early stages of the disease. Gantenerumab is currently being tested in an international Phase II/III trial in prodromal AD. Also for this compound, earlier studies resulted in a dose-dependent reduction in brain amyloid level, possibly through an effector cell-mediated mechanism of action [30].

Rachelle S. Doody, MD, PhD, Director of the Alzheimer's Disease and Memory Disorders Center at Baylor College of Medicine in Houston, Texas, pointed out that [31] "...there are at least seven other antibody-related infusion treatments under development and in human stages of testing, and none of them have so far been proven to benefit patients clinically."

6.2.3.1 *Active Vaccination*

A study led by the Karolinska Institute in Sweden reported, for the first time, positive effects of an active vaccine against AD with the new vaccine, CAD106 [32]. The treatment involves active immunization triggering the body's immune defense against A-beta. In this second clinical trial on humans, the vaccine was modified to affect only the harmful beta-amyloid; 80% of the patients involved in the trials developed their own protective antibodies against A-beta without suffering any side effects over the three years of the study.

Some answers as to whether the described situation of negative or failed studies is due to a "wrong target or wrong timing" may come from the long-term results of a prematurely ended A-beta 42 active immunization study in AD. The study was stopped early for safety reasons with patients developing meningoencephalitis.

Of 372 patients treated in the initial Phase IIa study (300 active; 72 placebo), a total of 264 (71.0%) were contacted to determine interest in follow-up study participation [33]. 159 agreed to participate in the follow-up study (30 placebo; 129 treated with AN1792). Of the original 59 subjects who were classified in the Phase IIa study as antibody responders, 25 (42.4%) agreed to participate in the follow-up study compared with 30/72 (41.7%) of the placebo-treated patients.

The majority of patients enrolled in this follow-up study were taking concomitant acetylcholinesterase inhibitors or memantine. The proportion of patients taking concomitant medications was similar between antibody responders and placebo-treated patients. After approximately 4.6 years of follow-up, antibody responders demonstrated a 25.0% lower decline in activities of daily living as determined by the Disability and Dementia (DAD) scale compared with placebo-treated patients. Comparisons of cognitive function in this follow-up study may not be representative of the entire placebo-treated group, and may favor the assessment of placebo-treated patients who were less impaired and capable of undergoing cognitive testing. The neuropsychologic test battery (NTB) was attainable in only 10/30 placebo-treated patients (33.3%) and 13/25 antibody responders (52.0%). No significant differences were observed in the change from baseline for the overall NTB nine-component z-score between antibody responders and placebo-treated patients. The ADAS-Cog was attainable in 11/30 placebo-treated patients

86   6. LESSONS LEARNED FROM MAJOR CLINICAL TRIALS

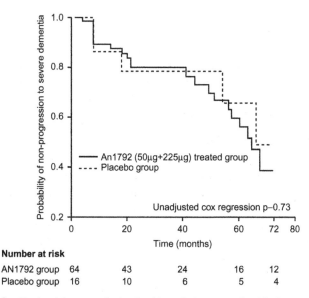

FIGURE 6.2   Kaplan-Meyer analysis of subjects being treated with the vaccine versus placebo. No clinical effect was observed, even though vaccination effectively cleared amyloid plaques [31].

(36.7%) and 16/25 antibody responders (64.0%). No significant differences in ADAS-Cog score were observed between placebo-treated patients and antibody responders after approximately 4.6 years of follow-up.

In a six-year follow-up post vaccination in 80 subjects [34], including post-mortem analysis of subjects that underwent immunization to clear plaques from the brain, A-beta clearance did not prevent the progression of neurodegeneration and dementia. The authors claim that:

> presence of A-beta plaques might be necessary to initiate, but not to maintain, progressive neuro-degeneration [...]. Second [...] the removal of plaques after AN1792 immunization could be a slow process [...]. Third, [...] immunization could fail to reduce the concentration of oligomeric A-beta and the concentration might even be increased during the active phase of disintegration of A-beta plaques. According to this view, aggregated A-beta in the form of plaques is harmless, or could even be protective [...].

See also Figure 6.2.

6.3 ALTERNATIVE TARGETS

It therefore seems to be crucial to focus on targets other than A-beta, such as tau-protein. In AD, the brain contains two types of aggregates: intracellular

III. CHALLENGES AND OPPORTUNITIES TO CONDUCT GLOBAL AD TRIALS

neurofibrillary tangles (tau protein) and extracellular senile or "amyloid" plaques consisting of the A-beta peptide, a cleavage product of the membrane protein APP [35].

Tau proteins are highly organized protein aggregates and are considered to be mediators of cellular toxicity and thus attract a great deal of attention from investigators. The last decade has witnessed a renaissance of interest in inhibitors of tau aggregation as potential disease-modifying drugs for AD and other "tauopathies" [36].

Tau, however, is an intracellular protein. Even though there are drugs under development to inhibit tau activation, these drugs need to be intra-cellulary active—with a risk of unexpected adverse reactions on brain cell metabolism [37].

So far, the situation with compounds that are targeted at tau protein is not much more promising: Tideglusib, an irreversible inhibitor of GSK-3 which inhibits tau protein phosphorylation in neuronal cultures and in pertaining transgenic mice models, showed disappointing results in Phase III studies.

Nonetheless, another innovative concept was linked to a drug development focused on tau: The patient recruitment company Medici Global developed a Facebook page to help those living with AD and to help bring new medicines to market [11], by attempting to promote a Phase III study in 21 countries with LMTX, a compound which shall dissolve tangles.

As disease-modifying drugs are still an option but expensive to develop, what else can be done?

6.4 ALTERNATIVE APPROACHES AND STUDY DESIGNS

In case one favors a treatment approach based on the concept of "the earlier the better," the question arises as to "how early should early be?" When considering this approach, one needs, according to Selkoe [38], to differentiate between primary and secondary prevention on the one hand and early symptomatic treatment on the other (Figure 6.3). Such outcome studies would need to follow non-symptomatic patients at risk of developing AD over several years. The hypothesis is to lower conversion into AD with active therapy.

The design of such projects would in principle follow recently published studies in vascular primary and secondary prevention (e.g., primary prevention of stroke in patients with ventricular fibrillation) [39]. Such projects may only be feasible under certain conditions:

• They require a well-defined and pre-selected patient population at the highest possible risk of conversion to AD in the not too distant future.

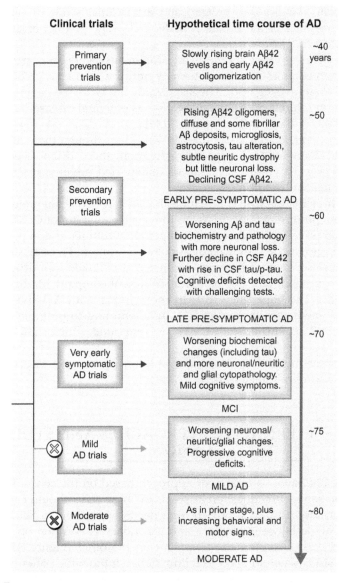

FIGURE 6.3 Aligning potential disease-modifying agents for AD with the course of the disease. Boxes on the left: clinical trial categories dependent on the stage of AD. "X" in bottom left box: trials in moderate AD not recommended. "X" in second-bottom box on left: trials in mild AD recommended with caution. Boxes on the right: speculative stages in the long pre-symptomatic and symptomatic phases of AD in a hypothetical individual who undergoes A-beta build-up. *Figure adapted from [38].*

- Therapy needs to be well tolerated to be acceptable for a still healthy population.
- Therapy needs to be easy to use (e.g., once daily oral application) to allow adherence to therapy in a preventive setting over months and years.
- Assessments need to be most non-invasive to pass IEC/IRB approval.

This concept was already agreed on in 2006 [40].

An in-depth discussion about the potential use of markers to "enrich" the population enrolled for follow-up can be found in [41].

The dilemma is that there is no agreement on what are the most sensitive and specific biomarkers that may predict later AD onset—and that biomarkers from CSF require an invasive lumbar puncture.

Non-invasive biomarkers would be beneficial in spotting those patients at highest risk for developing AD. In a longitudinal evaluation of the available data in "Alzheimer's disease neuroimaging initiative" (ADNI), Gomar et al. [42] studied patients with mild cognitive impairment who converted to AD (n = 116) and those who did not convert (n = 204) within a two-year period. They determined the predictive utility of 25 variables from all classes of markers, biomarkers, and risk factors in a series of logistic regression models and effect size analyses. Various types of markers were included, such as regional brain volumes, CSF measures of pathological A-beta 42 and total tau, cognitive measures, and individual risk factors. The results indicated that cognitive markers at baseline were more robust predictors of conversion than most biomarkers. A similar proof for cognitive markers was provided by the German Competence Network Dementia in a prospective study of subjects with MCI [43].

Another possible answer could be provided by performing such studies in AD patients who suffer from a hereditary variant of AD (dominantly inherited AD). Autosomal dominant AD follows a different time course with disease onset around the age of 48 years in patients with the most prevalent presenilin mutations, but has similar neuropathological findings and symptomatology.

The Dominantly Inherited Alzheimer Network (DIAN) [44] tries to address this concept by currently enrolling and thoroughly evaluating about 400 such patients in the USA, Australia, and Europe. In the case of a successful outcome, this study could be the basis for proof-of-concept studies in a well-defined and pre-selected patient population.

Other strategies to use enriched samples with people with a high genetic risk are to evaluate new treatments in cohorts of ApoE4-positive persons with further genetic markers [45]. This means that identifying people at risk of developing the disease may provide a more promising population for future studies. They may get identified by a genetic predisposition or by measuring biomarkers, such as the recently reported CSF measurement of a mix of A-beta 1–42 and phosphorylated tau protein.

In an attempt to find early pre-dementia patients for its gamma-secretase inhibitor avagacesat study, BMS screened 1,350 potential subjects. Only 550 of those met the criteria of MCI, and of those, only 48% met the biomarker criteria in CSF after lumbar puncture, creating an overall screen failure rate of 81% [46].

The situation described raises a very practical question: which company would be willing to identify, enroll, and follow up over nearly a decade thousands of subjects at an even earlier stage of the disease— with the need to screen many more subjects?

The FDA tried to address this dilemma by providing new guidance for industry with a focus on early stages of the disease [47], which is also summarized in [48]. The main change is to accept cognitive endpoints only, since daily functioning may not yet be affected in early stages. The FDA is open to considering the argument that a positive biomarker result (generally included as a secondary outcome measure in a trial) in combination with a positive finding on a primary clinical outcome measure may support a claim of disease modification in AD. Until there is widespread evidence-based agreement in the research community that an effect on a particular biomarker is reasonably likely to predict clinical benefit, the FDA will not be in a position to consider an approval based on the use of a biomarker as a surrogate outcome measure in AD (at any stage of the illness).

A recent study added further doubt to the "need to treat early" concept. The symptomatic therapies donepezil and memantine showed positive effects at advanced stages of the disease; 295 patients with a Mini Mental status of 5–13 points (indicating progressed stage of the disease), and already on therapy with donepezil, were randomized to one of four treatment groups: continue donepezil therapy, end therapy, switch to memantine, and add memantine to donepezil. After one year of observation, patients statistically significantly benefited from active treatment [49]. If symptomatic therapy requiring neuronal and synaptic response is still effective in later stages of the disease, why should other therapies that also require a remaining "critical mass" of neurons not work at all in even earlier stages?

An alternative approach could thus be the re-evaluation of mechanisms identified as relevant for the therapy of AD prior to the era of disease-modifying research. The list of drugs used prior to the introduction of cholinergics is as long as the assumed modes of action of these compounds. Pyritinole, meclofenoxate, co-dergocrine, pentoxifylline, nimodipine, gingko biloba, naftidrofuryl, nicergoline, and memantine shall act via impact on various neurotransmitters such as acetycholine, norepinephrine, dopamine, glutamate, and serotonine (for details see [50]).

1. Activation of neuro-metabolism (e.g., by activation of hexokinase, glucose-6-phosphat dehydrogenase, cytochrom-c-reductase, adenylatkinase, and facilitation of oxygen-uptake.
2. Increase cerebral microcirculation.
3. Reduction of free radicals in the brain and of oxidative stress, e.g., activation of superoxiddismutase, gluthathionperoxidase, and gluthathionreductase.
4. Immunomodulation such as inhibition of tumor-necrosis-factor alpha (TNF-alpha).
5. Limit calcium load of (neuronal) cells.

Orion Pharma disclosed the results of a 100 pts Phase II proof-of-concept study with the new selective alpha 2C adrenoreceptor antagonist, ORM 12741, as add-on therapy to a cholinesterase inhibitor drug. After three months, the memory scores for those who received the placebo pill had worsened by 33%, whereas the scores improved by 4% for those who took the active drug at two dose levels [51]. Another potential target for new AD drugs was recently re-evaluated: The aluminum hypothesis of the 1980s got new support with the observation that ferritin molecules are not only found in unusually high concentration in AD brains, but that these ferritin molecules do not contain iron but on average contain 62% aluminum. Even though this is a small study of only 21 AD patients compared with 200 healthy subjects, the results may be the "missing link" to explain how neurotoxic aluminum can pass the blood–brain barrier and why high aluminum exposure can thus trigger neuronal death [52].

Once any of these potentially symptomatic and disease-modifying mechanisms manage to provide proof-of-concept, it would be best to apply more advanced drug-design methodologies such as the "Delayed-Start Study Design", also called "Randomized-Start Design." The FDA also supports this approach, saying:

> We have not yet reached a conclusion that a comparison of the rate of change in key clinical efficacy parameters (based on slopes) between active treatment and control groups, using a standard parallel-arm study design, could provide the sole support for a claim of disease modification. A randomized-start or randomized-withdrawal trial design (with clinical outcome measures) appears to be a more convincing means of demonstrating such an effect. For ethical reasons, a randomized-start design would be most appropriate for use in AD [47].

In step 1 of this design, patients receive the assigned treatment (active or placebo) and are followed over an extended period of time; this allows the effects of the treatment on symptoms to be observed. In step 2, all

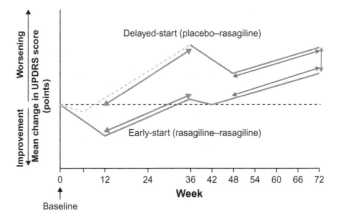

FIGURE 6.4 Schematic drawing of a delayed-start study design. Dotted line indicates the provision of placebo. The vertical arrow at the far right-hand side of the figure is seen as an indication for a disease-modifying effect. A purely symptomatic effect would not have endured after switching both treatment arms on active. One has to assume that during treatment Step 1 the progression of the disease was slowed down, also providing these patients with a benefit later on at the study end [47].

patients receive the active treatment, and the data obtained during this phase are used to evaluate the disease-modifying effects of the active drug [53]. This advanced design would allow the assessment of a symptomatic and a potential disease-modifying effect in one study. This design was only applied once with partial success in a related disorder; in Parkinson's disease [54]. See also Figures 6.4–6.6.

These innovative study designs can be even further developed, up to a complete two-period design [55] (Figure 6.7).

6.5 CONCLUSIONS

A-beta and related targets have consistently showed negative results in Phase III studies in this first decade of the 21st century, after showing promising trends in Phase II. This could be due to three major reasons:

1. The wrong patient population was observed, e.g., therapy started too late in the progression of the disease.
2. The effects of these therapeutics on A-beta were not large enough (potentially because of too low doses) or did not target the most toxic species of A-beta.
3. A-beta is the wrong target.

All of the above reasons may be true. Which of these main alternatives is correct cannot be finally determined, yet. Since so far no pivotal study

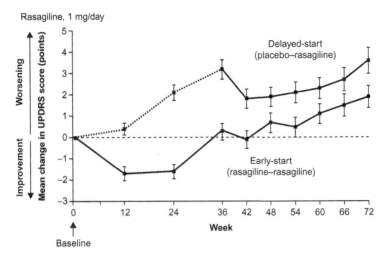

FIGURE 6.5   Real data from the rasagiline study: 1 mg/day dose arm. These results have a very similar shape as in the hypothetical concept displayed in Figure 6.2 above [47].

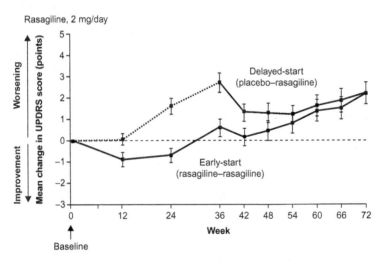

FIGURE 6.6   Real data from the rasagiline study: 2 mg/day dose arm. This is a result you would expect from a purely symptomatic therapy, with no enduring benefit after switching all study subjects to active drug [47].

targeting A-beta has shown clinical effects, it is fairly improbable that there is any true effect that so far could not have been demonstrated. The post-hoc identification of some trend in some less progressed disease is similar to trends observed in (also underpowered) Phase II studies and could also be explained by random fluctuations.

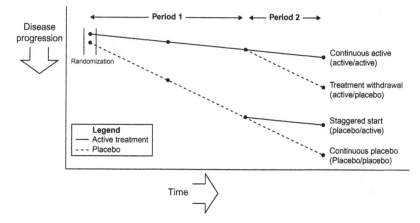

FIGURE 6.7   Schematic flow of a complete two-period design: A combination of a randomized delayed-start and a randomized withdrawal design [49].

Even if earlier therapy provides a disease-modifying effect, the studies confirming that hypothesis would be expensive and last several years, probably even decades.

In a cross-sectional study using a new PET tracer to visualize aggregated A-beta in dominantly inherited AD [56], A-beta accumulation started at a median age of 28.2 years, which is about 16 years prior to first AD symptoms and 21 years prior to full AD symptoms. Only very well-tolerated and easy-to-use therapies would be eligible for such a long-lasting prophylactic treatment.

As an alternative, better symptomatic therapies, with or without potential additional disease-modifying effects, should again find more attention to provide therapeutic alternatives to the existing cholinergic therapies and memantine. In future, effective disease management will also require multiple approaches.

References

[1] Alzheimer A. Ueber eine eigenartige Erkrankung der Hirnrinde. [An unusual disease of cerebral cortex] Allgemeine Zeitschrift für Psychiatrie und Psychisch-Gerichtl Med 1907;64:146–8.

[2] Hodger JR. Alzheimer's centennial legacy: origins, landmarks and the current status of knowledge concerning cognitive aspects. Brain 2006;129:2811–22.

[3] Drachman DA, Leavitt J. Human memory and the cholinergic system: a relationship to ageing? Arch Neurol 1974;30:113–21.

[4] Vogels OJ, Broere CA, ter Laak HJ, ten Donkelaar HJ, Nieuwenhuys R, Schulte BP. Cell loss and shrinkage in the nucleus basalis Meynert complex in Alzheimer's disease. Neurobiol Aging 1990;11:3–13.

[5] Selkoe DJ. The molecular pathology of Alzheimer's disease. Neuron 1991;6(4):487–98.

[6] Motter R, Vigo-Pelfrey C, Kholodenko D, et al. Reduction of beta-amyloid peptide42 in the cerebrospinal fluid of patients with Alzheimer's disease. Ann Neurol 1995;38:643–8.

[7] Maddalena A, Papassotiropoulos A, Müller-Tillmanns B, Jung HH, Hegi T, Nitsch RM, et al. Biochemical diagnosis of alzheimer's disease by measuring the cerebrospinal fluid ratio of phosphorylated tau protein to β-Amyloid peptide42. Arch Neurol 2003;60(9):1202–6.

[8] Braak H, Braak E. Neuropathological staging of Alzheimer-related changes. Acta Neuropathol 1991;82:239–59.

[9] Frackowiak RSJ, Pozzilli C, Legg NJ, Duboulay GH, Marshall J, Lenzi GL, et al. Regional cerebral oxygen supply and utilization in dementia. A clinical and physiological study with oxygen 15 and positron emission tomography. Brain 1981;104:753–78.

[10] [***author name]. Alzheimer's Research—Setbacks and Stepping Stones. Pharmaceutical Research and Manufacturers of America (PhRMA) [internet]. (April 2012) [***cited–year month day] Available from: <http://phrma.org/media/releases/setbacks-stepping-stones-alzheimers-disease>.

[11] Rosenberg R. Medici global says its Alzheimer's Facebook page demonstrates the need for more early detection trials. Center Watch Weekly 2012;16(50):1–4.

[12] The Lancet Why are drug trials in Alzheimer's disease failing? Lancet 2010;376:658.

[13] Smith DA. Why are drug trials in Alzheimer's disease failing? Lancet 2010;376:1466.

[14] Medicines in Development for Alzheimer's Disease. Pharmaceutical Research and Manufacturers of America (PhRMA). Available from: <http://www.phrma.org/research/medicines-development-alzheimers-disease>; 2012.

[15] Simons M, Schwärzler F, Lütjohann D, von Bergmann K, Beyreuther K, Dichgans J, et al. Treatment with simvastatin in normocholesterolemic patients with Alzheimer's disease: A 26-week randomized, placebo-controlled, double-blind trial. Ann Neurol 2002;52(3):346–50.

[16] Haag MDM, Hofman A, Koudstaal PJ, Stricker BHC, Breteler MMB. Statins are associated with a reduced risk of Alzheimer disease regardless of lipophilicity: The Rotterdam Study. J Neurol Neurosurg Psychiatry 2009;80:13–17.

[17] Lesser GT, Haroutunian V, Purohitm DP, Schnaider Beeri M, Schmeidler J, Honkanen L, et al. Serum lipids are related to Alzheimer's pathology in nursing home residents. Dementia Geriatr Cognit Disord 2009;27:42–9.

[18] Lesser GT, Beeri MS, Schmeidler J, Purohit DP, Haroutunian V. Cholesterol and LDL relate to neuritic plaques and to APOE4 presence but not to neurofibrillary tangles. Curr Alzheimer Res 2011;8(3):303–12.

[19] Matsuzaki T, Sasaki K, Hata J, Hirakawa Y, Fujimi K, Ninomiya T, et al. Association of Alzheimer's disease pathology with abnormal lipid metabolism. Neurology 2011;77(11):1068–75.

[20] Sano M, Bell KL, Galasko D, Galvin JE, Thomas RG, van Dyck CH, et al. A randomized, double-blind, placebo-controlled trial of simvastatin to treat Alzheimer's disease. Neurology 2011;77(6):556–63.

[21] Feldman HH, Doody RS, Kivipelto M, Sparks DL, Waters DD, Jones RW, et al. LEADe Investigators. Randomized controlled trial of atorvastatin in mild to moderate Alzheimer disease: LEADe. Neurology 2010;74(12):956–64.

[22] Trompet S, van Vliet P, de Craen AJ, Jolles J, Buckley BM, et al. Results of the PROSPER study. J Neurol 2010;257(1):85–90.

[23] Hermann D. Comment. Info Neurologie & Psychiatrie 2010;12:26.

[24] Green RC, Schneider LS, Amato DA, Beelen AP, Wilcock G, Swabb EA, et al. Effect of tarenflurbil on cognitive decline and activities of daily living in patients with mild Alzheimer disease: a randomized controlled trial. JAMA 2009;302(23):2557–64.

[25] Hermann D. Comment. Info Neurologie & Psychiatrie 2010;12:32.

III. CHALLENGES AND OPPORTUNITIES TO CONDUCT GLOBAL AD TRIALS

[26] Smith DA. Why are drug trials in Alzheimer's disease failing? Lancet 2010;376:1466.
[27] Presentation at American Neurological Society 2011.
[28] Anderson P. Hope for Bapineuzumap in Alzheimer's? Medscape Medical News 2012 Available from: <http://www.medscape.com/viewarticle/771210>[19.09.2012].
[29] Rinne JO, Brooks DJ, Rossor MN, Fox NC, et al. 11C-PiB PET assessment of change in fibrillar amyloid-beta load in patients with Alzheimer's disease treated with bapineuzumab: a phase 2, double-blind, placebo-controlled, ascending-dose study. Lancet Neurol 2010;9(4):363–72.
[30] Ostrowitzki S, Deptula D, Thurfjell L, Barkhof F, Bohrmann B, Brooks DJ, et al. Mechanism of amyloid removal in patients with Alzheimer's disease treated with gantenerumab. Arch Neurol 2012;69(2):198–207.
[31] Johnson K. Gantenerumab reduces brain amyloid in Alzheimer's. Medscape Medical News 2011 Available from: <http://www.medscape.com/viewarticle/751500>; [13.10.2011].
[32] Winblad B, Andreasen N, Minthon L, et al. Safety, tolerability, and antibody response of active Aβ immunotherapy with CAD106 in patients with Alzheimer's disease: randomized, double-blind, placebo-controlled, first-in-human study. Lancet Neurol 2012 10.1016, 1474–4422.
[33] Vellas B, Black R, Thal LJ, for the AN1792 (QS-21)-251 Study Team Long-term follow-up of patients immunized with AN1792: reduced functional decline in antibody responders. Curr Alzheimer Res 2009;6(2):144–51.
[34] Holmes C, Boche D, Wilkinson D, Yadegarfar G, et al. Long-term effects of Aβ42 immunisation in Alzheimer's disease: follow-up of a randomised, placebo-controlled phase I trial. Lancet 2008;372(9634):216–23.
[35] Haass C, Selkoe DJ. Soluble protein oligomers in neurodegeneration: lessons from the Alzheimer's amyloid beta-peptide. Nat Rev Mol Cell Biol 2007;8:101–12.
[36] Bulic B, Pickhardt M, Schmidt B, Mandelkow E, Waldmann H, Mandelkow E. Development of Tau aggregation inhibitors for Alzheimer's Disease. Angew Chem Int Ed 2009;48:2–15.
[37] Hu S, Begum AN, Jones MR, Oh MS, Beech WK, et al. GSK3 inhibitors show benefits in an Alzheimer's disease (AD) model of neurodegeneration but adverse effects in control animals. Neurobiol Dis 2009;33(2):193–206.
[38] Selkoe DJ. Preventing Alzheimer's disease. Science 2012;337:1448–92.
[39] Granger CB, Alexander JH, McMurray J, et al. Apixaban versus warfarin in patients with atrial fibrillation. N Engl J Med 2011;365:981–92.
[40] Frank RA, Galasko D, Hampel H, Hardy J, de Leon MJ, Mehta PD, et al. Biological markers for therapeutic trials in Alzheimer's disease. Proceedings of the biological markers working group; NIA initiative on neuroimaging in Alzheimer's disease. Neurobiol Aging 2003;24(4):521–36.
[41] European Medicines Agency Qualification opinion of Alzheimer's disease novel methodologies/biomarkers for PET amyloid imaging (positive/negative) as a biomarker for enrichment for use – in predementia AD clinical trials. Cited June 2013. Available from: <http://www.ema.europa.eu/docs/en_GB/document_library/Regulatory_and_procedural_guideline/2011/12/WC500118364.pdf>.
[42] Gomar JJ, Bobes-Bascaran MT, Conejero-Goldberg C, et al. Utility of combinations of biomarkers, cognitive markers, and risk factors to predict conversion from mild cognitive impairment to AD in patients in the AD neuroimaging initiative. Arch Gen Psychiatry 2011;68:961–9.
[43] Wagner M, Wolf S, Reischies FM, Daerr M, Wolfsgruber S, Jessen F, et al. Biomarker validation of a cued recall memory deficit in prodromal Alzheimer's disease. Neurology 2012;78(6):379–86.

[44] Dominantly Inherited Alzheimer Network (DIAN). Cited June 2013. Available at <www.dian-info.org>.

[45] Crenshaw DG, Gottschalk WK, Lutz MW, Grossman I, Saunders AM, et al. Using genetics to enable studies on the prevention of Alzheimer's disease. Clin Pharmacol Ther 2013;93(2):177–85.

[46] Rosenberg R. Medici global says its Alzheimer's Facebook page demonstrates the need for more early detection trials. Center Watch Weekly 2012;16(50):1–4.

[47] Federal Drug Administration. Draft Guidance for Industry. Alzheimer's Disease: Developing Drugs for the Treatment of Early Stage Disease 2013.

[48] Kozauer N, Katz R. Regulatory innovation and drug development for early-stage Alzheimer's disease. NEJM 2013;368(13):1169–71.

[49] Howard R, McShane R, Lindesay J, et al. Donepezil and memantine for moderate-to-severe Alzheimer's disease.. N Engl J Med 2012;366:893–903.

[50] Riederer P, Laux G, Pöldinger W, editors. Neuro-psychopharmaka 5: Parkinsonmittel und Antidementiva. [Anti-Parkinson's drugs and anti-dementia drugs] New York: *Springer*; 1999. pp. 543–705.

[51] Rouru J, Wesnes K, Hänninen J. et al. Safety and efficacy of ORM-12741 on cognitive and behavioral symptoms in patients with Alzheimer's disease: A randomized, double-blind, placebo-controlled, parallel group, multicenter, proof-of-concept 12 week study. Poster #002 at 65th AAN Meeting, San Diego, March 16–23, 2013.

[52] De Sole P, et al. Possible relationship between Al/ferritin complex and Alzheimer's disease. Clin Biochem 2013;46:89–93.

[53] D'Agostino RB. The delayed-start study design. N Engl J Med 2009;361:1304–6.

[54] Olanow CW, Rascol O, Hauser R, Feigin PD, Jankovic J, Lang A, et al. A double-blind, delayed-start trial of rasagiline in Parkinson's disease. N Engl J Med 2009;361:1268–78.

[55] Mohr E, Barclay CL, Anderson R, Constant J. Clinical trial design in the age of dementia treatments: challenges and opportunities Gauthier S, Scheltens P, Cummings J, editors. Alzheimer Disease and Related Disorders Annual 2004. United Kingdom: Martin Dunitz Ltd.; 2004. p. 99–125.

[56] Todd S, Stallard N. A new clinical trial design combining phases II and III: Sequential designs with treatment selection and a change of endpoint. Drug Inf J 2005;39:109–18.

[57] Fleisher AS, Chen K, Quiroz YT. Florbetapir PET analysis of amyloid-beta deposition in the presenilin 1 E280A autodomal dominant Alzheimer's disease kindred: a cross-sectional study. Lancet 2012;11:1057–65.

7

Why the Negative Studies in Alzheimer's Disease?

Hans J. Möbius

EnVivo International B.V., The Netherlands

7.1 INTRODUCTION

This chapter attempts to critically analyze the reasons why there have been so many negative studies and so few successes in developing drugs to treat Alzheimer's disease (AD) during the last 20 years. During this period a variety of treatment principles were successfully tested in animal models but only two have currently achieved approval as clinical therapies—acetylcholinesterase inhibition and uncompetitive N-methyl d-aspartate (NMDA) antagonism. To date, there have been more than 200 clinical development failures for various reasons and all completed Phase III trials on disease modifying compounds in AD during the past decade have failed to demonstrate a cognitive or clinically relevant improvement.

Of even greater concern are the discrepancies between the positive results seen in animal models, e.g., removal of brain amyloid and failure to show benefit in clinical trials when targeting the same mechanism. Despite major investments and increased understanding of pathophysiology, proof of disease modification remains elusive today. This is in stark contrast to progress in other therapeutic areas where considerable advances have been made, e.g., diabetes or cancer.

This chapter asks fundamental questions about the reasons for the series of negative studies:

• Why has there been so much focus on amyloid in AD?
• Has there been a too simplistic view of the pathophysiology of the disease and the temporal nature of the pathological processes?

M. Bairu & M.W. Weiner (Eds):
Global Clinical Trials for Alzheimer's Disease.
DOI: http://dx.doi.org/10.1016/B978-0-12-411464-7.00007-9

- How have issues in the use of preclinical models and their translation compounded the situation?
- Have the methods used in clinical drug development and the refinement of its tools contributed to the lack of success?
- Have researchers failed to consider the impact of demographic characteristics (medical comorbidities, concomitant medications) on course of illness and response to interventions?
- Have researchers failed to learn from previous mistakes in earlier AD drug development programs?
- Has regulatory guidance or lack thereof contributed to the situation?

7.2 WHY HAS THERE BEEN SO MUCH FOCUS ON AMYLOID IN AD?

Historically, the pathophysiology has progressed from initial metabolic considerations ("lecithin depletion") through regional post-mortem neurotransmitter reduction to the first neurotransmitter-based rational therapy (tacrine) and then the amyloid hypothesis [1], followed by Braak's paired helical filament (PHF) start and spread law [2]. It has long been generally accepted that the two AD hallmark lesions consist of Aβ plaques and neurofibrillary tangles build up from tau.

However, the publication of the first transgenic mouse model of AD [3] was based on the amyloid hypothesis, and amyloid precursor protein (APP) transgenic mouse models became key to the subsequently intensified search for a rational, causal therapy. Transgenic mouse models of tau were also published but did not lead to a comparable drug screening effort—or less success. In the following years, drug screening and development into late stages was mainly focused on the amyloid cascade hypothesis, with some on inflammation pathways and little on tau alteration. Ten years after the initial publication of the Braak PHF spread and staging approach [2] was correlated to clinical status, Giannakopoulos et al. [4] reported that tangle and neuron numbers, but not amyloid load, predict cognitive status in AD. Yet such reports did not change the mainstay of research and development (R&D). Recent neuropathological data point to tau formation in the olfactory bulb and brainstem even prior to Braak Stage I [5]. It has been shown that Aβ toxicity is tau dependent, although the mechanistic link is unclear [6,7]. Ittner et al. [8] described a less-known dendritic function of tau in postsynaptic targeting of the Src kinase Fyn, which is disrupted by truncated tau, and go on to suggest that tau and tau-dependent mechanisms might thus mediate Aβ toxicity at the post-synapse via NMDA receptor excitotoxicity. To date, not all these mechanisms are fully understood, although this kind of research points to an attempt of a more integrated understanding of the etiopathogenesis as opposed to a predominant focus on amyloid.

The key question of the relationship of "drugable" targets to the course of human disease remains to be better defined. AD is clearly polygenetic and multi-factorial and involves several different etiopathogenic mechanisms—but do researchers and scientists really take this fact sufficiently into account? While it is generally accepted that Aβ oligomers are toxic, it is still not known which "toxic species" of Aβ is/are the appropriate target, how much lowering is required, and in which phase of the illness.

Likewise, it proved very difficult to identify a "drugable" target to stop the formation of toxic tau oligomers and PHF formation; for example, memantine was shown to inhibit hyperphosphorylation of tau [9], but whether that contributes to its clinical effects at all is unclear, and the relevance of tau hyperphosphorylation to PHF formation has been debated [10].

So, 22 years after Hardy and Allsop [1], has the amyloid hypothesis matured into a theory? Increasing evidence points to the fact that amyloid is only part of the picture; how key to the whole picture remains to be elucidated—hence a theory is as yet unavailable. The recent Aβ-directed Phase III failures should not be considered proof of falsification due to the very specific nature of the interventions. Are we any closer to a unifying hypothesis of AD than we were 10 years ago? Probably not. Therefore, the lack of therapeutic progress is in large part due to the lack of a better understanding of the pathophysiological basis and complex nature of AD. This needs to be addressed by basic science not drug development. Only progress on the root causes of AD can lead to a unified theory that in turn can be proven or falsified by further research, both at the preclinical and clinical level.

7.3 HAS THERE BEEN A TOO SIMPLISTIC VIEW OF THE PATHOPHYSIOLOGY OF THE DISEASE AND THE TEMPORAL NATURE OF THE PATHOLOGICAL PROCESSES?

Problems with cognitive impairment, especially executive function, are often signs that patients first notice. These clinical symptoms occur when the pathology has already been present for a decade or longer. Amyloid deposits are accompanied by other changes, for example neurofribrillary tangles, marked synaptic loss, oxidative stress, elevation of cytokines, or mitochondrial dysfunction (Figure 7.1).

AD is a complex disorder that has long been reduced to a one-focus pathology. For the majority of long-term disorders, scientists/researchers/clinicians look at all the processes involved and treat with symptopmatic and protective/prophylactic therapies, e.g., diabetes, asthma. In AD research, the focus has been largely on impaired cognition, which likely is the end result of multiple upstream processes involving, for example,

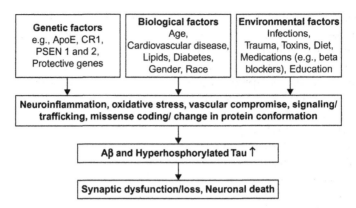

FIGURE 7.1   Potential mechanisms of AD pathology. *Adapted from [10] and [11].*

genetic factors, oxidative stress, neuroinflammation, and vascular compromise that in turn result in increased amyloid and tau (see Figure 7.1 [11,12]). It has been hypothesized that one of the main culprits could be cerebrovascular compromise that increases oxidative stress which in turn stimulates neuroinflammation, ultimately leading to a pathway of disease development with plaque and tangle formation in sporadic AD.

Epidemiological evidence suggesting the potential benefit of non-steroidal anti-inflammatory drugs (NSAIDs), oestrogen, statins, and vitamin E in AD has proved disappointing in randomized clinical trials [13] but supports the multi-factorial nature of sproadic AD and the need for diverse interventions and deeper considerations of patient comorbidities and concomitant medications when evaluating response/non-response in clinical trials.

Another source of the perceived failure may be due to direct translation of results from animal models that reflect familial AD whilst the majority of patients in clinical trials have sporadic late-onset AD (LOAD) and one or more physical co-morbidites (see biological factors in Figure 7.1). These other pathogenetic factors that we cannot adequately model are likely to be highly relevant but are often neglected in trial data analyses, or trials are too small or too short to allow for meaningful analyses. Large post-mortem series have repeatedly shown that a significant proportion (>50%) of subjects diagnosed clinically as AD actually had mixed dementia [14]. Likewise, there is still little established insight into the more granular pathogenesis of post-stroke dementia and possible relations to AD. Future preclinical research should aim to combine genetically defined targets with aging (e.g., wt APP in old mice) and include cerebrovascular factors (spontaneously hypertensive rats, diabetic rats, rats with other vascular lesions).

7.4 HOW HAVE ISSUES IN THE USE OF PRECLINICAL MODELS AND THEIR TRANSLATION ADDED TO THIS SITUATION?

There are no animal models of AD that meet all human disease criteria—so there is no actual model of AD. None reflects the structural, connective, functional, and immune system complexities of the human brain; neither can they reflect the time differences that are months in animals versus the decades for human disease to develop. All available animal models aim only to mimic certain aspects of human disease.

There are models of brain aging, brain amyloidosis, tau abnormalities (mutated tau and kinases, tau over-expression), cellular models of tau trans-synaptic and -neuronal transfection, and some combinations of the above. There are no models of altered mitochondrial function, immune response or microglial function, all of which appear to play a tangible role in AD pathophysiology.

So while models have been useful for, for example, understanding a compound's mode of action, target engagement, and initial dose selection, why is it that out of the treatment principles tested successfully in animal models only the first two in Table 7.1 have resulted in licensed medications?

Animal models of brain aging and AD are often based on defined mechanisms of action, for example the cholinergic deficit in human AD post-mortem tissue or the excitotoxicity theory. These models are based on well-known receptor systems, and pharmacological tools have been

TABLE 7.1 Treatment Principles Promoted Based on Animal Models

Successful NDAs/MAAs	Unsuccessful NDAs/MAAs or Never Filed	Still in Development or Never/Not Yet Applied
Acetyl cholinesterase inhibition (donepezil, galantamine, rivastigmine, tacrine) Uncompetitive NMDA antagonism (memantine)	Aβ aggregation inhibition (tramiprosate) Active immunization* Passive immunization (Monoclonal antibodies) β secretase inhibition* γ secretase inhibition* Gingko biloba GSK 3β inhibitors Muscarinic, Nicotinic agonists NSAIDs Statins Vit E, Coenzyme Q	Active/passive immunization (FAD) β secretaseinhibiton γ secretaseinhibiton and modulation Tau aggregation inhibition Iron chelation Nicotinic agonism 5HT$_6$ antagonism

Failed disease modification/slowing of disease progression strategy
FDA: New drug application (NDA); EMA: Marketing authorization application (MAA).

available to validate the mode of action of the research drugs at hand. Memantine has so far been the only drug with a clear effect at the NMDA receptor and a clinical benefit in human disease. Other uncompetitive NMDA antagonists with a similar receptor profile have failed to replicate memantine's success in the clinic [15,16]. The reasons for this failure remain unclear, as is the relevance of the excitotoxicity hypothesis to human AD. Hence, clear relationships between receptor level lesions and the core symptom cognition were always preferred, for example, in the human sco-polamine model of impaired cognition. Obviously, the complex cognitive impairment seen in human AD is only partially mimicked by scopolamine and AD-specific pathology was not important in selecting cholinergic drugs. In this early instance, the phenotypic screening for the core impairment cognition worked, but it has so far failed for all the other approaches.

The "time factor" may further play an important role in the predictability of animal models. Mice allow for a treatment period of about 16 months; this corresponds to 75% of the lifespan of a wild type mouse. In contrast, the human illness duration is 10–20 years, and in addition, clinical trials usually range from 6 to 18 months, which is a fraction of the human lifespan. Clinico-pathological correlation studies have established that there is a continuum between "normal" aging and AD dementia. Build-up of amyloid plaques occurs primarily before the onset of cognitive deficits, whilst neurofibrillary tangles, and neuron and synaptic loss, parallel the progression of cognitive decline [17]. These neuropathological data have been largely confirmed using longitudinal *in vivo* neuroimaging biomarkers such as amyloid positron emission tomography (PET) and volumetric magnetic resonance imaging [17]. This is a much more complicated picture than that portrayed in the often quoted article by Jack et al. [18]. As summarized in the paper by Kuller and Lopez [19], there are three major hypotheses relating to dementia: amyloid deposition and secondary synaptic loss, vascular injury, and aging.

The importance of, and the potential interaction between these hypotheses is not currently addressed in preclinical research. Other aspects of preclinical research that should be addressed include:

- Gender differences are known in most APP tg mice but their impact on expression of APP and production of Aβ, brain pathology, and behavior remain insufficiently addressed.
- Many transgenic animal models lack precise characterization (e.g., sub-strains with different features).
- The variability of behavioral results is often unknown and power analyses are not used for statistically significant and reproducible "treatment" effects.
- The induction of handling effects on behavioral and learning outcomes is poorly understood and adequate controls not commonly used.

- Too much emphasis is put on study of mode of action and downstream impact on metabolism; too little attention is paid to the investigation of effects on cognition in various models, particularly in the longer term.
- In animal modeling, the same quality principles should be adhered to as in good clinical research, for example data should be scrutinized regarding relevance for human disease, cross-model comparisons, replication in at least one additional model, and relevant safety findings [20]. In a quality survey study of methodology employed in tg mouse models of AD and other neurological conditions, Egan et al. [21] reported randomization in 15%, a blinded outcome assessment in 21%, and a prospective sample size and power calculation in 0%.
- There is a propensity to ignore (and not report) negative data and to embrace positive data without careful replication.

Other factors that potentially contribute to the failure of translation from preclinical to clinical research are:

- Lack of knowledge about the exact toxic species of Aβ and therefore lack of a common functional outcome measure in animal research.
- Blood–brain-barrier pharmacokinetics and pharmacodynamics (in both animals and/or humans) do not support availability of the molecule for treatment of central nervous system (CNS) disorders (e.g., tarenflurbil, pGP substrates).
- Insufficient target engagement at the achieved brain concentrations.
- The pharmacodynamics of the molecule are such that animal tests may show short-term effects but long-term benefits will be lacking and/ or detrimental effects will be produced (e.g. segamacestat vs. gamma secretase modulators (GSMs)).

For example, tarenflurbil achieves only low brain levels after nine days of treatment in young Tg2576 mice [22]. Furthermore, short-term treatment with tarenflurbil did not reduce brain Aβ 1–42 and 1–40 levels [23]. Therefore, the preclinical data for tarenflurbil hardly justified the move into clinical trials, at least from an amyloid hypothesis perspective.

In the case of γ secretase inhibitors, whilst acute dosing with both segamacestat and BMS-708163 improved memory deficits in APP tg and non-tg mice, the effects disappeared after eight days of sub-chronic dosing. The authors [24] suspect that synaptic accumulation of beta-C-terminal fragments in the hippocampus caused this loss of benefit. They go on to show that second generation GSMs ameliorate memory deficits in tg mice and wild type, both acutely and sub-chronically. Should the different functional consequences of gamma secretase inhibition (GSI) versus modulation (GSM) have been predicted?

Although animal models certainly cannot reliably predict (serious) adverse effects, researchers need to be alert to preliminary evidence of potential side effects in their work. The brain-specific adverse event vasogenic edema, now summarized under the term "Amyloid Related Imaging Abnormalities with Parenchymal Edema (ARIA-E)," was predicted from the tg mouse model [25]. This is thought to be due to the accumulation of monoclonal antibody antigen complexes in the brain vasculature. However, such effects when they do occur require serious investigations and consideration. Should the increased risk of skin cancer with segamacestat have been anticipated because of potential "off target" effects at Notch [26]?

7.5 HAVE THE METHODS USED IN CLINICAL DRUG DEVELOPMENT AND THE REFINEMENT OF ITS TOOLS CONTRIBUTED TO THE LACK OF SUCCESS?

Why do we still employ trial designs from the early nineties (placebo-controlled, double-blind, parallel group) instead of advancing the field by innovative trial designs that were proposed over a decade ago [27]? Instead, discussion has focused on "secular change" supposedly causing loss of placebo decline, which was shown not to be the case [28]. Pharmaceutical companies have also shown a "herd mentality," i.e., a reluctance to change their approach despite the increasing number of failed trials.

A recent review by Cummings et al. [29] outlines alternative trial designs and their merits. For example, Bayesian adaptive clinical trials could be particularly useful in Phase II as they allow the use of data collected in the trial to modify doses, sample size, trial duration, and entry criteria in an ongoing way. Futility designs permit the use of historical controls and may shorten the duration of trials of potential disease-modifying or -slowing agents. In complex disorders combination therapy is the rule rather than the exception; trial designs need to allow for investigation of potential additive or synergistic treatment effects.

Despite the availability of a wide range of scales to assess cognition, functional ability quality of life, behavioral and psychological symptoms, caregiver costs and reducing costs of illness, many of these measures have significant shortcomings [30]. Aspects of cognition that are infrequently addressed by current scales include misidentification, learning aptitude, decision making, self-determination, and disturbed/slowed response to external stimuli. Equally, issues with communication and social interaction such as responsiveness, correct use and interpretation of gestures, implementation of commands, cooperation in care and daily living, social involvement, adaptability, relationships with family and friends, and intimacy of contacts (informal/formal) are also rarely addressed. The majority of instruments have significant limitations with respect to sensitivity to stages of disease and changes over time. Ideally one would like to have a new instrument that can assess multiple domains at all stages of AD whilst remaining sensitive to changes and therapy effects. Scales such as the Clinical Dementia Rating Sum of Boxes (CDR-SB) that combine cognitive and functional assessments and have sensitivity across stages of disease are a step in this direction [31]. However, there is still a need for a new multi-domain and easy-to-administer AD scale for the assessment of disease progression and response to therapy.

With the increasing trend for multinational clinical trials has come the need for more attention to consistency across sites for all aspects of the trial. This includes patient recruitment and assessment, interpretation of outcomes that have been translated into different languages, standardization of assessment techniques (psychometric scales as well as electrocardiograms, laboratory tests, neuroimaging), and interpretation of tests. Many companies now specialize in rater training and translation of scales but no one body ensures that training, application, and data analysis are consistent with one another.

The availability of new tools also influences the research focus. With the recent approval of the amyloid imaging agent, florbetapir, for research purposes, there has been renewed emphasis on the amyloid hypothesis. If we are to make progress, researchers need to be mindful of the complexity of AD and the need for equivalent investment and development of assessment tools and biomarkers for other aspects of the disease.

In this era of personalized medicine there is a move towards individualized therapies. This approach is inconsistent with the current considerations in Phase III clinical trials where generalization to as wider population as possible is the aim. Most clinical programs aim to study one potential aspect of the pathophysiology, but it is clear that AD as defined and captured by our current diagnostic systems is not a uniform disease and rather consists of mixed neuropathologies.

7.6 HAVE RESEARCHERS FAILED TO CONSIDER THE IMPACT OF IMPORTANT DEMOGRAPHIC CHARACTERISTICS ON THE COURSE OF ILLNESS AND RESPONSE TO INTERVENTIONS?

There is a growing body of data from clinical trials, epidemiological studies, and studies in clinical practice that demonstrate that a range of patient factors (comorbid conditions, concomitant medications) can impact on cognitive decline and its rate of progression. Evidence from pharmaceutical research suggests that most of these factors are not considered in recruitment to clinical trials, prospective stratification, or in analyses of the efficacy and risk–benefit.

Physiological impairment of renal function is a function of age and is common in the elderly. There is a growing body of evidence showing that even mild renal impairment is associated with increased risk of cardiovascular and cerebrovascular events with a more rapid rate of cognitive decline in the elderly [32], a factor that is rarely accounted for in clinical trial analyses.

Using a modification of the Cardiovascular Health Study Criteria to define frailty that includes weight loss, exhaustion, weakness, slowness, and low physical activity, the Italian Study of Aging showed that frailty is a short-term predictor of overall dementia and vascular dementia [33]. Another aspect to consider is the growing body of data linking vascular risk factors (diabetes, hypertension, raised cholesterol, smoking) with increased susceptibility for AD and other factors (angina, atrial fibrillation, hypertension) with increased rate of decline [34]. Clinico-pathological data also show that people with both vascular disease and AD pathology show either more severe cognitive impairment during life than those with pure AD. The relationship between vascular risk factors is not fully understood. It is thought that vascular and neurodegenerative mechanisms develop in parallel and that vascular disease acts synergistically with AD pathology. The degree to which vascular factors contribute to dementia will vary from individual to individual, giving the likely scenario of a continuum from relatively pure AD through mixed dementia to vascular dementia. The inter-relationship between vascular factors, dementia sub-type, and progress of cognitive decline has important implications for clinical trials, especially for patient recruitment and assessment of efficacy. To date most trial sponsors have not paid much attention to these aspects that are likely to have contributed to the reasons for failure.

When looking at the standard primary outcome variable in AD clinical trials, the Alzheimer's Disease Assessment Scale-cognitive portion (ADAS-Cog), it is interesting to note the factors that can influence rate of change or progression [35]. Covariate analyses indicate that baseline Mini-Mental State Examination (MMSE) score, education, age, and apolipoprotein3/4 genotype had a significant effect on the level and shape of the trajectories of the mean model predicted ADAS-Cog change from baseline. It has been appreciated previously that cognitive decline is not linear. What has been less appreciated is that analysis in different patient sub-populations is warranted to confirm and generalize the findings of the present analysis to consider the indirect response model as a reference model for characterizing the time course of AD.

It is now generally recognized that there is considerable overlap between the risk factors for AD and vascular dementia (VaD). Indeed AD, VaD, and mixed dementias are generally regarded as discreet diagnostic entities. However, the risk factors such as cardiovascular and cerebrovascular disease, and metabolic disorders (diabetes, obesity), are features of all these dementias. It would seem more relevant to focus on determining the mechanisms by which vascular and neurodegenerative mechanisms jointly contribute to the development and progression of aging-related cognitive disorders rather than considering them as separate diseases. In these respects the degree of control of physical co-morbidities (hypertension, diabetes mellitus) and the impact of long-term treatments by medications to treat these disorders needs more detailed consideration in the selection of study participants and in the sub-group analyses of response to interventions.

7.7 HAVE RESEARCHERS FAILED TO LEARN FROM PREVIOUS MISTAKES IN EARLIER AD DRUG DEVELOPMENT PROGRAMS?

An important aspect of learning from previous experience is to consider both the positive and the negative aspects. However, in research there is the longstanding issue of failure to disclose negative trial results. In preclinical research, Li et al. [36] report on a data mining effort covering the years 2001 to 2011 in which they identified more than 146 substances and treatment modalities tested in 11 transgenic mouse models including APP, tau, double- and triple-cross transgenic mice. Far from all of the results have been published. Irrespective of that fact, while research compounds test positive in such models, there is a widespread perception that animal models appear to have little if any predictive value, because drugs continue to fail in clinical trials.

The history of the vaccination therapy approach in AD is a clear example of where detailed evaluation of the reasons for failure of translation is warranted. Total $A\beta$ deposition as shown by immunohistochemistry was markedly reduced in tg mice after eight weeks of systemic anti-$A\beta$ antibody administration [37]. The same principle was evidenced in humans not only by the initial active vaccination trial with AN1792 in postmortem data from patients that died due to encephalitis [38], but later also using 11C-PIB PET *in vivo* after 78 weeks of bapineuzumab treatment. So the mechanistic basis for the elimination of $A\beta$ deposits appeared confirmed. Moreover, Morgan et al. [39] showed that tg mice benefited significantly from $A\beta_{1-42}$ immunization at the age of 7.5 months when tested later in the radial water maze at the age of 15.5 months, suggesting that also the functional proof of concept was established before the start of late-phase clinical trials.

As known today, cognitive improvement was neither shown in the follow-up of AN1792 survivors nor in the bapineuzumab Phase III trials.

In the two solanezumab Phase III trials (Expedition 1 and 2) for mild to moderate AD patients, benefit on the primary endpoints (cognition and function) did not differ significantly from placebo. However, in a pre-specified secondary analysis, slowing of cognitive decline was shown in patients with mild AD and a number of biomarkers showed an effect of solanezumab. The results of trials with monoclonal antibodies deserve more detailed scrutiny to determine the potential implications for further evaluation in early AD.

There is also evidence of a continued reluctance to look critically at data from early-phase clinical trials, with the result that programs are progressed to later-phase development with inadequate evidence of efficacy and/or safety, and then fail. Such late-stage failures make a major contribution to the high cost of drug development [40]. In 2011, these concerns prompted the Alzheimer's Association to convene a Roundtable discussion involving scientists from academia, industry, and government regulatory agencies to review the lessons learnt and discuss strategies for improving Go–No go decision making about the probability of Phase II trial results predicting success in Phase III [41].

In summary, the following lessons are learnt:

- Phase II trials should explore the dose/exposure–response relationships and show proof of mechanism (i.e., that the target has been engaged in the CNS).
- The target must be active and relevant with respect to therapeutic manipulation in the phase of the disease being studied.
- Biomarker selection and outcomes should be consistent with expected actions of drugs, or pathways related to the target.
- Pharmacokinetics and pharmacodynamic modeling should be used to optimize dose and dosing regimen selection.
- Phase II trials would demonstrate that clinical endpoints are affected, although the difficulties in assessing clinical effects in small Phase II trials with short durations are acknowledged.
- In planning for studies of earlier-stage disease, the goal remains to demonstrate efficacy that is clinically beneficial.
- Data from failed proof-of-concept trials should be rapidly fed back to the drug discovery process to improve the understanding of mechanisms.
- Data from all clinical sub-groups, post hoc, or other types of secondary analyses are important, but they are also potentially misleading when not subsequently tested prospectively.

The focus has been on development programs that target the largest possible market with the broadest labeling when smaller, more focused target labels were likely to be more successful; for example, there was more success in Parkinson's disease dementia and Lewy body dementia with cholinesterase inhibitors. A recent article by Boxer et al. [42] suggested that Frontotemporal dementia (FTD) should be considered an attractive target for developing therapies for the following reasons:

- The clinical and molecular features of FTD, including rapid disease progression and relatively pure molecular pathology.
- Consensus diagnostic criteria will facilitate the identification of patients.
- A variety of neuropsychological, functional, and behavioral scales have been shown to be sensitive to disease progression.
- Quantitative neuroimaging measurements demonstrate progressive brain atrophy in FTD at rates that may surpass AD.
- The similarities between FTD and other neurodegenerative diseases suggest that FTD researchers will be able to draw on this experience to create a road map for FTD drug development.

7.8 HAS REGULATORY GUIDANCE OR LACK THEREOF CONTRIBUTED TO THE SITUATION?

While the Food and Drug Administration (FDA) issued a first AD Guidance in 1990 [43], its status has not been elevated from "draft" since then. The first European Medicines Agency guidelines on dementia were issued in 2005 and revised in 2008 [44] to include, for the first time, important advice for clinical researchers on how to translate drugs with a disease-modifying potential into feasible trial designs—of note, introducing of a two-staged approach where "delay of disability" could represent an earlier, and "disease modification" a later, labeling target. In 2013, and in keeping with the broader understanding of AD as a continuum spanning decades until initial clinical symptoms become apparent, the FDA issued a new draft guideline for early or prodromal AD [45], overcoming some of the trial design limitations of the past. Given the proportion of required investments into late-stage clinical development in AD, these later regulatory guidances are very welcome as, due to the many prior failures, "Big Pharma" as well as venture capital is asking for more "investment security." For all the reasons listed above, it appears highly debatable whether regulatory history has had any tangible influence on progressing the current situation.

7.9 SUMMARY AND CONCLUSIONS

In light of the demographic "AD tsunami" ahead of all developed societies, the medical need for effective symptomatic and disease-modifying drugs could not be higher. After two decades of chief focus on the amyloid hypothesis, and the large failures of amyloid-based Phase III programs, there is clearly a momentum for broadening the horizon to refine the amyloid approach and to include a wider range of modes of action, alone and in combination, particularly tau, neuroinflammation, oxidative, and metabolic stress.

There is an increased interest in tau immunotherapy as it was shown to reduce tau pathology, facilitate p-tau clearance, improve cognition in animal models, and potentially delay progression [46], and might serve an integrated approach at combined Aβ and tau toxicity mediated via NMDA receptor excitotoxicity [47].

Scientists are taking a wider view of dementia and demonstrating a greater appreciation of the impact of the similarities and differences both within and between dementias. Different factors influence the age of onset and rate of progress of familial and sporadic AD. The increased appreciation of AD as a syndromal diagnosis rather than a single distinct entity will support the identification of targeted therapies, e.g., against familial AD.

Meanwhile, available opportunities for designing prevention trials that target modification of risk factors for dementia, such as aggressively treating raised blood pressure and poorly controlled diabetes, should receive greater consideration. Such trials are not without their own set of challenges, i.e., which patients, which intervention(s), what duration of follow-up, etc. Even then life is not simple, as illustrated by the effect of age on the risk of dementia associated with raised blood pressure; this risk *decreases* with increasing age. Therefore, if one was designing a trial looking at the impact of improved blood pressure control on dementia risk, one would want to enroll younger patients (say, 65 to 75 years) rather than older patients.

Over and above patient heterogeneity, another factors that has undermined the potential success of clinical trials for AD is the lack of standardized methodologies. The Alzheimer's Disease Neuroimaging Initiative (ADNI) is an excellent example of how collaboration among researchers and scientists in academia and the pharmaceutical industry can result in major advances in the understanding of AD [48]. The group has not only developed standardized methodologies for assessments (clinical tests, cerebrospinal fluid analysis, neuroimaging) but has also improved diagnostic categorization, advanced the understanding of biomarkers and genetics, and determined how the rate of change of outcomes differs between controls and patients with AD. Importantly, the group also developed a platform for data and information sharing that will hopefully stimulate more research and help clarify competing hypotheses and answer as yet unresolved questions about AD.

Biomarker development and validation will be ever-more important in a number of potential ways, for example to define susceptible populations, to confirm interaction with the selected target, to determine response/non-response, and to determine liability to safety issues. In their paper about the development of biomarkers to chart all AD stages, Hampel et al. [49] describe the need for biomarkers that could address the sources of "systems failure" during the entire course of AD as a prerequisite to:

- Improving and accelerating drug development;
- Facilitating the identification of biochemical effects of a drug in short-term pilot studies;
- Selecting, enriching, and stratifying specific patient and target populations;
- Assessing the effects of treatment on disease progression and outcome.

Such markers should enable better selection of drug candidates, better verification of the mechanism of action, clearer definition of dose effects, shortening of trial durations, reduction in sample sizes and costs, and improvement in recruitment and retention of study participants.

None of the known AD susceptibility variants were shown to be significantly associated with the rate of cognitive decline except for ApoE and CR1; last but not least, gene expression studies in conjunction with neuropathology and cognitive endophenotypes might become a more useful approach than genome-wide analyses to discover novel AD susceptibility genes and pathways [12].

Looking to the future, we cannot afford to falter. Through a broader, more integrated vision of dementia [50], remembering the appropriate use of animal models, consideration of wider demographic variables (co-morbid illnesses and genetic influences), critical evaluation of preclinical and clinical methodology and data, as well as learning from other therapeutic areas, and a greater collaborative effort (e.g., ADNI and the Coalition against Major Diseases), there is hope for greater success.

References

[1] Hardy J, Allsop D. Amyloid deposition as the central event in the aetiology of Alzheimer's disease. Trends Pharmacol Sci Oct 1991;12(10):383–8.
[2] Braak H, Braak E, Bohl J. Staging of Alzheimer cortical destruction. Eur Neurol 1993;33(6):403–8.
[3] Games D, Adams D, Alessandrini R, Barbour R, Berthelette P, Blackwell C, et al. Alzheimer-type neuropathology in transgenic mice overexpressing V717Fβ-amyloid precursor protein. Nature 1995;373:523–7.
[4] Giannakopoulos P, Herrmann FR, Bussiere T. Tangle and neuron numbers, but not amyloid load, predict cognitive status in Alzheimer's disease. Neurology 2003;60:1495–500.
[5] Attems J, Thomas A, Jellinger K. Correlations between cortical and subcortical tau pathology. Neuropathol Appl Neurobiol 2012;38:582–90.

[6] Götz J, Chen F, van Dorpe J, Nitsch RM. Formation of neuro-fibrillary tangles in P3011 tau transgenic mice induced by Abeta 42 fibrils. Science 2001;293:1491–5.

[7] Lewis J, Dickson DW, Lin WL, Chisholm L, Corral A, Jones G, et al. Enhanced neurofibrillary degeneration in transgenic mice expressing mutant tau and APP. Science 2001;293:1487–91.

[8] Ittner LM, Ke YD, Delerue F, Bi M, Gladbach A, Van Eersel J, et al. Dendritic function of tau mediates Amyloid-b Toxicity in Alzheimer's disease mouse models. Cell 2010;142:387–97.

[9] Li L, Sengupta A, Haque N, Grundke-Iqbal I, Iqbal K. Memantine inhibits and reverses the Alzheimer's type abnormal hyperphosphorylation of tau and associated neurodegeneration. FEBS Lett 2004;566(1–3):261–9.

[10] Bondareff W, Harrington CR, Wischik CM, Hauser DL, Roth M. Absence of abnormal hyperphosphorylation of tau in intracellular tangles in Alzheimer's disease. J Neuropathol Exp Neurol 1995;54(5):657–63.

[11] Brian B, McNaull A, Todd S, McGuinness B, Passmore AP. Inflammation and anti-inflammatory strategies for Alzheimer's Disease—A mini-review. Gerontology 2010; 56:3–14.

[12] Nilüfer ET, DeJager PL, Lei Y, Bennett DA. Alternative approaches in gene discovery and characterization in Alzheimer's disease. Curr Genet Med Rep 2013;1:39–51.

[13] Kawas CH. Medications and diet protective factors for AD. Alzheimer Dis Assoc Disord 2006;20(3 Suppl 2):S89–96.

[14] Jellinger KA, Attems J. Incidence of cerebrovascular lesions in Alzheimer's disease: a post mortem study. Acta Neuropathol 2003;105:14–17.

[15] Reisberg B, Doody R, Stöffler A, Schmitt F, Ferris S, Möbius HJ. Memantine in moderate-to-severe Alzheimer's Disease. N Engl J Med 2003;348:1333–41.

[16] Rammes G, Schierloh A. Neramexane. IDrugs 2006;9(2):128–35. PMID 16523403.

[17] Serrano-Pozo A, Frosch MP, Masliah E, Hyman BT. Neuropathological Alterations in Alzheimer's Disease. Cold Spring Harb Perspect Med 2011;1:a006189.

[18] Jack Jr CR, Knopman DS, Jagust WJ, Shaw LM, Aisen PS, Weiner MW, et al. Hypothetical model of dynamic biomarkers of the Alzheimer's pathological cascade. Lancet Neurol 2010;9(1):119–28. doi:10.1016/S1474-4422(09)70299-6.

[19] Kuller LH, Lopez OL. Dementia and Alzheimer's disease: a new direction. The 2010 Jay L. Foster memorial lecture. Alzheimers Dement 2011;7(5):540–50.

[20] Windisch M. (2013) Advanced Training Course For Drug Development In Neurodegenerative Disorders: Can We Increase The Success? In: AD/PD Conference; 8 March, Florence, Italy.

[21] Egan K.J, Sena E.S, Vesterinen H.M, McLeod M.R. (2011) AD/PD Conference. Barcelona, Spain.

[22] Imbimbo BP, Del Giudice E, Cenacchi V, Volta R, Villetti G, Facchinetti F, et al. In vitro and in vivo profiling of CHF5022 and CHF5074: Two beta-amyloid1–42 lowering agents. Pharmacol Res 2007;55(4):318–28. Epub 2007 Jan 16.

[23] Lanz TA, Fici GJ, Merchant KM. Lack of specific amyloid-β(1–42) suppression by non-steroidal anti-inflammatory drugs in young, plaque-free Tg2576 mice and in guinea pig neuronal cultures. J Pharmacol Exp Ther 2005;312:399–406.

[24] Mitani Y, Yarimizu J, Saita K, Uchino H, Akashiba H, Shitaka Y, et al. Differential Effects between γ-Secretase Inhibitors and Modulators on Cognitive Function in Amyloid Precursor Protein-Transgenic and Non-Transgenic Mice. J Neurosci 2012;32(6):2037–50.

[25] Goodman J, Freeman G, Angus W, Brown T, Cheng-te Chou P. Spontaneous amyloid-related imaging abnormalities of the microhemorrage and effusive/edematous types in aged APP+ presenilin 1 mice. Alzheimers Dement 2012;8:11–12. doi:10.1016/j.jalz.2012.05.035.

[26] Panelos J, Massi D. Emerging role of Notch signaling in epidermal differentiation and skin cancer. Cancer Biol Ther 2009;8(21):1986–93.

III. CHALLENGES AND OPPORTUNITIES TO CONDUCT GLOBAL AD TRIALS

[27] Leber P. Slowing the progression of Alzheimer's disease: methodologic issues. Alzheimer Dis Assoc Disord 1997;11:S10–21.

[28] Schneider LS, Sano M. Current Alzheimer's disease trials: methods and placebo outcomes. Alzheimers Dement 2009;5(5):388–97. doi:10.1016/j.jalz.2009.07.038.

[29] Cummings J, Gould H, Zhong K. Advances in designs for Alzheimer's disease clinical trials. Am J Neurodegener Dis 2012;1(3):205–16.

[30] Robert P, Ferris S, Gauthier S, Ihl R, Winblad B, Tennigkeit F. Review of Alzheimer's disease scales: Is there a need for a new multi-domain scale for therapy evaluation in medical practice? Alzheimer's Research & Therapy 2010;2(24):1–13.

[31] Cedarbaum JM, Jaros M, Hernandez C, Coley N, Andrieu S, Grundmann M, et al. Rationale for use of the clinical dementia rating sum of boxes as a primary outcome measure for Alzheimer's disease clinical trials. Alzheimers Dement 2012;9(1):45–55.

[32] Buchman AS, Tanne D, Boyle PA, Shah RC, Leurgans SE, Bennett DA. Kidney function is associated with the rate of cognitive decline in the elderly. Neurology 2009;73:920–7.

[33] Solfrizzi V, Scafato E, Frisardi V, Seripa D, Logroscino G, Maggi S, et al. Frailty syndrome and the risk of vascular dementia: The Italian Longitudinal Study on Aging. Alzheimers Dement 2013;9:113–22.

[34] Viswanathan A, Rocca WA, Tzourio C. Vascular risk factors and dementia: How to move forward. Neurology 2009;72:368–74.

[35] Gomeni R, Simeonib M, Zvartau-Hind M, Irizarry MC, Austin D, Gold M. Modeling Alzheimer's disease progression using the disease system analysis approach. Alzheimers Dement 2012;8:39–50.

[36] Li C, Ebrahimi A, Schluesener H. Drug pipeline in neurodegeneration based on transgenic mice models of Alzheimer's disease. Ageing Res Rev 2013;12(1):116–40.

[37] Wilcock DM, Rojiani A, Rosenthal A, Levkowitz G, Subbarao S, Alamed J, et al. Passive amyloid immunotherapy clears amyloid and transiently activates microglia in a transgenic mouse model of amyloid deposition. J Neurosci 2004;24:6144–51.

[38] Holmes C, Boche D, Wilkinson D, Yadegarfar G, Hopkins V, Bayer A, et al. Long-term effects of Abeta42 immunisation in Alzheimer's disease: follow-up of a randomised, placebo-controlled phase I trial. Lancet 2008;372(9634):216–23.

[39] Morgan D, Diamond DM, Gottschall PE, Ugen KE, Dickey C, Hardy J. A beta peptide vaccination prevents memory loss in an animal model of Alzheimer's disease. Nature 2000;408:982–5.

[40] Schachter A,D, Ramoni M,F. Clinical forecasting in drug development. Nat Rev Drug Discov 2007;6:107–8.

[41] Greenberg BD, Carrillo MC, Ryan JM, Gold M, Gallagher K, Grundman M, et al. Improving Alzheimer's disease phase II clinical trials. Alzheimers Dement 2013;9:39–49.

[42] Boxer AL, Gold M, Huey E, Hud W, Rosen H, Kramer J, et al. The advantages of frontotemporal degeneration drug development (part 2 of frontotemporal degeneration: The next therapeutic frontier. Alzheimers Dement 2013;9:189–98.

[43] Leber P. Guidelines for the Clinical Evaluation of Antidementia Drugs. United States Food and Drug Administration, Washington, DC; 1990. [First draft].

[44] European Medicines Agency. Guideline on Medicinal Products for the Treatment of Alzheimer's Disease and Other Dementias (2008). CPMP/EWP/553/95 Rev. 1 Jul.

[45] Administration Center for Drug Evaluation and Research. Guidance for Industry for Alzheimer's Disease: Developing Drugs for the Treatment of Early Stage Disease. US Department of Health and Human Services Food and Drug Administration Center for Drug Evaluation and Research (CDER). 2013, February.

[46] Iqbal K, Alonso Adel C, Chen S, Chohan MO, El-Akkad E, Gong CX, et al. Tau pathology in Alzheimer's disease and other tauopathies. Biochim Biophys Acta 2005;1739(2–3):198–210.

[47] Ittner LM, Ke YD, Delerue F, Bi M, Gladbach A, van Eersel J, et al. SourceDendritic function of tau mediates amyloid-beta toxicity in Alzheimer's disease mouse models. Cell 2010;142(3):387–97. doi:10.1016/j.cell.2010.06.036. Epub 2010 Jul 22.

III. CHALLENGES AND OPPORTUNITIES TO CONDUCT GLOBAL AD TRIALS

[48] Weiner M, Veitch DP, Aisen PS, Beckett LA, Cairns NJ, Green RC, et al. The Alzheimer's Disease neuroimaging initiative: a review of papers published since its inception. Alzheimers Dement 2012;8:S1–68.
[49] Hampel H, Lista S, Khachaturian ZS. Development of biomarkers to chart all Alzheimer's disease stages: The royal road to cutting the therapeutic Gordian Knot. Alzheimers Dement 2012;8:312–36.
[50] Korczyn AD. Why have we failed to cure Alzheimer's Disease? J Alzheimers Dis 2011;29:275–82.

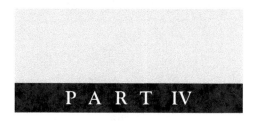

PART IV

GLOBAL REGULATORY ENVIRONMENT SURROUNDING ALZHEIMER'S DISEASE TRIALS

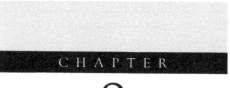

CHAPTER

8

The Regulatory Environment Surrounding Alzheimer's Disease Research: FDA and EMA Guidance

Muriel O' Byrne[1] and Menghis Bairu[2]

[1]Global Regulatory Affairs, Elan Pharma International Ltd, Treasury Building, Lower Grand Canal Street, Dublin 2, Ireland, [2]Elan Pharmaceuticals, Cambridge, Massachusetts, USA, and Speranza Therapeutics Corp, Dublin, Ireland

8.1 INTRODUCTION

The regulatory environment surrounding Alzheimer's disease (AD) research is set against a backdrop of disappointing clinical outcomes and late stage failures that have seen little meaningful progress in the treatment options available to patients for several years. Such is the challenge from a scientific and financial perspective that companies are becoming reluctant to view AD research as a viable target. Despite this, the unmet need remains significant. In the USA alone deaths from AD increased 68% between 2000 and 2010, while deaths from other major diseases, including the number one cause of death (heart disease), decreased [1]. Both the European Medicines Agency (EMA) and the US Food and Drug Administration (FDA) have historically provided guidance to sponsors of AD clinical research to direct their efforts in developing interventions against this disease, either by issuing specific guidelines or through regulatory approvals establishing the precedent of data requirements. With the shift in research from symptomatic interventions to now looking at the ability of newer treatments to modify the course of the disease, earlier preclinical stages of the disease are

M. Bairu & M.W. Weiner (Eds):
Global Clinical Trials for Alzheimer's Disease.
DOI: http://dx.doi.org/10.1016/B978-0-12-411464-7.00008-0

119

coming into play and the regulatory environment is again evolving to align with the clinical direction.

8.2 CURRENT EUROPEAN GUIDELINES

In the European Union (EU), all medicines for the treatment of diseases causing degeneration of the brain and nervous system, including dementia, are considered as "Mandatory Scope" [2], and so must be authorized for marketing centrally at a European level, rather than in each Member State separately.

In 2005, the EMA Efficacy Working Party recognized the need for a revision to the existing guideline to assist sponsors in the development of medicinal products to treat AD [3]. These updates included extending the guidance to cover other dementia types but also to address clinical endpoints, study duration, and the use of biomarkers. Following a period of consultation the new guideline came into effect in early 2009 [4]. This guideline delineated the varying requirements depending on the primary objective of the study, be it symptomatic treatment, disease-modifying treatment, or a primary prevention study. What was clear from the guidance was the continuing requirement for co-primary endpoints in studies of overt AD where symptomatic improvement of symptoms is the goal. Given the current use of symptomatic treatments as standard of care in many geographies, the provision of active comparator data was highlighted as a requirement in the EU to facilitate the benefit–risk assessment of new interventions.

Disease modification has become the focus of more recent clinical programs and the Committee for Medicinal Products for Human Use (CHMP) guidance addressed this through a requirement for evidence of improved clinical outcomes coupled with evidence of an effect on the underlying pathophysiology of the disease. This evidence, which would need to be compelling in order for the agency to consider such a claim, would be derived from a biomarker program. What remains unclear is exactly which biomarkers are indeed indicative of an underlying impact on the physiology of the disease that will translate into a meaningful clinical benefit for the patient. The recent findings from the bapineuzumab program revealed changes in biomarkers that included decreased CSF-tau [5] and improved amyloid burden versus placebo in carriers of the ApoE4 allele. However, these changes have not been associated with improvements in clinical outcomes as recorded on the Alzheimer's Disease Assessment Scale-cognitive portion (ADAS-Cog) and DAD as cognitive and functional endpoints, respectively. These conflicting data from clinical versus biomarker endpoints present a significant challenge for future studies seeking to demonstrate disease modification.

The final aspect of AD clinical development addressed in EU guidance is that of primary prevention studies. Trials in this area have been inconclusive to date and future studies are likely to be lengthy.

8.2.1 Shift Towards Earlier Disease Stages

The lack of alignment of the expected clinical outcomes with biomarker changes has led researchers to consider studying earlier stages of the disease, in which the introduction of anti-amyloid interventions may preserve neural integrity in a manner that can still yield clinical improvement to the patient. The EU guideline addressed early stages of the disease as mild cognitive impairment (MCI), a somewhat conceptual entity in which subjects would experience some cognitive deficits but without a complete presentation of dementia. The challenge surrounding this entity was the lack of progression of individuals with MCI to a dementia state over time, as well as some subjects actually reverting back to normal. The 2009 guideline called for additional efforts on diagnostic criteria to more clearly define a homogenous pre-dementia population. Subsequently, additional work on biomarkers as tools for clinical trial enrichment led the agency to adopt a clearer definition of how to diagnose the pre-dementia state.

8.2.2 Biomarker Qualification

In early 2009, the EMA Qualification of Novel Methodologies for Drug Development [6] was implemented. This qualification process was a new voluntary pathway leading to either a CHMP opinion or a Scientific Advice on innovative methods or drug development tools. The qualification opinion essentially represents EMA's endorsement of a particular tool or methodology for pharmaceutical research and development.

The EMA has issued a number of qualification opinions on biomarkers for AD that may enable the diagnosis of the disease before patients show signs of dementia. In the first of these adopted in April 2011 [7], the agency formally accepted a cerebrospinal fluid (CSF) biomarker signature based on a low Aβ1-42 and a high total-tau as qualified to identify MCI patients at the prodromal stage of AD (as defined by Dubois and colleagues [8]) and who are at risk to evolve into AD-dementia.

Subsequently, in November 2011, hippocampal atrophy detected by MRI was also adopted for use in clinical trials in the pre-dementia stage of AD [9]. Low hippocampal volume was considered a marker of progression to dementia in subjects with cognitive deficit compatible with the pre-dementia stage of AD, for the purposes of enriching a clinical trial population and serving as a marker of progression to full dementia.

Amyloid-related positive/negative PET imaging became the next signal qualified to identify patients, again with clinical diagnosis of pre-dementia AD who are at increased risk of having an underlying AD neuropathology, for the purposes of enriching a clinical trial population [10]. In this case however, the agency clarified that this biomarker could not yet be considered as predictive of the rate of such progression to dementia. Therefore, follow-up of patients until clinical diagnosis of mild AD is made was recommended.

These three qualification opinions related to subjects in the pre-dementia stage of AD as tools for enriching clinical studies and selecting patients with high probability of progression to AD over the course of a clinical study. The agency has also qualified the use of the CSF biomarker signature and PET imaging in patients with mild to moderate AD, as parameters associated with a high likelihood of having an underlying AD pathology [11].

It remains to be seen whether enriching clinical programs in such a fashion will translate into additional diagnostic criteria being applied in the final product labeling. However, the availability of clear diagnostic criteria that are pre-approved by the agency for application in this setting is of great help to sponsors looking to conduct research at the earlier stage of the disease process.

8.2.3 Revisions to the EU Guideline

With the publication of the qualification opinions described above, as well as the emerging data from a number of immunotherapy studies, a revision to the EU guidance was considered imminent. However, the agency issued a concept paper in 2012 indicating that it considered revisions to be premature at that time [12]. As new validated data on diagnostic criteria and potential biomarkers emerge, the agency indicated that these scientific developments and experience in scientific Advice procedures will be taken into consideration for a future update of the "Guideline on Medicinal Products for the Treatment of Alzheimer's Disease and Other Dementias."

8.3 FDA GUIDANCE

Historically, approval of the cholinesterase inhibitors and other symptomatic interventions defined the requirements for FDA approval of such interventions in AD, as well as the recognized standards for regulatory evidence of safety and efficacy, including for example the completing of two adequate and well-controlled clinical trials. More recently, the FDA issued draft guidance for industry with respect to drug development at early stage AD [13].

8.3.1 Draft Guidance on Early Disease Stages

In this earlier stage of disease, a shift away from the traditional co-primary cognitive and functional endpoints was warranted due to the lack of available tools that are sensitive enough to detect subtle functional changes in patients. The guidance addresses a number of aspects of clinical research in this population, including selection of patients, but also the categorizing of patients into prodromal or preclinical disease.

8.3.2 Preclinical versus Prodromal AD

In terms of selecting patients for AD studies at the early stage of the disease, FDA see two stages of disease prior to overt dementia; preclinical AD is the earliest stage whereby subjects will be identified purely on their biomarker profile, although future development of more sensitive clinical tools may be able to detect the very subtle cognitive changes also displayed in these patients. Prodromal AD, or MCI, equates to a further stage of progression where increasing effects on cognition are accompanied by mild changes in some functional abilities.

Although FDA also has a biomarker qualification process available [14], it has yet to issue formal endorsement of the biomarkers accepted by EMA and discussed above. However, this is likely in the near future. Importantly from a drug development perspective, the agency recognizes that standard outcome measures have major limitations when being applied to these early stages of AD.

In prodromal AD, the standard assessment tools for cognitive and functional improvements have not been validated for use. Therefore the agency considers the use of a composite scale such as the Clinical Dementia Rating–Sum of Boxes (CDR–SB), which has been validated for earlier stage patients, to represent a suitable outcome measure. In the earlier preclinical patients, only very subtle cognitive changes are evident in the absence of functional impairment. The agency has therefore suggested that in this population, an accelerated approval pathway [15] would be available to assess programs showing an effect on a valid and reliable cognitive measure used as a single outcome assessment. Further post approval studies to verify the clinical benefit would be expected.

While some reports have indicated this to represent an "easing" of FDA requirements for approval, the accelerated pathway has been established at the FDA for some time and allows the FDA to grant the marketing approval of certain drugs based on an effect on a clinical endpoint that is reasonably likely to predict the ultimate clinical outcome of interest (e.g., persistent improvement in cognition). Substantial evidence will still be required, as reiterated by the FDA in a recent webinar on the subject [16].

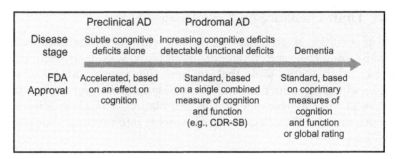

FIGURE 8.1   FDA guidance on early AD stages *(Adapted from [18]).*

8.3.2.1 Disease Modification?

The FDA draft guidance also addresses the demonstration of disease modification. Use of a biomarker as a surrogate endpoint (single primary) is not accepted at any stage of AD, as there is thought to be insufficient evidence to correlate the effect on any biomarker with clinical improvement. The agency will however consider the argument for disease modification when biomarker data are provided in support of clinical outcomes. As discussed earlier, the current challenge is identifying which biomarker is indicative of an impact on the pathophysiology of the disease while also aligning with clinical improvement. In the absence of a consensus amongst the scientific community on this topic sponsors are encouraged to gather data on multiple biomarkers and to analyze these independently, rather than applying a hierarchy to the statistical assessment. In light of the absence of approved treatments for disease modification in AD, an agent in development for such an indication is likely to qualify for fast-track designation [17].

The FDA guidance (summarized in Figure 8.1) remains as a draft at present, but when finalized will represent a major reference for sponsors of early AD clinical programs.

8.4 ACCEPTANCE OF FOREIGN CLINICAL DATA

Traditionally, clinical studies in the area of AD at the Phase III stage are global in nature with patients from multiple territories being included in efficacy and safety analyses. As competition for patients grows among the various trials, as well as cost factors being considered, it is becoming standard practice to expand the clinical program to beyond the typical US, Canada and western EU territories. The question therefore arises as to the acceptance of foreign clinical data in marketing applications in both the USA and EU.

In the EU, the EMA adopted a reflection paper in 2010 [19] to address the agency's thinking on the acceptability of data from clinical studies conducted outside the EU. This reflection paper suggests, similar to ICH E5 [20], that extrinsic factors, such as medical practice, disease definition, and study population, may influence the applicability of foreign data to an EU setting. Interestingly, foreign data in this sense include data from North America. The paper indicates that differences in concomitant medications and so-called "standard of care" of patients can impact the outcome of certain parameters. The paper calls for an:

> in-depth, prospective analysis of potential extrinsic and/or intrinsic factors when conducting a clinical trial in a certain region. The outcome of such analyses may facilitate for regulatory assessors the decision whether certain clinical trials conducted in a specific area of the world are relevant to the EU setting or if there are reasons to perform additional clinical trials within the EU.

In terms of studies of AD it is therefore advisable to ensure that a representative sample of patients in a Phase III program is sourced from EU geographies and can therefore serve as an internal reference for ex-EU sourced data and facilitate the comparative sub-analyses that would be expected within the marketing authorization application (MAA).

When a study is being conducted under a US investigational new drug (IND), the required investigator documentation and financial disclosure forms will be required irrespective of the geography in which the study is being conducted. The FDA, however, also accepts data from foreign clinical trials not conducted under an IND when in compliance with 21 CFR 312.120 [21]. In this case adherence to good clinical practice (CGP) is critical and the sponsor must provide the agency with a description of the steps taken to ensure adherence was effectively implemented. Importantly for any late stage clinical development, full adherence to the principles of ICH GCP, in particular E6 [22] will safeguard the regulatory acceptability of the study data. It is feasible, however, to submit a new drug application (NDA) based solely on data derived from outside of the USA [23], but again the relevance of the data to the US population and US medical practice will need to be evident, and the competence of the clinical investigators will also need to be demonstrated.

References

[1] Alzheimer's Association. Alzheimer's disease facts and figures [Internet]. 2013. [cited June 2013]. Available from: <http://www.alz.org/alzheimers_disease_facts_and_figures.asp#quickFacts>.
[2] Scientific aspects and working definitions for the mandatory scope of the centralized procedure [Regulation (EC) No 726/2004 of the European Parliament and of the Council of 31 March 2004] [Internet]. Doc. Ref. EMEA/CHMP/121944/2007. [cited June 2013]. Available from: <http://www.ema.europa.eu/docs/en_GB/

document_library/Regulatory_and_procedural_guideline/2009/10/WC500004085. pdf>.

[3] Recommendation on the need for revision of the guideline on clinical investigation of medicinal products in the treatment of Alzheimer's disease (CPMP/EWP/553/95) [Internet]. Doc. Ref. EMEA/CHMP/EWP/369929/2005. [cited June 2013]. Available from: <http://www.ema.europa.eu/docs/en_GB/document_library/Scientific_guideline/2009/09/WC500003564.pdf>.

[4] Guideline on medicinal products for the treatment of Alzheimer's disease and other dementias [Internet]. Doc. Ref. CPMP/EWP/553/95 Rev. 1. [cited June 2013]. Available from: <http://www.emea.europa.eu/docs/en_GB/document_library/Scientific_guideline/2009/09/WC500003562.pdf>.

[5] Blennow K, Zetterberg H, Rinne JO, Salloway S, Wei J, Black R, et al. Effect of immunotherapy with bapineuzumab on cerebrospinal fluid biomarker levels in patients with mild to moderate Alzheimer Disease. Arch Neurol 2012;69(8):1002–10.

[6] Qualification of novel methodologies for drug development: guidance to applicants [Internet]. Ref. EMA/CHMP/SAWP/72894/2008 Rev.1. [cited June 2013]. Available from: <http://www.emea.europa.eu/docs/en_GB/document_library/Regulatory_and_procedural_guideline/2009/10/WC500004201.pdf>.

[7] Committee for Medicinal Products for Human Use (CHMP). Qualification opinion of novel methodologies in the pre-dementia stage of Alzheimer's disease: cerebro-spinal fluid related biomarkers for drugs affecting amyloid burden [Internet]. 14 April 2011; Ref. EMA/CHMP/SAWP/102001/2011. [cited June 2013]. Available from: <http://www.ema.europa.eu/docs/en_GB/document_library/Regulatory_and_procedural_guideline/2011/05/WC500106357.pdf>.

[8] Dubois B, Feldman HH, Jacova C, Dekosky ST, Barberger-Gateau P, Cummings J, et al. Research criteria for the diagnosis of Alzheimer's disease: 327 revising the NINCDS-ADRDA criteria. Lancet Neurol 2007;6(8):734–46.

[9] Committee for Medicinal Products for Human Use (CHMP). Qualification opinion of low hippocampal volume (atrophy) by MRI for use in clinical trials for regulatory purpose–in pre-dementia stage of Alzheimer's disease [Internet]. 17 November 2011; Ref. EMA/CHMP/SAWP/809208/2011. [cited June 2013]. Available from: <http://www.ema.europa.eu/docs/en_GB/document_library/Regulatory_and_procedural_guideline/2011/12/WC500118737.pdf>.

[10] Committee for Medicinal Products for Human Use (CHMP). Qualification opinion of Alzheimer's disease novel methodologies/biomarkers for PET amyloid imaging (positive/negative) as a biomarker for enrichment, for use in regulatory clinical trials in pre-dementia Alzheimer's disease [Internet]. 16 February 2012; Ref. EMA/CHMP/SAWP/892998/2011. [cited June 2013]. Available from: <http://www.ema.europa.eu/docs/en_GB/document_library/Regulatory_and_procedural_guideline/2012/04/WC500125018.pdf>.

[11] Committee for Medicinal Products for Human Use (CHMP). Qualification opinion of Alzheimer's disease novel methodologies/biomarkers for the use of CSF AB 1-42 and t-tau and/or PET-amyloid imaging (positive/negative) as biomarkers for enrichment, for use in regulatory clinical trials in mild and moderate Alzheimer's disease, 16 February 2012; Ref. EMA/CHMP/SAWP/893622/2011 [Internet]. [cited June 2013]. Available from: <http://www.ema.europa.eu/docs/en_GB/document_library/Regulatory_and_procedural_guideline/2012/04/WC500125019.pdf>.

[12] Committee for Medicinal Products for Human Use (CHMP). Concept paper on no need for revision of the guideline on medicinal products for the treatment of Alzheimer's disease and other dementias, 15 March 2012; Ref. EMA/CHMP/60715/2012 [Internet]. [cited June 2013]. Available from: <http://www.ema.europa.eu/docs/en_GB/document_library/Scientific_guideline/2012/03/WC500124534.pdf>.

[13] FDA Guidance for Industry–Alzheimer's Disease: Developing Drugs for the Treatment of Early Stage Disease [Internet]. 2013, February. [cited June 2013]. Available from: <http://www.fda.gov/downloads/Drugs/GuidanceComplianceRegulatoryInformation/Guidances/UCM338287.pdf>.

[14] FDA Biomarker Qualification program [Internet]. 2012, [cited June 2013]. Available from: <http://www.fda.gov/Drugs/DevelopmentApprovalProcess/·DrugDevelopmentToolsQualificationProgram/ucm284076.htm>.

[15] Food and Drug Administration, Code of Federal Regulations Title 21, Part 314, Subpart H Accelerated Approval of New Drugs for Serious or Life-Threatening Illnesses [Internet]. [cited June 2013]. Available from: <http://www.accessdata.fda.gov/scripts/cdrh/cfdocs/cfcfr/CFRSearch.cfm?CFRPart=314&showFR=1&subpartNode=21:5.0.1.1.4.8>.

[16] FDA Webinar: Draft Guidance For Industry On Alzheimer's Disease: Developing Drugs For The Treatment Of Early Stage Disease [Internet]. 2012, [cited March 2013]. Available from: <http://www.fda.gov/Training/GuidanceWebinars/ucm345077.htm>.

[17] Guidance for Industry, Fast Track Drug Development Programs–Designation, Development, and Application Review. [Internet] January 2006. [cited June 2013]. Available from: <http://www.fda.gov/downloads/Drugs/Guidances/ucm079736.pdf>.

[18] Kozauer N, Katz R. Regulatory innovation and drug development for early-stage Alzheimer's disease. N Engl J Med 2013;368:1169–71.

[19] Committee for Medicinal Products for Human Use (CHMP). Reflection paper on the extrapolation of results from clinical studies conducted outside the EU to the EU-population [Internet]. Doc. Ref. EMEA/CHMP/EWP/692702/2008. [cited June 2013]. Available from: <http://www.ema.europa.eu/docs/en_GB/document_library/Scientific_guideline/2009/11/WC500013468.pdf>.

[20] ICH Harmonized Tripartite Guideline E5: Ethnic factors in the acceptability of foreign clinical data [Internet]. February 1998. [cited June 2013]. Available from: <http://www.ich.org/fileadmin/Public_Web_Site/ICH_Products/Guidelines/Efficacy/E5_R1/Step4/E5_R1__Guideline.pdf>.

[21] Food and Drug Administration, Code of Federal Regulations Title 21, Part 312.120 Foreign clinical studies not conducted under an IND [Internet]. [cited June 2013]. Available from: <http://www.accessdata.fda.gov/scripts/cdrh/cfdocs/cfCFR/CFRSearch.cfm?fr=312.120>.

[22] ICH Harmonized Tripartite Guideline E6: Guideline for Good Clinical Practice [Internet]. June 1996. [cited June 2013]. Available from: <http://www.ich.org/fileadmin/Public_Web_Site/ICH_Products/Guidelines/Efficacy/E6_R1/Step4/E6_R1__Guideline.pdf>.

[23] Food and Drug Administration [Internet]. Code of Federal Regulations Title 21, Part 314.106 Foreign Data. [cited June 2013]. Available from: <http://www.accessdata.fda.gov/scripts/cdrh/cfdocs/cfCFR/CFRSearch.cfm?fr=314.106>.

IV. GLOBAL REGULATORY ENVIROMENT SURROUNDING AD TRIALS

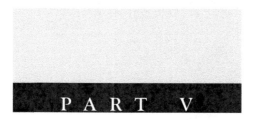

STANDARDIZATION OF DIAGNOSTIC AND OUTCOME MEASURES IN GLOBAL ALZHEIMER'S DISEASE TRIALS

9

Standardization of MRI and Amyloid Imaging

Michel Grothe[1], Jens Kurth[2], Harald Hampel[3], Bernd J. Krause[2] and Stefan Teipel[1,4]

[1]DZNE, German Center for Neurodegenerative Diseases, Rostock, Germany [2]Department of Nuclear Medicine, University of Rostock, Rostock, Germany [3]Department of Psychiatry, University of Frankfurt, Frankfurt, Germany [4]Department of Psychosomatic Medicine, University of Rostock, Rostock, Germany

9.1 INTRODUCTION

Accumulating evidence for a long and differentiated pre-dementia phase of Alzheimer's disease (AD) has motivated the current revision of NINCDS-ADRDA criteria for the diagnosis of AD [1], which aims to implement the use of imaging-derived biomarkers to improve specificity of AD diagnosis [2] and to detect AD pathology before the emergence of dementia [3]. The new diagnostic entities of preclinical and pre-dementia AD are intended to serve the early diagnosis in clinical diagnostic studies and the enrichment and stratification of samples for testing effects of potential disease modification in clinical trials of AD. In this context, molecular markers of abnormal amyloid accumulation are employed to define the presence of AD pathology, whereas structural lesion markers allow tracking disease progression and may be used for predicting stage transitions from preclinical over pre-dementia to clinically manifest stages of AD [4,5].

While abnormal levels of amyloid molecules in the cerebrospinal fluid (CSF) have widely been used as an indirect marker of cerebral amyloid deposition [6], the recent development of radioactively labeled amyloid tracers suitable for positron emission tomography (PET) [7] now allows a direct *in-vivo* visualization of abnormal amyloid aggregates. On the other

M. Bairu & M.W. Weiner (Eds):
Global Clinical Trials for Alzheimer's Disease.
DOI: http://dx.doi.org/10.1016/B978-0-12-411464-7.00009-2

hand, lesion markers of ongoing neurodegeneration can be derived from multimodal magnetic resonance imaging (MRI) protocols. Thus, volumetric measures from structural MRI acquisitions have been found to correlate well with the extent of neurofibrillary degeneration and cell loss in AD brains at autopsy, motivating their application as surrogate markers of neuronal atrophy [8,9]. Diffusion tensor imaging (DTI) is a novel MRI-based technology which provides a measure of the microstructural integrity of white matter fiber tracts, rendering it a promising biomarker candidate for subtle tissue changes affecting the integrity of the brain's structural connections and interregional information transfer [10].

Neuroimaging measurements are increasingly being incorporated into large-scale multicenter clinical studies to be used as diagnostic markers or potential outcome markers to assess treatment effects. For this, the measures should (i) show validity in respect to underlying pathology and clinical outcome, (ii) they should be easily applicable, i.e., the test should be non-invasive, widely available, and pose low patient burden, and finally (iii) the measures should be reliable both within one center (test–retest reliability) and across centers [11]. While PET-based imaging of amyloid deposits has been demonstrated to reliably detect molecular AD pathology [12], MRI-based lesion markers of neuronal degeneration are more closely related to clinical outcome measures such as cognitive decline [13,14]. Structural MRI is non-invasive, can easily be applied even to more handicapped patients, and is widely available through its common use in clinical settings. Although a wide clinical applicability of the first amyloid-sensitive PET ligands was hindered by the short half-life of the attached radioprobe (^{11}C), this limitation has recently been overcome by the development of ^{18}F-labeled amyloid ligands [15]. Due to the substantially slower decay rate, these ligands can be transported across sites, thus enabling their use in clinical centers that do not have an on-site cyclotron.

While large-scale multicenter study designs allow the recruitment of large numbers of subjects in relatively short periods of time, the biomarker criterion of reliability is of particular importance in these settings. Thus, multi-centric variability in the outcome measure may lead to a corresponding loss of diagnostic accuracy or decreased power to detect treatment effects, which may cancel out the gains of increased sample sizes. Recent multicenter network studies, such as the North-American Alzheimer's Disease Neuroimaging Initiative (ADNI) or the European ADNI (E-ADNI) [16] have greatly advanced the development of imaging biomarkers for AD. These and other large-scale national and international multisite networks provide a platform on which experimental markers can be tested for practicability and multicenter stability along fast acquisition and analysis protocols in large and well-defined clinical cohorts.

In this chapter we will give an overview of widely used molecular and structural neuroimaging markers, as well as the extent of multi-center variability in these measures and its most common sources. This overview will be followed by a description of strategies for dealing with multicenter variability, including recommendations for multi-centric collection and quality control of imaging data, as well as techniques to account for multicenter variability by means of post-acquisition image processing and analytic design.

9.2 AMYLOID PET IN GLOBAL CLINICAL TRIALS

9.2.1 Amyloid PET as *In-Vivo* Indicator of the Molecular Pathology of AD

Following the amyloid cascade hypothesis, abnormal processing of amyloid precursor protein (APP) with subsequent formation of amyloid-beta oligomers and amyloid plaques is a key event in the pathogenesis of AD [17]. The sequence of pathogenetic events has been derived from findings in autosomal-dominantly inherited cases of familial AD that are caused by a mutation in the APP or the APP degrading enzymes prese-niline 1 and preseniline 2 (PS1 and PS2) [18]. Based on these findings, transgenic mouse models of AD have been created exhibiting mutations of APP and/or PS1/PS2. These models replicate essential features of AD pathology, including amyloid plaques and decline in memory function [19]; however, they cannot serve as a comprehensive model of AD pathology.

Recent evidence in sporadic AD underscores the role of neurofibrillary pathology, the second pathological characteristic of AD upon autopsy. The formation of fibrillary bundles from abnormally phosphorylated microtubule-associated tau protein has been described in the brains of adolescent and young adults, suggesting that sporadic AD may be characterized by the parallel convergence of amyloid and tau pathology into a common end-stage of AD pathology [20]. Still, the detection of molecular amyloid *in vivo* using ^{11}C-labeled radioligands with PET was a major breakthrough in the diagnosis of early stages of AD pathology *in vivo* [7]. Convergent evidence from ^{11}C-labeled compound PIB and ^{18}F-labeled compounds florbetaben, florbetapir, and flutemetamol suggests that the large majority of patients with a clinical diagnosis of AD dementia, about 50% of subjects with a clinical diagnosis of MCI, and even a fraction of up to 25% of cognitively healthy subjects aged 70 and higher exhibit significant levels of amyloid binding in their brains. Moreover, the presence of amyloid in the brain of MCI subjects predicts subsequent conversion to AD dementia with more than 90%

accuracy [21], whereas cognitively healthy subjects have a 25% risk of developing cognitive decline if they present with increased amyloid accumulation in their brains at baseline [22].

Amyloid PET has also been employed to detect effects of amyloid lowering treatments in AD [23]. Interestingly, effects are often heterogeneous over time with sudden increases or declines that are difficult to explain on a neurobiological basis. These phenomena suggest that methodological problems may interfere with the quantification of results. But in addition to cross-sectional analysis, multicenter effects need to be taken into account when considering amyloid PET as a future biomarker for clinical trials and diagnosis in defined clinical samples.

9.2.2 Sources and Extent of Multicenter Variability of Amyloid PET Measurements

There are two main categories that cause differences in human PET scans: i) inter-subject variability due to anatomical and functional differences, and ii) systematic differences that are related to scanner hardware and software and other technical equipment that is necessary for quantitative PET imaging. Because the goal of PET is to determine the functional differences between individuals or groups of individuals, in a multicenter setup it is necessary to eliminate both the anatomic differences that exist between subjects and the systematic differences across diverse scanner models.

Data on variability and standardization of multicenter amyloid PET are still scarce. However, lessons can be learned from the widely distributed fluorodeoxyglucose (FDG)-PET approach. The use of FDG is based on the close coupling of neuronal glucose metabolism with neuronal function [24]. Studies in human subjects have demonstrated a close relation between FDG uptake and cerebral glucose metabolism [25]. The coupling is mediated by the neuron-astrocyte, glutamate shuttle [26,27]. Although the relative contributions of neurons and astrocytes to functional coupling are still under debate [28], the coupling of glucose consumption in functional units with neuronal function has not been challenged. Interestingly, cerebral glucose metabolism is less variable than blood flow, which is influenced by systemic parameters such as arterial PCO_2.

FDG-PET can gauge neuronal activity at a resting state without the need for cognitive activation. Normal regional variability is in the order of 5–10%. There is good reproducibility of regional values and the coefficients of variability are 16.5% for absolute values. About half of the regional variation is due to variation of global metabolism. Thus, the variability of normalized regional values is typically less than 10%. Use of arterial blood sampling and normalization of values to global metabolism can thus decrease between-center variability. Multivariate post-processing approaches such as principal component analysis in the context of the European NEXT-DD study have shown that effects of center can at least partly be separated from effects of age or AD [29]. Another more clinically oriented approach is the definition of predefined areas of interest for individual PET data analysis and the derivation of a z-standardized deviation score relative to a center- or study-specific comparison sample for a given individual [30].

Analysis of amyloid PET scans across sites is well established using visual reading of scans, where rater experience takes multicenter variation into account [31]. Quantitative analysis of amyloid PET data, although widely used, has rarely explicitly addressed the issue of multicenter effects. Large multicenter networks such as the ADNI study take multicenter variability into account by downgrading PET images according to the scanner with the lowest spatial resolution and standardizing image intensity within sites. However, this limits the available resolution to the lowest common denominator.

Factors that influence the signal estimation in amyloid PET (and PET in general) are the selection of reference regions (if no absolute quantification is used or possible) [32], the duration of image sampling, time interval of data acquisition after tracer injection [33,34], and the strategy of image reconstruction [35]. Systematic differences in the reconstructed images across different PET scanners are related primarily to differences in spatial resolution, image uniformity, and the applied corrections for attenuation and scatter during reconstruction. Differences in the uniformity of the PET scanner may manifest as changes in contrast, i.e., ratios of uptake within gray matter (GM) compared with white matter (WM) [36].

An additional source of uncertainty is the use of partial volume correction methods, because PET images suffer from poor resolution due to the finite resolution of the tomographic systems, which is described by the point-spread function (PSF) of the system, modeling the loss of resolution in the reconstruction by a convolution of the true activity with PSF. This results in edge smoothing and degradation of small structures in the reconstructed images as well as bias in quantification. If the concerned region is small with respect to the PSF, then the activity in this region spills out to the surrounding regions and the activity of the neighboring regions spills in. This phenomenon is known as partial volume effect (PVE). Confounding factors in PVE can often be spatial and temporal variation, because the cerebral cortex is no more than a few millimeters thick and suffers from severe PVE when imaged using PET. Further PVEs are caused by atrophic changes in cerebral tissue such as those caused by neurodegenerative diseases [37].

To take into account these systematic effects of atrophy on estimated PET signal per volume GM, a valid correction of the partial volume effect is necessary [38,39]. Partial volume correction (PVC) could in theory be achieved by some kind of inverse filtering technique, reversing the effect of the system PSF. However, these methods are limited, and usually lead to noise-amplification or image artifacts. Some form of regularization is therefore needed, and this can be achieved using information from co-registered anatomical images, such as CT or MRI [39–41]. The accuracy of these anatomically guided PVE correction algorithms mainly depends on the performance of MRI segmentation algorithms partitioning the brain into its main classes, namely GM, WM, and CSF [42].

For FDG-PET it has been shown that PVE correction reduces the apparent difference in cortical metabolism between AD patients and controls, but still maintains between-group differences [43–45]. Physical phantom and clinical data suggest that atrophy correction can increase accuracy of estimates of regional signal distribution with ^{18}F-flutemetamol as amyloid tracer [46]. Again, multicenter studies assessing the effect of atrophy correction on between-site variability are still lacking.

In quantitative analysis of amyloid PET, the increase of neocortical uptake shows little regional differences and therefore a global average is normally expressed as a ratio relative to a reference uptake (usually cerebellum or pons). Due to the non-specific tracer uptake within WM in controls, techniques for distinction between GM and WM are required. The use of MRI-based or PET template-based approaches to define GM and WM influences the classification of amyloid PET scans [47]. Also, the threshold applied to discriminate between "amyloid positive" and "amyloid negative" scans is intrinsically linked with the data processing approach used in a specific study [48]. A systematic comparison of all these parameters within a multicenter framework is still lacking.

9.2.3 Reducing Multicenter Variability of PET Measurements

The first and most important point in reducing multicenter variability of PET data is to standardize patient preparation for all participating sites as well as acquisition-, reconstruction-, and post-processing parameters for every dedicated PET or PET/CT scanner used in the study on a very high level.

Therefore it is necessary to check the image quality of all participating sites. However, evaluation and validation of clinical PET images is inherently difficult. Sometimes examples of patient studies displaying brain PET images are used as indicators of image quality, but experimentally measured or simulated data are often used for a more objective analysis. The Hoffman 3D-phantom closes the gap between the images usually obtained with simple geometric test phantoms and activity distributions seen in *in-vivo* images. It allows the evaluation of the accuracy of measurements with PET systems in the brain [49]. The main idea behind the scanning of the Hoffman 3D-phantom is to produce images of a uniform isotropic spatial resolution over a variety of different scanners. If the minimal criteria for image quality are met by the participating centers, acquisition and reconstruction parameters for the PET should be optimized for the different PET- or PET/CT scanners to achieve similar image qualities (spatial resolution and homogeneity) across participating sites.

An interesting methodology to reach this goal is the use of high frequency corrections, where a smoothing kernel for each scanner model is estimated to smooth all images to a common resolution, and low frequency corrections, where smooth affine correction factors are obtained to reduce the attenuation and scatter correction errors. Multi-centric PET studies have already shown that high frequency correction can reduce the variability by 20–50% [36]. It is mandatory that patients participating in a clinical study are scanned using the same protocol that was used for the phantom scan.

It should also be kept in mind that any hard- or software upgrade of the PET- or PET/CT scanner might have an influence on the imaging performance of the system. Therefore, ideally, any hardware or software upgrades of the imaging system should be avoided during the duration of a study.

Another important requirement in quantitative PET imaging is the proper calibration of the PET scanner and that peripheral devices (i.e., dose calibrator and well counter) are cross calibrated to the scanner, also in terms of absolute activity. This becomes even more important when data are collected and analyzed in multi-centric settings [50,51]. The recommended procedure is to cross calibrate against a cylindrical phantom containing a solution of a short-lived positron emitter, such as F-18, of known activity and volume in which activity is measured using the on-site dose calibrator. The well counter is then checked using a set of samples from this phantom. This type of calibration procedure depends on the accuracy of the on-site dose calibrator. However, if the same dose calibrator is used to determine the activity administered to the patient, any deviation in accuracy will be canceled out, assuming that deviation is constant and the complete cross calibration procedure has been followed, including nuclide-specific corrections for branching ratio and decay. Using such a procedure, an accuracy of at least 5–10% could be achieved for nearly all the dedicated PET scanners [50].

However, measurements and readjustments performed reflect the status of the PET scanner and associated devices at that specific time point. Therefore a permanent monitoring by participating institutions is needed to maintain this condition. This includes a continued quality monitoring of the PET- or PET/CT scanner and the ancillary equipment (i.e., blood glucose meter, dose calibrator, well counter, and pipette) during the execution phase of a study. As pointed out already, patient preparation also needs to be standardized with respect to the uptake period, the room's ambient conditions, the administered activity, etc. It is also necessary to inspect the data for subject motion, and the inter-frame motion has to be corrected using a more extensive registration procedure on a frame-by-frame basis [52,53].

There is a clear need for guidelines to evaluate reconstruction techniques and other image processing issues in brain PET. Further research and development efforts are therefore still required to establish a standardized framework for optimized data acquisition, reconstruction, and quantification in 3D brain PET.

9.3 MRI-BASED MEASUREMENTS IN GLOBAL CLINICAL TRIALS

9.3.1 Quantitative MRI Indices as *In-Vivo* Markers for Neurodegeneration

The neurodegeneration in AD leads to a marked reduction of brain tissue in patients with AD dementia, which is most striking in medial temporal lobe (MTL) structures, such as the hippocampus, and can be clearly distinguished on structural MRI scans. Thus, assessment of MTL atrophy on structural MRI, either by visual ratings [54] or by quantitative volumetric measurements [55], was proposed many years ago as a complementary diagnostic tool in AD. Since then, considerable progress has been made regarding both improvements in MRI technology and development of advanced quantitative image analysis methods. Automated voxel-based and atlas-based image parcelation techniques now allow a fast and rater-independent measurement of not just a single structure like the hippocampus but of multiple brain regions simultaneously [56,57].

One of the most commonly used automated volumetry approaches is voxel-based morphometry (VBM). In its original implementation, structural MRI scans are segmented into GM, WM, and CSF partitions and globally normalized into a common reference space to control overall differences in brain size and shape. Local differences in GM volume (or other types of brain tissue) that are not modeled by the global normalization are then examined using voxel-wise univariate statistics [56]. Using VBM to study atrophic changes in AD patients compared with healthy controls, several studies have revealed consistent spatial atrophy patterns that match up well with earlier findings from neuropathological autopsy studies [58]. Modern computational methods for automated volumetry expand the original VBM approach by the implementation of high-dimensional image deformation algorithms [59]. These algorithms achieve a highly accurate match between the native images and the template image, thereby eliminating spatial differences among the individual scans. The information on inter-individual spatial variability then resides entirely in the deformation functions, which can be used to extract volumetric information from the individual deformation fields themselves [60] or to automatically segment the individual brains into regions of interest based on inverse warping of detailed atlases in the template space [57]. Automatically segmented regions of interest show high anatomic accuracy when compared with manual volumetry techniques [59,61] and even allow for the detailed structural analysis of brain regions that are less amenable to manual delineation.

DTI is a novel MRI-based technology that can detect changes in the microstructural integrity of white matter fiber tracts, which are widely independent of macroscopic (i.e., volumetric) changes and not readily identifiable by visual inspection [62]. Through the simultaneous assessment of several diffusion-weighted images along uniformly distributed diffusion gradient directions, tissue-specific indices of water mobility can be derived from DTI acquisitions. Whereas an increase in general water mobility (mean diffusivity) is indicative of a microscopic disruption of tissue integrity, a decreased directional mobility (fractional anisotropy) within the brain's white matter points to a microstructural decline in fiber tract integrity [63]. Similar to the volumetric analysis of structural MRI scans, quantitative measures can be derived from DTI acquisitions by measuring indices of diffusivity in manually or automatically determined regions of interest, or by using voxel-based methods [10]. Furthermore, diffusion-weighted acquisitions can also be used to automatically reconstruct individual fiber tracts from selected seed points based on the inter-voxel continuation of the principal diffusion direction. Quantitative measures derived from such reconstructed fiber tracts account more precisely for the inter-individual variability in fiber tract anatomy and are less contaminated by signals from brain tissue surrounding the tract of interest [64,65].

Due to their non-invasive character and their experimentally verified association with underlying disease-related neuronal changes [8,9,66,67], MRI measurements are ideally suited to be employed as diagnostic markers for early and differential diagnosis of AD, as well as for the assessment of neurobiological effects of medical treatments in clinical trials. Given the severe atrophy of the MTL in AD, even simple visual rating scales of MTL atrophy can distinguish AD patients from healthy controls with high diagnostic accuracies of approximately 85% [54,68]. Manual as well as automated measurements of hippocampus volume yield diagnostic accuracies ranging from 70% for pre-dementia stages of AD to complete group separation for advanced stages of AD dementia [55,69,70]. These quantitative volumetry methods are also sensitive enough to track disease progression over time [71,72]. Microstructural fiber tract alterations as quantified by DTI carry complementary information of the disease process and were found to benefit the diagnosis of early-stage AD by significantly improving diagnostic accuracies when combined with markers of GM degeneration [73,74]. While quantitative measures of global and regional brain atrophy from serially acquired MRI scans have already been widely employed as outcome measures in AD clinical trials [75–77], longitudinal changes in DTI-derived metrics are only beginning to be considered as surrogate markers for the disease-modifying effects of medical interventions [78].

Despite the promising findings for the clinical utility of quantitative MRI measurements reported by controlled single-center studies, a widespread clinical use of these structural imaging biomarkers has so far been hampered by the lack of standardized acquisition and analysis methods in multi-centric settings. In recent years, an increasing number of national and international collaborations have been established to investigate how variability in multi-centric data acquisitions affects quantitative imaging measurements and their clinical utility.

9.3.2 Multicenter Variability of Quantitative MRI Measurements

9.3.2.1 Sources and Extent of Multicenter Variability of Volumetric MRI Measurements

Variability of MRI acquisitions is caused by multiple scanner- and subject-related factors. These include variations in voxel size due to differences in scanner calibration [79,80], but also image intensity inhomogeneities and image geometry distortions due to imaging gradient non-linearities, susceptibility effects, and subject-specific noise such as motion artifacts and differences in head positioning [81–83]. Furthermore, variability in scanner hardware, field strengths, and imaging protocols affects the image quality in various ways, including differences in spatial resolution and signal-to-noise ratios, as well as tissue-specific voxel intensities and tissue contrasts [84–86].

With respect to within scanner variability, several studies have shown that the test–retest reliability of repeated manual and automated volumetric measures from the same scanner is generally high [85,87–89]. The intra-scanner between session variability of these measurements does not usually exceed 5%, even when the sessions are separated by upgrades of the scanner software [88,89]. However, modifications of the acquisition protocol can introduce a significant bias in automated measurements even within the same scanner [85,88]. In the context of multicenter comparability of MRI measurements, it has to be considered that differing scanner models and inter-vendor differences in acquisition protocols significantly increase the variability of quantitative MRI estimates [88–92]. This is particularly the case for automated measurements, such as voxel-based methods which rely on intensity-based segmentations of brain tissue into GM, WM, and CSF compartments.

While an experienced radiologist can identify and disregard minor image artifacts for visual ratings or manual segmentation of brain structures, automated methods are less robust against image imperfections, such as differing contrast-to-noise levels or spatially varying intensity inhomogeneities. In one study, the variability of automated volumetric measures of global GM, WM, and CSF compartments across 12 different MRI scanners was below 5% [90], and the variability of manual volumetric measurements of the hippocampus was only 3.5%. This is in the range of accuracy of repeated manual or automated volumetric measurements on the same scanner in a single-center approach [87,89]. However, the mean inter-center coefficient of variation for voxel-intensities within the GM maps was 13% [90], indicating considerably higher multi-centric variability of automated methods at local scales compared with global measurements [91,92]. Interestingly, multicenter imaging studies of AD have shown that the center differences in volume measurements did not interact with diagnosis and were in general substantially lower compared with the volumetric differences between patients and healthy control subjects [93]. Accordingly, manual and automated volumetric measurements in multi-centric AD data revealed similar regional atrophy patterns and effect sizes for group separation compared with single-center studies [90,93,94].

A similar independence from center effects has also been found for brain-behavior relationships between quantitative measures of regional brain atrophy and decline in cognitive task performance [95]. Although these findings from cross-sectional comparisons of multi-centric MRI data are encouraging for a wider application of quantitative MRI measures as diagnostic tools for AD, they may not be easily transferable to longitudinal assessments of brain atrophy in the individual subject, which is necessary for monitoring treatment effects in clinical trials. Intra-individual volumetric changes in AD patients that occur over typical follow-up times of one to two years are usually substantially smaller than the absolute volume differences relative to healthy controls. The use of a visual rating scale to determine rates of atrophy over time only reached accuracy at chance level relative to volumetric hippocampus measures, suggesting that this approach may not be usefully employed as a secondary endpoint in clinical trials [68]. Reliable quantification of subtle volumetric changes over short time intervals may be improved by automated volumetry methods, which further overcome the inter-rater variability of manual measurements [72,96], but these automated methods are in general also more susceptible to variations in image quality [84,97].

9.3.2.2 *Sources and Extent of Multicenter Variability of DTI Measurements*

Compared with conventional structural MRI, DTI acquisitions have lower signal-to-noise ratios and resolution is more susceptible to thermal noise and motion [98]. DTI acquisitions usually employ echo planar imaging (EPI) sequences, which are especially sensitive to susceptibility-induced inhomogeneities of the static magnetic field resulting in local geometric distortions (EPI-distortions) [99]. The rapid changes in the magnetic field associated with the large field gradients applied in DTI acquisitions further result in the induction of eddy currents, which vary with the applied diffusion gradient direction and lead to image distortions and misalignment among the individual diffusion-weighted images [100]. Acquisition of a DTI sequence requires the selection of a range of additional acquisition parameters, most notably the number of applied diffusion gradient directions and the amount of diffusion weighting, i.e., the intensity and duration of the applied gradient pulse (characterized by the b-value).

Several studies assessing the reproducibility of DTI-derived diffusion indices have shown that these metrics are sensitive to the choice of diffusion-weighting schemes, but no generally agreed upon criteria for parameter selection have yet emerged [98,101–103]. Given the wide heterogeneity in the implementation of DTI acquisitions and their general vulnerability to noise, it is not surprising that DTI-derived diffusion indices were found to show considerable variability across scanner models and imaging sites [104–108]. Only recently have DTI-derived measures of tissue integrity entered the state of multicenter clinical studies. Within the framework of the European DTI Study in Dementia (EDSD), a clinical and physical phantom study across 12 European centers suggested around 50% higher variability of multicenter-acquired DTI data compared with classical anatomical MRI scans, significantly limiting its applicability in the wider clinical setting [107]. Multi-centric measurement variability was further found to vary across different types of fiber tracts and diffusion metrics.

The multicenter variability of DTI-derived diffusion indices is particularly high in WM regions that show low values of directed water diffusivity, such as those caused by constellations of crossing fibers or by partial volume effects in small structures bordering GM or CSF spaces. Quantitative metrics from relatively large fiber bundles that are characterized by highly organized fiber tract architectures, such as the corpus callosum, generally show the best reproducibility across centers [107,108]. With respect to clinical application across 300 subjects in the EDSD cohort, voxel-based analysis of diffusion indices showed relatively lower diagnostic accuracy for discriminating AD patients from healthy controls compared with anatomical MRI data [109]. Likewise, diffusion metrics derived from individual tractography reconstructions of the cingulate bundle showed considerable variation across centers and relatively low effect sizes for group differences between AD patients and controls [110].

9.3.2.3 Variability in Analytic Methods

Besides multi-centric variability in MRI-based acquisitions related to differences in scanner hardware and parameter settings for scanning sequences, comparability of quantitative imaging measures in a wider clinical context is further limited by a lack of standards in analytic methods. For example, a recent review on methods for defining the hippocampus in structural MRI scans revealed over 70 published manual segmentation protocols in the neuroimaging literature, with protocols differing widely in the use and definition of anatomical landmarks [111]. Even within the narrower field of AD research, 12 different widely used segmentation protocols could be identified, leading to up to 2.5-fold volume differences in reported group means for hippocampus volume [112]. This variability in hippocampus definition equally affects automated segmentation methods, which depend on accurate hippocampus labels in template space [113]. Beyond hippocampus volumetry, a wide variety of automated methods for the quantitative assessment of regional volumetric changes in AD has been proposed, mainly differing in the selection of assessed brain regions [60,114–118]. Outcome measures of automated processing pipelines further depend on the technical implementation of the method, including dependencies on algorithms for tissue-class segmentation [119], spatial normalization [59,115], and template selection [120].

For DTI data, several methods for the reconstruction of diffusion indices from the multiple diffusion-weighted images have been proposed, the choice of which can also bias the diffusivity estimates [121]. Once the diffusion metrics are reconstructed, the DTI data can be analyzed using a variety of methods, including extraction of diffusivity values from manually or automatically labeled regions/tracts-of-interest as well as whole-brain voxel-based methods [10]. Tractography analysis provides an alternative and anatomically more precise definition of individual fiber tracts, but there is also considerable heterogeneity regarding fiber tracking algorithms as well as seed-point selection and tract termination criteria [121].

9.3.3 Reducing Multicenter Variability of MRI Measurements

9.3.3.1 Standardization of Acquisition Protocols

Probably the most important step for achieving comparability of multi-centric MRI measurements lies in the standardization of the acquisition protocol across scanner platforms. A first evaluation of scanning compatibility across multi-centric scanner platforms can be achieved by scanning a physical phantom at all participating sites. For structural MRI acquisitions a physical phantom can be used to assess accuracy of the scanner performance, such as accuracy of slice positioning and geometric measurements, intensity uniformity, and minimum spatial resolution under controlled signal-to-noise ratios [80,90]. For the assessment of DTI acquisitions, uniform liquid phantoms that resemble the diffusion characteristics of the human body have been developed for calibration of the gradient coils [98]. In addition, anisotropic phantoms based on synthetic fibers can be used to evaluate the accuracy of tract reconstructions and scalar diffusivity measures of directed water mobility [107,108].

Once minimal criteria for scanner quality are met by the participating centers, acquisition parameters for the MRI-based sequences should be optimized for the different scanner models to achieve similar image qualities across sites in terms of tissue contrast, spatial resolution, and resistance to artifacts [122]. The standardization process can include restrictions to a selected number of scanner models and software versions, specification of the permitted types of pulse-sequences (typically magnetization prepared rapid gradient echo [MP-RAGE] or spoiled gradient echo [SPGR] for structural MRI and EPI-sequences for DTI), as well as vendor-specific tuning of parameter settings [98,122]. Given that quantitative analysis methods differ in their requirements on image quality and tissue contrast, optimization of the acquisition protocol should be evaluated with regard to the intended outcome measures of the study [97,123]. In DTI data, for example, robust estimates of fiber orientation for tractography usually require a higher number of unique gradient directions compared with the reconstruction of scalar diffusion indices [101,102].

Prospective protocols for acquisition of multicenter DTI data for the study of neurodegenerative disorders have been suggested already [124] and will be evaluated in future studies. Interestingly, the effect of standardization of machines and acquisition parameters across sites had only a moderate effect on between-center variability of DTI data, decreasing the coefficient of variation from 7% across platforms and parameters to 5% with standardized platforms and parameters in a physical phantom study [107]. These data suggest that within a reasonable selection of parameters, variation of DTI data across sites is only partly driven by differences in acquisition protocols and imaging platforms.

An important factor in the selection and optimization of standardized acquisition sequences is the total scan time. While signal-to-noise ratios of MRI-based acquisitions can be substantially increased by within-session scan repetition and averaging, this can rapidly increase total scan times to levels that are not easily tolerated by elderly and demented participants. For ethical considerations research protocols should also include sequences that enable a customary clinical evaluation of the imaging exam. Thus, in multi-centric research protocols more experimental sequences aimed for research purposes are usually combined with common sequences that are suitable for general diagnostic purposes, including clinical lesion detection and evaluation of vascular disease. Several

advanced scanning options exist to reduce acquisition times, such as parallel imaging techniques using phased-array head coils [125], but these
techniques would have to be supported by all the scanners in the study to
assure uniformity of acquisition settings and total scan times.

A central component of multi-centric imaging studies should be a rigorous quality control, including visual and/or automated tests for typical MR
imaging artifacts, such as partial coverage of the brain, blurring due to subject motion, severe image non-uniformities or irregularities in tissue contrast [122,126]. Most common artifacts specific to DTI acquisitions include
large signal dropouts due to susceptibility effects, geometric distortions
and misalignment among the diffusion-weighted images [63]. Although
some of these artifacts can be attenuated by post-processing techniques, an
initial quality control can detect severely corrupted images that have to be
repeated (on-site quality control) or excluded from the study (central quality control) [126]. Besides direct quality control of the imaging output, phantom-based monitoring of individual scanner performance is an effective way
to control for consistency of image quality over the course of the study [80].

9.3.3.2 *Post-acquisition Image Processing*

Even in the face of standardized acquisition protocols and quality
assurance procedures, scanner dependent imaging artifacts and differences in image quality cannot be removed completely across different types of scanning platforms in multi-centric settings. Furthermore,
in some studies the imaging data cannot be acquired prospectively but
already existing datasets are pooled across centers.

In order to further increase signal uniformity across multicenter scanner platforms, several computational image processing steps have been
developed to correct for various types of typically encountered image
artifacts. For structural MRI data the most important processing steps
include image-distortion corrections due to gradient nonlinearity [81,127]
and corrections for intensity non-uniformity, such as caused by non-
uniform receiver coil sensitivity or wave effects at higher field strengths
[83,97,128]. Particularly important for longitudinal MRI acquisitions are
geometric scaling corrections that account for small differences in voxel
size caused by scanner drift, either using drift estimates derived from
phantom-based scanner monitoring [80] or by means of inter-scan registration [79]. In addition, serial MRI scans should undergo some form of
inter-scan intensity normalization as global or, even worse, tissue-specific
intensity differences can significantly affect the estimates of automated
algorithms for tissue segmentation and spatial registration [86].

Typical post-processing steps for DTI acquisitions include corrections
for eddy-current distortions and motion artifacts as well as corrections
for local EPI-distortions. Eddy-current distortions and motion-related
misalignments among the individual diffusion-weighted images can be

corrected in the same step through affine registrations to the non-diffusion-weighted (B0) reference image [100]. In contrast, corrections of the more severe EPI-distortions, which affect all the images of the DTI sequence equally, usually require non-linear registrations to a structural MRI reference scan or additional information about local gradient field inhomogeneities from field maps acquired during the scanning session [99].

9.3.3.3 Accounting for Multicenter Variance in the Statistical Model

The statistical framework for the analysis of multicenter cross-sectional and intra-individual longitudinal data can largely influence the obtained results. For modeling multicenter variability based on ROI or voxel-based data, one can employ mixed effects regression models (random effects models, 2nd level models) [129]. These approaches allow explicitly modeling the effect of center as a random variable [94]. Compared with more widely used fixed effects models, random effects models allow generalization of the results from a specific set of centers to all possible centers in general because the centers are treated as a random sample out of the population of all centers. Similarly, this approach can usefully be employed to assess rates of volumetric decline, where time of observation is treated as a random variable, and it has shown to yield higher effect sizes of estimates of change compared with linear fixed effects models [130]. Another approach to explicitly take multicenter variability into account is the use of center-based meta-analysis. With this approach, effect size estimates of regional pattern of atrophy are determined within each center and pooled across centers using a meta-analytical approach [90]. These methods can be assumed to be less prone to false positive findings compared with the simple pooling of data across centers and treating center as a fixed effect covariate.

The limited accuracy of multicenter DTI data using simple linear approaches, such as tractography-based measurements or voxel-based analysis of pooled data across sites, requires an extension of statistical frameworks. One approach which was usefully employed in voxel-based analysis of multicenter DTI data was the use of random effects models and voxel-based meta-analysis across centers. These methods yielded more specific results in terms of spatial distribution of effects, but increased accuracy of group separation only by a few percent compared with fixed effects linear models [109]. In contrast, the use of multivariate machine-learning algorithms, including support vector machines, increased diagnostic accuracy by about 9%. However, DTI data was at best as accurate as structural MRI in detecting AD dementia [131]. Presently, studies are underway to assess the potential added value of DTI over structural MRI for the identification of pre-dementia AD in MCI subjects based on multicenter data and machine-learning classification.

9.3.3.4 Standardization of Quantitative Measures and Analytic Design

A widespread clinical use of quantitative MRI measures as imaging markers for AD requires that these measures be comparable across sites. This calls for an international standardization of measurement protocols for those imaging markers that have proven clinical utility in controlled mono- and multicenter studies. A first step in this direction has been initiated by the international project for harmonization of hippocampus protocols [112,132]. In this combined research effort of the European Alzheimer's Disease Consortium (EADC) and the ADNI, a task force of international experts on hippocampus volumetry has been founded to define standards for anatomical landmarks and boundaries to be employed for manual hippocampus segmentation.

Based on manual delineation of the hippocampus following the harmonized protocol in a representative sample of AD patients and elderly controls with varying degrees of hippocampus atrophy, a set of standardized benchmark labels and probabilistic hippocampus maps have been produced to serve as a publicly available reference standard. In addition, an interactive web-based interface has been developed which enables remote training and qualification for manual hippocampus segmentation based on the standardized criteria.

The standardization of manual hippocampus delineation in structural MRI scans will also benefit harmonization of automated segmentation algorithms because of their dependence on a-priori models of hippocampal shape [113]. As an extension of the harmonization project, a larger dataset of benchmark labels covering a wide physiological variability across healthy and diseased brains is currently being produced by qualified human tracers to produce a comprehensive set of gold standard labels suitable for proper training of automated segmentation algorithms. Although several multiregional structural imaging markers for AD have been suggested that cover the AD-specific atrophy pattern in a more comprehensive way than simple hippocampus measurements [60,114–118], these automated methods so far lack internationally agreed upon standards for the employed metrics and automated image processing routines.

Several DTI-derived measures have shown to capture AD-specific neuronal changes, indicating their utility in a clinical context, but no clear recommendations for DTI-based imaging markers of AD have emerged so far [10,78]. This is related to both the generally less robust performance of DTI-derived measures within multicenter settings [107,108], but also to the high variability in analytic methods, including region-of-interest analysis, voxel-based methods, and tractography approaches [10]. In this regard, the variability in the reproducibility of regional DTI-derived metrics across multi-centric acquisitions should be taken into account for the design of DTI-based imaging markers to be used in clinical settings

[107]. The generation of manually drawn [133] or tractography-based atlases [134] of the brain's major WM fiber tracts in standardized stereotaxic space, as well as the publication of stereotaxic coordinates suitable for automated tractography [65], are first steps towards standardization of analytic methods for DTI acquisitions.

9.4 CONCLUSIONS

In summary, the existing data indicate that acceptable precision of manual and automated volumetric MRI measures can be achieved in multi-centric settings, as long as the multi-centric variance is controlled by standardized acquisition protocols, stringent quality control, and computational post-processing of common imaging artifacts. The utility of multi-centric quantitative MRI measures as imaging markers for AD-related neuronal changes in therapeutic trials, and for diagnostic purposes in clinical settings, can be further increased by the use of appropriate statistical models. When analyzed by the same computational methods, quantitative volumetric measures are highly comparable between different international studies on AD using standardized acquisition protocols [135,136].

DTI-derived metrics are promising imaging markers to provide complementary information on neuronal changes in AD, but compared with volumetric MRI measures the standardization and establishment of DTI-derived measures within a multicenter context is less well developed. Even for volumetric MRI, quantitative methods are only beginning to be standardized on an international level. Widespread clinical use of quantitative MRI as an AD biomarker will finally depend on the establishment of internationally agreed upon standards for image acquisition, quality assurance, and employed quantitative metrics.

Amyloid PET has become one of the key diagnostic markers for AD. Despite its wide use in multicenter settings, the systematic exploration of sources of variability across sites and on measures to reduce multicenter effects is still underdeveloped. Presently, areas of research can be identified that need to be explored for the future employment of amyloid PET as a diagnostic marker for AD in clinical trials and even in routine care. The availability of ^{18}F-labeled amyloid binding compounds (one is already approved in the USA and Europe) will enhance the application of amyloid diagnostics at least in large university diagnostic centers worldwide even outside of clinical studies. The provision of a firm methodological basis to ensure comparability of results across sites will be an important prerequisite for the valid use of these markers in future dementia care.

References

[1] Jack Jr CR, Albert MS, Knopman DS, McKhann GM, Sperling RA, Carrillo MC, et al. Introduction to the recommendations from the National Institute on aging-Alzheimer's association workgroups on diagnostic guidelines for Alzheimer's disease. Alzheimers Dement 2011;7(3):257–62.

[2] McKhann GM, Knopman DS, Chertkow H, Hyman BT, Jack Jr CR, Kawas CH, et al. The diagnosis of dementia due to Alzheimer's disease: recommendations from the National Institute on Aging-Alzheimer's Association workgroups on diagnostic guidelines for Alzheimer's disease. Alzheimers Dement 2011;7(3):263–9.

[3] Sperling RA, Aisen PS, Beckett LA, Bennett DA, Craft S, Fagan AM, et al. Toward defining the preclinical stages of Alzheimer's disease: recommendations from the National Institute on Aging-Alzheimer's Association workgroups on diagnostic guidelines for Alzheimer's disease. Alzheimers Dement 2011;7(3):280–92.

[4] Jack Jr CR, Knopman DS, Jagust WJ, Shaw LM, Aisen PS, Weiner MW, et al. Hypothetical model of dynamic biomarkers of the Alzheimer's pathological cascade. Lancet Neurol 2010;9(1):119–28.

[5] Teipel SJ, Sabri O, Grothe M, Barthel H, Prvulovic D, Buerger K, et al. Perspectives for multimodal neurochemical and imaging biomarkers in Alzheimer's disease. J Alzheimers Dis 2013;33(Suppl. 1):S329–47.

[6] Blennow K, Vanmechelen E, Hampel H. CSF total tau, Abeta42 and phosphorylated tau protein as biomarkers for Alzheimer's disease. Mol Neurobiol 2001;24(1–3):87–97.

[7] Klunk WE, Engler H, Nordberg A, Wang Y, Blomqvist G, Holt DP, et al. Imaging brain amyloid in Alzheimer's disease with Pittsburgh Compound-B. Ann Neurol 2004;55(3):306–19.

[8] Bobinski M, de Leon MJ, Wegiel J, Desanti S, Convit A, Saint Louis LA, et al. The histological validation of post mortem magnetic resonance imaging-determined hippocampal volume in Alzheimer's disease. Neuroscience 2000;95(3):721–5.

[9] Whitwell JL, Josephs KA, Murray ME, Kantarci K, Przybelski SA, Weigand SD, et al. MRI correlates of neurofibrillary tangle pathology at autopsy: a voxel-based morphometry study. Neurology 2008;71(10):743–9.

[10] Oishi K, Mielke MM, Albert M, Lyketsos CG, Mori S. DTI analyses and clinical applications in Alzheimer's disease. J Alzheimers Dis 2011;26(Suppl. 3):287–96.

[11] Hampel H, Frank R, Broich K, Teipel SJ, Katz RG, Hardy J, et al. Biomarkers for Alzheimer's disease: academic, industry and regulatory perspectives. Nat Rev Drug Discov 2010;9(7):560–74.

[12] Fleisher AS, Chen K, Liu X, Roontiva A, Thiyyagura P, Ayutyanont N, et al. Using positron emission tomography and florbetapir F18 to image cortical amyloid in patients with mild cognitive impairment or dementia due to Alzheimer disease. Arch Neurol 2011;68(11):1404–11.

[13] Grothe M, Zaborszky L, Atienza M, Gil-Neciga E, Rodriguez-Romero R, Teipel SJ, et al. Reduction of basal forebrain cholinergic system parallels cognitive impairment in patients at high risk of developing Alzheimer's disease. Cereb Cortex 2010;20(7):1685–95.

[14] Deweer B, Lehericy S, Pillon B, Baulac M, Chiras J, Marsault C, et al. Memory disorders in probable Alzheimer's disease: the role of hippocampal atrophy as shown with MRI. J Neurol Neurosurg Psychiatry 1995;58(5):590–7.

[15] Herholz K, Ebmeier K. Clinical amyloid imaging in Alzheimer's disease. Lancet Neurol 2011;10(7):667–70.

[16] Frisoni GB. Alzheimer's disease neuroimaging initiative in Europe. Alzheimers Dement 2010;6(3):280–5.

[17] Selkoe DJ. The genetics and molecular pathology of Alzheimer's disease: roles of amyloid and the presenilins. Neurol Clin 2000;18(4):903–22.

[18] Pera M, Alcolea D, Sanchez-Valle R, Guardia-Laguarta C, Colom-Cadena M, Badiola N, et al. Distinct patterns of APP processing in the CNS in autosomal-dominant and sporadic Alzheimer's disease. Acta Neuropathol 2013;125(2):201–13.

[19] Bryan KJ, Lee H, Perry G, Smith MA, Casadesus G. Transgenic mouse models of alzheimer's disease: behavioral testing and considerations Buccafusco JJ, editor. Methods of behavior analysis in neuroscience (2nd ed.). Boca Raton (FL): CRC Press; 2009. Chapter 1.

[20] Braak H, Del Tredici K. The pathological process underlying Alzheimer's disease in individuals under thirty. Acta Neuropathol 2011;121(2):171–81.

[21] Zhang S, Han D, Tan X, Feng J, Guo Y, Ding Y. Diagnostic accuracy of 18F-FDG and 11C-PIB-PET for prediction of short-term conversion to Alzheimer's disease in subjects with mild cognitive impairment. Int J Clin Pract 2012;66(2):185–98.

[22] Villemagne VL, Pike KE, Chetelat G, Ellis KA, Mulligan RS, Bourgeat P, et al. Longitudinal assessment of Abeta and cognition in aging and Alzheimer disease. Ann Neurol 2011;69(1):181–92.

[23] Rinne JO, Brooks DJ, Rossor MN, Fox NC, Bullock R, Klunk WE, et al. 11C-PiB PET assessment of change in fibrillar amyloid-beta load in patients with Alzheimer's disease treated with bapineuzumab: a phase 2, double-blind, placebo-controlled, ascending-dose study. Lancet Neurol 2010;9(4):363–72.

[24] Sokoloff L. Relation between physiological function and energy metabolism in the central nervous system. [Review]. J Neurochem 1977;29(1):13–26.

[25] Reivich M, Kuhl D, Wolf A, Greenberg J, Phelps M, Ido T, et al. The [18F]fluorodeoxyglucose method for the measurement of local cerebral glucose utilization in man. Circ Res 1979;44(1):127–37.

[26] Kasischke KA, Vishwasrao HD, Fisher PJ, Zipfel WR, Webb WW. Neural activity triggers neuronal oxidative metabolism followed by astrocytic glycolysis. Science 2004;305(5680):99–103.

[27] Pellerin L, Magistretti PJ. Glutamate uptake into astrocytes stimulates aerobic glycolysis: a mechanism coupling neuronal activity to glucose utilization. Proceedings of the National Academy of Sciences of the United States of America 1994;91(22):10625–9.

[28] Haydon PG, Carmignoto G. Astrocyte control of synaptic transmission and neurovascular coupling. Physiol Rev 2006;86(3):1009–31.

[29] Zuendorf G, Kerrouche N, Herholz K, Baron JC. Efficient principal component analysis for multivariate 3D voxel-based mapping of brain functional imaging data sets as applied to FDG-PET and normal aging. Hum Brain Mapp 2003;18(1):13–21.

[30] Mosconi L, Tsui WH, Herholz K, Pupi A, Drzezga A, Lucignani G, et al. Multicenter standardized 18F-FDG PET diagnosis of mild cognitive impairment, Alzheimer's disease, and other dementias. J Nucl Med 2008;49(3):390–8.

[31] Cohen AD, Mowrey W, Weissfeld LA, Aizenstein HJ, McDade E, Mountz JM, et al. Classification of amyloid-positivity in controls: comparison of visual read and quantitative approaches. Neuroimage 2013;71:207–15.

[32] Edison P, Hinz R, Ramlackhansingh A, Thomas J, Gelosa G, Archer HA, et al. Can target-to-pons ratio be used as a reliable method for the analysis of [11C]PIB brain scans? Neuroimage 2012;60(3):1716–23.

[33] Aalto S, Scheinin NM, Kemppainen NM, Nagren K, Kailajarvi M, Leinonen M, et al. Reproducibility of automated simplified voxel-based analysis of PET amyloid ligand [11C]PIB uptake using 30-min scanning data. Eur J Nucl Med Mol Imaging 2009;36(10):1651–60.

[34] McNamee RL, Yee SH, Price JC, Klunk WE, Rosario B, Weissfeld L, et al. Consideration of optimal time window for Pittsburgh compound B PET summed uptake measurements. J Nucl Med 2009;50(3):348–55.

[35] Wong KP, Kepe V, Dahlbom M, Satyamurthy N, Small GW, Barrio JR, et al. Comparative evaluation of Logan and relative-equilibrium graphical methods for parametric imaging of dynamic [18F]FDDNP-PET determinations. Neuroimage 2012;60(1):241–51.

[36] Joshi A, Koeppe RA, Fessler JA. Reducing between scanner differences in multi-center PET studies. Neuroimage 2009;46(1):154–9.

[37] Frisoni GB, Laakso MP, Beltramello A, Geroldi C, Bianchetti A, Soininen H, et al. Hippocampal and entorhinal cortex atrophy in frontotemporal dementia and Alzheimer's disease. Neurology 1999;52(1):91–100.

[38] Meltzer CC, Kinahan PE, Greer PJ, Nichols TE, Comtat C, Cantwell MN, et al. Comparative evaluation of MR-based partial-volume correction schemes for PET. J Nucl Med 1999;40(12):2053–65.

[39] Erlandsson K, Buvat I, Pretorius PH, Thomas BA, Hutton BF. A review of partial volume correction techniques for emission tomography and their applications in neurology, cardiology and oncology. Phys Med Biol 2012;57(21):R119–59.

[40] Bousse A, Pedemonte S, Thomas BA, Erlandsson K, Ourselin S, Arridge S, et al. Markov random field and Gaussian mixture for segmented MRI-based partial volume correction in PET. Phys Med Biol 2012;57(20):6681–705.

[41] Muller-Gartner HW, Links JM, Prince JL, Bryan RN, McVeigh E, Leal JP, et al. Measurement of radiotracer concentration in brain gray matter using positron emission tomography: MRI-based correction for partial volume effects. J Cereb Blood Flow Metab 1992;12(4):571–83.

[42] Gutierrez D, Montandon ML, Assal F, Allaoua M, Ratib O, Lovblad KO, et al. Anatomically guided voxel-based partial volume effect correction in brain PET: impact of MRI segmentation. Comput Med Imaging Graph 2012;36(8):610–9.

[43] Samuraki M, Matsunari I, Chen WP, Yajima K, Yanase D, Fujikawa A, et al. Partial volume effect-corrected FDG-PET and grey matter volume loss in patients with mild Alzheimer's disease. Eur J Nucl Med Mol Imaging 2007;34(10):1658–69.

[44] Ibanez V, Pietrini P, Alexander GE, Furey ML, Teichberg D, Rajapakse JC, et al. Regional glucose metabolic abnormalities are not the result of atrophy in Alzheimer's disease. Neurology 1998;50(6):1585–93.

[45] Bokde AL, Teipel SJ, Drzezga A, Thissen J, Bartenstein P, Dong W, et al. Association between cognitive performance and cortical glucose metabolism in patients with mild Alzheimer's disease. Dement Geriatr Cogn Disord 2005;20(6):352–7.

[46] Thomas BA, Erlandsson K, Modat M, Thurfjell L, Vandenberghe R, Ourselin S, et al. The importance of appropriate partial volume correction for PET quantification in Alzheimer's disease. Eur J Nucl Med Mol Imaging 2011;38(6):1104–19.

[47] Edison P, Carter SF, Rinne JO, Gelosa G, Herholz K, Nordberg A, et al. Comparison of MRI-based and PET template-based approaches in the quantitative analysis of amyloid imaging with PIB-PET. Neuroimage 2013;70:423–33.

[48] Lopresti BJ, Klunk WE, Mathis CA, Hoge JA, Ziolko SK, Lu X, et al. Simplified quantification of Pittsburgh compound B amyloid imaging PET studies: a comparative analysis. J Nucl Med 2005;46(12):1959–72.

[49] Hoffman EJ, Cutler PD, Guerrero TM, Digby WM, Mazziotta JC. Assessment of accuracy of PET utilizing a 3-D phantom to simulate the activity distribution of [18F]fluorodeoxyglucose uptake in the human brain. J Cereb Blood Flow Metab 1991;11(2):A17–25.

[50] Geworski L, Knoop BO, de Wit M, Ivancevic V, Bares R, Munz DL. Multicenter comparison of calibration and cross calibration of PET scanners. J Nucl Med 2002;43(5):635–9.

[51] Boellaard R. Standards for PET image acquisition and quantitative data analysis. J Nucl Med 2009;50(Suppl. 1):11S–20S.

[52] Buhler P, Just U, Will E, Kotzerke J, van den Hoff J. An accurate method for correction of head movement in PET. IEEE Trans Med Imaging 2004;23(9):1176–85.

[53] Bloomfield PM, Spinks TJ, Reed J, Schnorr L, Westrip AM, Livieratos L, et al. The design and implementation of a motion correction scheme for neurological PET. Phys Med Biol 2003;48(8):959–78.

[54] Scheltens P, Leys D, Barkhof F, Huglo D, Weinstein HC, Vermersch P, et al. Atrophy of medial temporal lobes on MRI in "probable" Alzheimer's disease and normal ageing: diagnostic value and neuropsychological correlates. J Neurol Neurosurg Psychiatry 1992;55(10):967–72.

[55] Seab JP, Jagust WJ, Wong ST, Roos MS, Reed BR, Budinger TF. Quantitative NMR measurements of hippocampal atrophy in Alzheimer's disease. Magn Reson Med 1988;8(2):200–8.

[56] Ashburner J, Friston KJ. Voxel-based morphometry—the methods. Neuroimage 2000;11(6 Pt 1):805–21.

[57] Heckemann RA, Keihaninejad S, Aljabar P, Gray KR, Nielsen C, Rueckert D, et al. Automatic morphometry in Alzheimer's disease and mild cognitive impairment. Neuroimage 2011;56(4):2024–37.

[58] Busatto GF, Diniz BS, Zanetti MV. Voxel-based morphometry in Alzheimer's disease. Expert Rev Neurother 2008;8(11):1691–702.

[59] Klein A, Andersson J, Ardekani BA, Ashburner J, Avants B, Chiang MC, et al. Evaluation of 14 nonlinear deformation algorithms applied to human brain MRI registration. Neuroimage 2009;46(3):786–802.

[60] Teipel SJ, Born C, Ewers M, Bokde AL, Reiser MF, Moller HJ, et al. Multivariate deformation-based analysis of brain atrophy to predict Alzheimer's disease in mild cognitive impairment. Neuroimage 2007;38(1):13–24.

[61] Barnes J, Foster J, Boyes RG, Pepple T, Moore EK, Schott JM, et al. A comparison of methods for the automated calculation of volumes and atrophy rates in the hippocampus. Neuroimage 2008;40(4):1655–71.

[62] Canu E, McLaren DG, Fitzgerald ME, Bendlin BB, Zoccatelli G, Alessandrini F, et al. Microstructural diffusion changes are independent of macrostructural volume loss in moderate to severe Alzheimer's disease. J Alzheimers Dis 2010;19(3):963–76.

[63] Tournier JD, Mori S, Leemans A. Diffusion tensor imaging and beyond. Magn Reson Med 2011;65(6):1532–56.

[64] Taoka T, Iwasaki S, Sakamoto M, Nakagawa H, Fukusumi A, Myochin K, et al. Diffusion anisotropy and diffusivity of white matter tracts within the temporal stem in Alzheimer's disease: evaluation of the "tract of interest" by diffusion tensor tractography. AJNR Am J Neuroradiol 2006;27(5):1040–5.

[65] Zhang Y, Zhang J, Oishi K, Faria AV, Jiang H, Li X, et al. Atlas-guided tract reconstruction for automated and comprehensive examination of the white matter anatomy. Neuroimage 2010;52(4):1289–301.

[66] Gouw AA, Seewann A, Vrenken H, van der Flier WM, Rozemuller JM, Barkhof F, et al. Heterogeneity of white matter hyperintensities in Alzheimer's disease: postmortem quantitative MRI and neuropathology. Brain 2008;131(Pt. 12):3286–98.

[67] Schmierer K, Wheeler-Kingshott CA, Boulby PA, Scaravilli F, Altmann DR, Barker GJ, et al. Diffusion tensor imaging of post mortem multiple sclerosis brain. Neuroimage 2007;35(2):467–77.

[68] Ridha BH, Barnes J, van de Pol LA, Schott JM, Boyes RG, Siddique MM, et al. Application of automated medial temporal lobe atrophy scale to Alzheimer's disease. Arch Neurol 2007;64(6):849–54.

[69] Teipel SJ, Pruessner JC, Faltraco F, Born C, Rocha-Unold M, Evans A, et al. Comprehensive dissection of the medial temporal lobe in AD: measurement of hippocampus, amygdala, entorhinal, perirhinal and parahippocampal cortices using MRI. J Neurol 2006;253(6):794–800.

[70] Mak HK, Zhang Z, Yau KK, Zhang L, Chan Q, Chu LW. Efficacy of voxel-based morphometry with DARTEL and standard registration as imaging biomarkers in Alzheimer's disease patients and cognitively normal older adults at 3.0 Tesla MR imaging. J Alzheimers Dis 2011;23(4):655–64.

[71] Barnes J, Bartlett JW, van de Pol LA, Loy CT, Scahill RI, Frost C, et al. A meta-analysis of hippocampal atrophy rates in Alzheimer's disease. Neurobiol Aging 2009;30(11):1711–23.

[72] van de Pol LA, Barnes J, Scahill RI, Frost C, Lewis EB, Boyes RG, et al. Improved reliability of hippocampal atrophy rate measurement in mild cognitive impairment using fluid registration. Neuroimage 2007;34(3):1036–41.

[73] Wang L, Goldstein FC, Veledar E, Levey AI, Lah JJ, Meltzer CC, et al. Alterations in cortical thickness and white matter integrity in mild cognitive impairment measured by whole-brain cortical thickness mapping and diffusion tensor imaging. AJNR Am J Neuroradiol 2009;30(5):893–9.

[74] Zhang Y, Schuff N, Jahng GH, Bayne W, Mori S, Schad L, et al. Diffusion tensor imaging of cingulum fibers in mild cognitive impairment and Alzheimer disease. Neurology 2007;68(1):13–19.

[75] Hashimoto M, Kazui H, Matsumoto K, Nakano Y, Yasuda M, Mori E. Does donepezil treatment slow the progression of hippocampal atrophy in patients with Alzheimer's disease? Am J Psychiatry 2005;162(4):676–82.

[76] Wilkinson D, Fox NC, Barkhof F, Phul R, Lemming O, Scheltens P. Memantine and brain atrophy in Alzheimer's disease: a 1-year randomized controlled trial. J Alzheimers Dis 2012;29(2):459–69.

[77] Fox NC, Black RS, Gilman S, Rossor MN, Griffith SG, Jenkins L, et al. Effects of Abeta immunization (AN1792) on MRI measures of cerebral volume in Alzheimer's disease. Neurology 2005;64(9):1563–72.

[78] Kilimann I, Likitjaroen Y, Hampel H, Teipel S. Diffusion tensor imaging to determine effects of antidementive treatment on cerebral structural connectivity in Alzheimer's disease. Curr Pharm Des 2013.

[79] Clarkson MJ, Ourselin S, Nielsen C, Leung KK, Barnes J, Whitwell JL, et al. Comparison of phantom and registration scaling corrections using the ADNI cohort. Neuroimage 2009;47(4):1506–13.

[80] Gunter JL, Bernstein MA, Borowski BJ, Ward CP, Britson PJ, Felmlee JP, et al. Measurement of MRI scanner performance with the ADNI phantom. Med Phys 2009;36(6):2193–205.

[81] Jovicich J, Czanner S, Greve D, Haley E, van der Kouwe A, Gollub R, et al. Reliability in multi-site structural MRI studies: effects of gradient non-linearity correction on phantom and human data. Neuroimage 2006;30(2):436–43.

[82] Preboske GM, Gunter JL, Ward CP, Jack Jr. CR. Common MRI acquisition non-idealities significantly impact the output of the boundary shift integral method of measuring brain atrophy on serial MRI. Neuroimage 2006;30(4):1196–202.

[83] Sled JG, Zijdenbos AP, Evans AC. A nonparametric method for automatic correction of intensity nonuniformity in MRI data. IEEE Trans Med Imaging 1998;17(1):87–97.

[84] Kruggel F, Turner J, Muftuler LT. Impact of scanner hardware and imaging protocol on image quality and compartment volume precision in the ADNI cohort. Neuroimage 2010;49(3):2123–33.

[85] Wonderlick JS, Ziegler DA, Hosseini-Varnamkhasti P, Locascio JJ, Bakkour A, van der Kouwe A, et al. Reliability of MRI-derived cortical and subcortical morphometric measures: effects of pulse sequence, voxel geometry, and parallel imaging. Neuroimage 2009;44(4):1324–33.

[86] Leung KK, Clarkson MJ, Bartlett JW, Clegg S, Jack Jr CR, Weiner MW, et al. Robust atrophy rate measurement in Alzheimer's disease using multi-site serial MRI: tissue-specific intensity normalization and parameter selection. Neuroimage 2010;50(2):516–23.

[87] Byrum CE, MacFall JR, Charles HC, Chitilla VR, Boyko OB, Upchurch L, et al. Accuracy and reproducibility of brain and tissue volumes using a magnetic resonance segmentation method. Psychiatry Res 1996;67(3):215–34.

[88] Han X, Jovicich J, Salat D, van der Kouwe A, Quinn B, Czanner S, et al. Reliability of MRI-derived measurements of human cerebral cortical thickness: the effects of field strength, scanner upgrade and manufacturer. Neuroimage 2006;32(1):180–94.

[89] Jovicich J, Czanner S, Han X, Salat D, van der Kouwe A, Quinn B, et al. MRI-derived measurements of human subcortical, ventricular and intracranial brain volumes: Reliability effects of scan sessions, acquisition sequences, data analyses, scanner upgrade, scanner vendors and field strengths. Neuroimage 2009;46(1):177–92.

[90] Ewers M, Teipel SJ, Dietrich O, Schonberg SO, Jessen F, Heun R, et al. Multicenter assessment of reliability of cranial MRI. Neurobiol Aging 2006;27(8):1051–9.

[91] Schnack HG, van Haren NE, Brouwer RM, van Baal GC, Picchioni M, Weisbrod M, et al. Mapping reliability in multicenter MRI: voxel-based morphometry and cortical thickness. Hum Brain Mapp 2010;31(12):1967–82.

[92] Reig S, Sanchez-Gonzalez J, Arango C, Castro J, Gonzalez-Pinto A, Ortuno F, et al. Assessment of the increase in variability when combining volumetric data from different scanners. Hum Brain Mapp 2009;30(2):355–68.

[93] Stonnington CM, Tan G, Kloppel S, Chu C, Draganski B, Jack Jr CR, et al. Interpreting scan data acquired from multiple scanners: a study with Alzheimer's disease. Neuroimage 2008;39(3):1180–5.

[94] Teipel SJ, Ewers M, Wolf S, Jessen F, Kolsch H, Arlt S, et al. Multicentre variability of MRI-based medial temporal lobe volumetry in Alzheimer's disease. Psychiatry Res 2010;182(3):244–50.

[95] Dickerson BC, Fenstermacher E, Salat DH, Wolk DA, Maguire RP, Desikan R, et al. Detection of cortical thickness correlates of cognitive performance: Reliability across MRI scan sessions, scanners, and field strengths. Neuroimage 2008;39(1):10–18.

[96] Hua X, Gutman B, Boyle CP, Rajagopalan P, Leow AD, Yanovsky I, et al. Accurate measurement of brain changes in longitudinal MRI scans using tensor-based morphometry. Neuroimage 2011;57(1):5–14.

[97] Leow AD, Klunder AD, Jack Jr CR, Toga AW, Dale AM, Bernstein MA, et al. Longitudinal stability of MRI for mapping brain change using tensor-based morphometry. Neuroimage 2006;31(2):627–40.

[98] Jones DK. Precision and accuracy in diffusion tensor magnetic resonance imaging. Top Magn Reson Imaging 2010;21(2):87–99.

[99] Jezzard P. Correction of geometric distortion in fMRI data. Neuroimage 2012;62(2):648–51.

[100] Jezzard P, Barnett AS, Pierpaoli C. Characterization of and correction for eddy current artifacts in echo planar diffusion imaging. Magn Reson Med 1998;39(5):801–12.

[101] Jones DK. The effect of gradient sampling schemes on measures derived from diffusion tensor MRI: a Monte Carlo study. Magn Reson Med 2004;51(4):807–15.

[102] Ni H, Kavcic V, Zhu T, Ekholm S, Zhong J. Effects of number of diffusion gradient directions on derived diffusion tensor imaging indices in human brain. AJNR Am J Neuroradiol 2006;27(8):1776–81.

[103] Wang JY, Abdi H, Bakhadirov K, Diaz-Arrastia R, Devous Sr. MD. A comprehensive reliability assessment of quantitative diffusion tensor tractography. Neuroimage 2012;60(2):1127–38.

[104] Pfefferbaum A, Adalsteinsson E, Sullivan EV. Replicability of diffusion tensor imaging measurements of fractional anisotropy and trace in brain. J Magn Reson Imaging 2003;18(4):427–33.

[105] Cercignani M, Bammer R, Sormani MP, Fazekas F, Filippi M. Inter-sequence and inter-imaging unit variability of diffusion tensor MR imaging histogram-derived metrics of the brain in healthy volunteers. AJNR Am J Neuroradiol 2003;24(4):638–43.

[106] Vollmar C, O'Muircheartaigh J, Barker GJ, Symms MR, Thompson P, Kumari V, et al. Identical, but not the same: intra-site and inter-site reproducibility of fractional anisotropy measures on two 3.0T scanners. Neuroimage 2010;51(4):1384–94.

[107] Teipel SJ, Reuter S, Stieltjes B, Acosta-Cabronero J, Ernemann U, Fellgiebel A, et al. Multicenter stability of diffusion tensor imaging measures: a European clinical and physical phantom study. Psychiatry Res 2011;194(3):363–71.

[108] Zhu T, Hu R, Qiu X, Taylor M, Tso Y, Yiannoutsos C, et al. Quantification of accuracy and precision of multi-center DTI measurements: a diffusion phantom and human brain study. Neuroimage 2011;56(3):1398–411.

[109] Teipel SJ, Wegrzyn M, Meindl T, Frisoni G, Bokde AL, Fellgiebel A, et al. Anatomical MRI and DTI in the diagnosis of Alzheimer's disease: a European multicenter study. J Alzheimers Dis 2012;31(Suppl. 3):S33–47.

[110] Fischer FU, Scheurich A, Wegrzyn M, Schermuly I, Bokde AL, Kloppel S, et al. Automated tractography of the cingulate bundle in Alzheimer's disease: a multi-center DTI study. J Magn Reson Imaging 2012;36(1):84–91.

[111] Konrad C, Ukas T, Nebel C, Arolt V, Toga AW, Narr KL. Defining the human hippocampus in cerebral magnetic resonance images—an overview of current segmentation protocols. Neuroimage 2009;47(4):1185–95.

[112] Boccardi M, Ganzola R, Bocchetta M, Pievani M, Redolfi A, Bartzokis G, et al. Survey of protocols for the manual segmentation of the hippocampus: preparatory steps towards a joint EADC-ADNI harmonized protocol. J Alzheimers Dis 2011;26(Suppl. 3):61–75.

[113] Nestor SM, Gibson E, Gao FQ, Kiss A, Black SE. A direct morphometric comparison of five labeling protocols for multi-atlas driven automatic segmentation of the hippocampus in Alzheimer's disease. Neuroimage 2012;66C:50–70.

[114] Cuingnet R, Gerardin E, Tessieras J, Auzias G, Lehericy S, Habert MO, et al. Automatic classification of patients with Alzheimer's disease from structural MRI: a comparison of ten methods using the ADNI database. Neuroimage 2011;56(2):766–81.

[115] Matsuda H, Mizumura S, Nemoto K, Yamashita F, Imabayashi E, Sato N, et al. Automatic voxel-based morphometry of structural MRI by SPM8 plus diffeomorphic anatomic registration through exponentiated lie algebra improves the diagnosis of probable Alzheimer's Disease. AJNR Am J Neuroradiol 2012;33(6):1109–14.

[116] Davatzikos C, Xu F, An Y, Fan Y, Resnick SM. Longitudinal progression of Alzheimer's-like patterns of atrophy in normal older adults: the SPARE-AD index. Brain 2009;132(Pt. 8):2026–35.

[117] Vemuri P, Whitwell JL, Kantarci K, Josephs KA, Parisi JE, Shiung MS, et al. Antemortem MRI based STructural Abnormality iNDex (STAND)-scores correlate with postmortem Braak neurofibrillary tangle stage. Neuroimage 2008;42(2):559–67.

[118] Dickerson BC, Stoub TR, Shah RC, Sperling RA, Killiany RJ, Albert MS, et al. Alzheimer-signature MRI biomarker predicts AD dementia in cognitively normal adults. Neurology 2011;76(16):1395–402.

[119] Eggert LD, Sommer J, Jansen A, Kircher T, Konrad C. Accuracy and reliability of automated gray matter segmentation pathways on real and simulated structural magnetic resonance images of the human brain. PLoS One 2012;7(9):e45081.

[120] Shen Q, Zhao W, Loewenstein DA, Potter E, Greig MT, Raj A, et al. Comparing new templates and atlas-based segmentations in the volumetric analysis of brain magnetic resonance images for diagnosing Alzheimer's disease. Alzheimers Dement 2012;8(5):399–406.

[121] Jones DK, Cercignani M. Twenty-five pitfalls in the analysis of diffusion MRI data. NMR Biomed 2010;23(7):803–20.

[122] Jack Jr CR, Bernstein MA, Fox NC, Thompson P, Alexander G, Harvey D, et al. The Alzheimer's disease neuroimaging initiative (ADNI): MRI methods. J Magn Reson Imaging 2008;27(4):685–91.

V. STANDARDIZATION OF DIAGNOSTIC AND OUTCOME MEASURES

[123] Chalavi S, Simmons A, Dijkstra H, Barker GJ, Reinders AA. Quantitative and qualitative assessment of structural magnetic resonance imaging data in a two-center study. BMC Med Imaging 2012;12:27.

[124] Turner MR, Grosskreutz J, Kassubek J, Abrahams S, Agosta F, Benatar M, et al. Towards a neuroimaging biomarker for amyotrophic lateral sclerosis. Lancet Neurol 2011;10(5):400–3.

[125] Brau AC, Beatty PJ, Skare S, Bammer R. Comparison of reconstruction accuracy and efficiency among autocalibrating data-driven parallel imaging methods. Magn Reson Med 2008;59(2):382–95.

[126] Simmons A, Westman E, Muehlboeck S, Mecocci P, Vellas B, Tsolaki M, et al. MRI measures of Alzheimer's disease and the AddNeuroMed study. Ann N Y Acad Sci 2009;1180:47–55.

[127] Goto M, Abe O, Kabasawa H, Takao H, Miyati T, Hayashi N, et al. Effects of image distortion correction on voxel-based morphometry. Magn Reson Med Sci 2012;11(1):27–34.

[128] Acosta-Cabronero J, Williams GB, Pereira JM, Pengas G, Nestor PJ. The impact of skull-stripping and radio-frequency bias correction on grey-matter segmentation for voxel-based morphometry. Neuroimage 2008;39(4):1654–65.

[129] Littell RC, Milliken GA, Stroup WW, Wolfinger RD. SAS System for Mixed Models. Cary, NC, USA: SAS Institute Inc; 1996.

[130] Teipel SJ, Peters O, Heuser I, Jessen F, Maier W, Froelich L, et al. Atrophy outcomes in multicentre clinical trials on Alzheimer's disease: effect of different processing and analysis approaches on sample sizes. World J Biol Psychiatry 2011;12(Suppl. 1):109–13.

[131] Dyrba M, Ewers M, Wegrzyn M, Kilimann I, Plant C, Oswald A, et al. Automated detection of structural changes in Alzheimer's disease using multicenter DTI. PLoS One 2013 in press.

[132] Frisoni GB, Jack CR. Harmonization of magnetic resonance-based manual hippocampal segmentation: a mandatory step for wide clinical use. Alzheimers Dement 2011;7(2):171–4.

[133] Mori S, Oishi K, Jiang H, Jiang L, Li X, Akhter K, et al. Stereotaxic white matter atlas based on diffusion tensor imaging in an ICBM template. Neuroimage 2008;40(2):570–82.

[134] Thiebaut de Schotten M, Ffytche DH, Bizzi A, Dell'Acqua F, Allin M, Walshe M, et al. Atlasing location, asymmetry and inter-subject variability of white matter tracts in the human brain with MR diffusion tractography. Neuroimage 2011;54(1):49–59.

[135] Frisoni GB, Henneman WJ, Weiner MW, Scheltens P, Vellas B, Reynish E, et al. The pilot European Alzheimer's disease neuroimaging initiative of the european Alzheimer's disease consortium. Alzheimers Dement 2008;4(4):255–64.

[136] Westman E, Simmons A, Muehlboeck JS, Mecocci P, Vellas B, Tsolaki M, et al. AddNeuroMed and ADNI: similar patterns of Alzheimer's atrophy and automated MRI classification accuracy in Europe and North America. Neuroimage 2011;58(3):818–28.

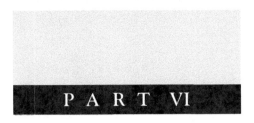

PART VI

OPERATIONALIZATION OF GLOBAL ALZHEIMER'S DISEASE TRIALS

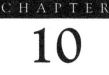

CHAPTER 10

Operationalization of Global Alzheimer's Disease Trials

Lynne Hughes[1] and Spencer Guthrie[2]

[1]Quintiles, Reading, Berkshire, UK [2]Genentech, Elan, Jansen Alzheimer's Immunotherapy and Ultragenyx Pharmaceutical, Novato, California, USA

10.1 INTRODUCTION: OVERVIEW OF ALZHEIMER'S DISEASE

10.1.1 Incidence and Prevalence

Alzheimer's disease (AD) is a devastating, progressive neurological disease that affects millions of people across the world. Alzheimer's Disease International estimates that 35.6 million people are living with dementia worldwide and that this number will increase to 115.4 million by 2050 [1,2]. By 2050, an estimated 1 in 85 persons worldwide will be living with the disease. It is estimated that about 43% of cases need a high level of care equivalent to that of a nursing home. If interventions could delay both disease onset and progression by a modest 1 year, there would be nearly 9.2 million fewer cases of disease in 2050, with nearly all the decline attributable to decreases in persons needing a high level of care [3].

The reported worldwide prevalence of dementia is 0.3–1.0/100 people in individuals aged 60–64 years, and increases to 42.3–68.3/100 people in individuals 95 years and older [4]. The incidence varies from 0.8–4.0/1,000 person years in people aged 60–64 years, and increases to 35.7–49.8/1,000 person years when the population is older than 95 years.

AD is the most common cause of dementia, accounting for 60–80% of dementia cases. In the United States, it is estimated that 5.3 million Americans suffer from dementia caused by AD, and that by 2050 the prevalence will double or triple unless effective treatment is found [1].

AD poses possibly the largest future medical challenge to developed countries and the challenge is also increasing in developing countries

M. Bairu & M.W. Weiner (Eds):
Global Clinical Trials for Alzheimer's Disease.
DOI: http://dx.doi.org/10.1016/B978-0-12-411464-7.00010-9

TABLE 10.1 Projection of AD Prevalence by Region and Disease Stage [1]

	Prevalence (in millions)					
	2006			2050		
	Overall	Early Stage	Late Stage	Overall	Early Stage	Late Stage
Africa	1.33	0.76	0.57	6.33	3.58	2.75
Asia	12.65	7.19	5.56	62.85	34.84	28.01
Europe	7.21	4.04	3.17	16.51	9.04	7.47
Latin Am. / Caribbean	2.03	1.14	0.89	10.85	5.99	4.86
North America	3.10	1.73	1.37	8.85	4.84	4.01
Oceania	0.23	0.13	0.10	0.84	0.46	0.38
Total	26.55	14.99	11.56	106.23	58.75	47.48

(Tables 10.1 and 10.2). Most people with dementia live in developing countries (60% in 2001, rising to 71% by 2040). Rates of increase are not uniform; numbers in developed countries are forecast to increase by 100% between 2001 and 2040, but by more than 300% in India, China, and their south Asian and western Pacific neighbors [5]. Thus, the LAMIC—the "low and middle income countries"—are expected to see the largest increase in the number of new cases of AD reported, which presents an ever-increasing burden on their healthcare systems.

Evidence from well-planned, representative epidemiological surveys is scarce in many regions. It is estimated that 24.3 million people have dementia today, with 4.6 million new cases of dementia every year (one new case every 7 seconds) [5]. The number of people affected is forecast to double every 20 years to 81.1 million by 2040.

10.1.2 Clinical Characteristics

Clinically, AD is a progressive neurodegenerative disorder characterized by cognitive impairment, behavioral disturbances, psychiatric symptoms, and, eventually, impairment of the activities of daily living. These clinical manifestations constitute the dementia syndrome. The main pathological hallmarks of the disease are senile plaques in the brain, containing beta-amyloid ($A\beta$) and neurofibrillary tangles (NFTs) composed of hyperphosphorylated tau protein. Although the pathogenesis of these plaques and tangles, and how they contribute to the clinical syndrome, remains to be fully elucidated, the leading hypothesis—the "amyloid cascade"—proposes that the driving force behind the disease

TABLE 10.2 Prevalence of AD vs Total Dementia Cases per Country [3]

Country	Total Population Per Country 2008	Calculated Actual AD Cases in 2005	Prevalence Eurodem*	Country	Total Population Per Country 2008	Calculated Actual AD Cases in 2005	Prevalence Eurodem
India	1,142,780,000	3,542,618	0.003	Germany	82,127,000	1,116,927	0.014
Japan	127,704,000	1,711,234	0.013	France	64,473,140	876,835	0.014
Australia	21,550,000	172,400	0.008	Italy	59,619,290	757,165	0.013
New Zealand	4,293,500	19,321	0.005	UK	61,186,000	673,046	0.011
South Africa	47,850,700	NA		Spain	46,063,500	626,464	0.014
Turkey	70,586,256	1,270,553	0.018	Netherlands	16,490,950	209,435	0.013
Russia	145,500,000	1,091,250	0.008	Belgium	10,666,866	144,003	0.014
Ukraine	46,191,022	586,626	0.013	Portugal	10,617,600	134,844	0.013
Poland	38,115,967	484,073	0.013	Sweden	9,248,805	117,460	0.013
Romania	21,528,600	273,413	0.013	Austria	8,340,924	105,930	0.013
Greece	11,215,000	142,431	0.013	Switzerland	7,689,100	97,652	0.013
Hungary	10,035,000	127,445	0.013	Denmark	5,506,000	69,926	0.013
Serbia	9,527,100	120,994	0.013	Finland	5,327,490	67,659	0.013
Czech Rep	10,446,157	107,595	0.010	Norway	4,802,050	60,986	0.013
Israel	7,373,000	100,273	0.014	Ireland	4,422,100	56,161	0.013
Bulgaria	7,640,238	86,335	0.011	Luxembourg	483,800	6,144	0.013
Slovakia	5,404,784	68,641	0.013	Iceland	319,765	4,061	0.013
Lithuania	3,361,100	42,686	0.013	Brazil	188,453,000	1,507,624	0.008
Latvia	2,268,000	28,804	0.013	Mexico	106,682,500	949,474	0.009
Slovenia	2,041,050	25,921	0.013	Colombia	44,660,000	397,474	0.009

(Continued)

TABLE 10.2 (Continued)

Country	Total Population Per Country 2008	Calculated Actual AD Cases in 2005	Prevalence Eurodem*
Estonia	1,340,600	17,026	0.013
Malta	410,600	5,215	0.013
Croatia	4,435,400	NA	
China	1,335,740,000	5,209,386	0.004
Hong Kong	9,960,000	38,844	0.004
Egypt	75,730,000	204,471	0.003
Lebanon	4,099,000	30,743	0.008
Jordan	5,924,000	NA	
Kuwait	2,851,000	NA	
Morocco	31,343,359	NA	
Saudi Arabia	24,735,000	NA	
Tunisia	10,327,000	NA	
UAE	4,380,000	NA	
USA	306,070,000	4,591,050	0.015
Canada	33,512,000	360,000	0.011

Country	Total Population Per Country 2008	Calculated Actual AD Cases in 2005	Prevalence Eurodem
Peru	28,750,770	241,506	0.008
Chile	16,850,000	149,965	0.009
Ecuador	13,867,761	123,423	0.009
Argentina	39,745,613	55,246	0.001
Costa Rica	4,468,000	39,765	0.009
Puerto Rico	3,991,000	30,132	0.008
Indonesia	229,005,000	503,811	0.002
Philippines	90,457,200	90,457	0.001
Korea	72,014,000	82,816	0.001
Malaysia	27,757,000	31,921	0.001
Taiwan	23,027,672	26,482	0.001
Singapore	4,839,400	5,565	0.001
Thailand	63,038,247	NA	0.001

*Eurodem Prevalence Data and http://www.alz.co.uk/adi/pdf/prevalence.pdf

process is the accumulation of Aβ resulting from an imbalance between Aβ production and Aβ clearance in the brain [6]. Biomarker and clinicopathologic studies suggest that the disease process commences 10–20 years prior to the onset of symptoms, and some of the early pathological findings include the deposition of neocortical neuritic plaques and mesial temporal NFTs followed years later by neocortical NFTs [7].

Aβ peptides are generated from the amyloid precursor protein [8]. Several Aβ isoforms of up to 43 amino acids exist (e.g., Aβ40, Aβ42). These peptides have a variable tendency to aggregate into higher order forms, from soluble monomers and oligomers to insoluble plaques [9]. In particular, Aβ42 and pyroglutamate-Aβ, an amino-terminally truncated species beginning at glutamate 3 or 11, have a higher tendency to aggregate and account for the majority of the Aβ deposits found in the brains of patients with AD [10,11]. Evidence suggests that both soluble and insoluble forms of Aβ contribute to neuronal dysfunction [12,13].

Diagnosis of AD is discussed in detail in several major publications [14,15,16,17].

10.2 SIGNIFICANT CLINICAL TRIALS WITH POTENTIAL DISEASE-MODIFYING DRUGS

There have been a significant number of Phase II and Phase III trials testing potential disease-modifying drugs (DMDs) in AD over the past 8 to 10 years. These trials have tested thousands of patients across many countries.

Alzheimer's DMD development has been driven mainly by the amyloid hypothesis, and most trials conducted in the past 10 years have targeted Aβ. Aβ peptides derive from amyloid precursor protein (APP) by proteolytic cleavage (by β-secretases and γ-secretases) via the amyloidogenic pathway. The amyloid hypothesis has undergone an evolution in terms of the type of Aβ thought to play the most important role in AD. The focus was initially on removing the hard plaques, but studies have not shown that removing plaques will reverse the damage or stop the Alzheimer's dementia. The focus has shifted to oligomers, monomers and other forms of soluble Aβ. There have also been a number of Aβ approaches that have not shown meaningful clinical effects in trials.

10.2.1 Active Immunotherapy

The first of the approaches that garnered much attention was active vaccination against Aβ. In a Phase II trial of AN-1792 (QS-21), an anti-Aβ vaccine, in patients with mild-to-moderate AD, patients responded to immunization with Aβ1–42, developing significant Aβ-antibody titers.

However, this study was stopped because of aseptic meningoencepha-litis in some patients, which was attributed to cytotoxic T cells and/or autoimmune reactions to AN-1792.

Analyses of the z-score composite across the neuropsychological test battery (NTB) revealed differences favoring antibody responders (0.03 +/− 0.37 vs −0.20 +/− 0.45; p = 0.020). In the small subset of subjects who had cerebrospinal fluid (CSF) examinations, CSF tau was decreased in antibody responders (n = 11) vs placebo subjects (n = 10; p < 0.001). Upon autopsy, some of the AN-1792 subjects did show significant loss of amyloid plaque. However, due to the encephalitis, development was stopped.

Several other active vaccines are now in development. These treatments have developed strategies to induce Aβ-specific antibodies without stimulating T cells. ACC-001, CAD-106 and AD02 are three active vaccines that are currently being tested in Phase II trials.

A trial of AN1792 enrolled 290 subjects in the United States, and one involving ACC-001 enrolled >500 subjects across the US, Western Europe and Japan. A trial of CAD-106 enrolled around 200 subjects in US, Canada and Western Europe. One for AD02 enrolled about 350 subjects in Western and Eastern Europe. The vast majority of the subjects in active vaccines trials to date were enrolled in the US and Western Europe.

10.2.2 Passive Immunotherapy

Passive immunotherapy is based on monoclonal antibodies targeting Aβ to directly remove it or to promote its clearance. Several compounds have been or are being tested in patients with AD, such as: solanezumab (LY-2062430), bapineuzumab (AAB-001), gantenerumab (R-1450), cren-ezumab (MABT-5102A), AAB-003, GSK-933776, and several others in early phase.

Bapineuzumab is a humanized anti-Aβ monoclonal antibody that binds to all toxic forms of Aβ. A significant side effect, called vasogenic edema (VE) or amyloid related imaging abnormality (ARIA), was dis-covered in the bapineuzumab program. The side effect caused inflam-mation and brain swelling in 10–20% of subjects and is hypothesized to be caused by the leaking of vessels due to removal of amyloid plaque. This side effect was shown to be dose dependent and limited the dose of bapineuzumab that could be given to the subjects. The sponsor had to discontinue its highest dose during the Phase III trial. The Phase III tri-als did not meet their primary endpoints and the bapineuzumab intrave-nous administration program has been discontinued. One subcutaneous (SC) administration trial of bapineuzumab is still ongoing.

Carriers of ApoE—a genotype at increased risk of AD—and non-carriers were split into two separate development programs for bapineuzumab, making the development program double the size of other programs to date. Some 4,500 subjects were enrolled in the bapineuzumab program globally. Although most subjects were enrolled in North America and Western Europe, patients were also enrolled in Japan, Eastern Europe, South Africa and South America. The Phase III program utilized more than 400 clinical sites globally and took around three years to fully recruit.

Solanezumab has gone through a large development program that began in Phase I in 2004 and Phase III trials were completed and results announced in September 2012. Solanezumab is a monoclonal antibody that selectively binds to soluble Aβ to promote Aβ clearance. Solanezumab has also gone through a large development program that began in Phase I in 2006; Phase III trials were completed and results announced in October 2012. VE or ARIA was not a substantial side effect seen with solanezumab, although it was seen in the trials. The Phase III trials did not meet their primary endpoints. However, the study did meet its endpoints for a pre-specified mild AD meta-analysis, and the sponsor plans to continue the program.

Around 2,200 subjects were enrolled in the solanezumab program globally, including North and South America, Western and Eastern Europe, and Asia. The solanezumab Phase III program—which was initiated 18 months after the bapineuzumab program—used a more global strategy, utilizing fewer sites overall, a lower percentage of US and Western European sites, and utilizing emerging countries such as Taiwan, Korea, Brazil and Russia. The strategy appears to have paid off, as the studies completed enrollment in about 18 months and utilized fewer than 200 clinical sites globally.

Several other passive immunotherapies are now in development. Developers of these treatments have devised strategies to dose higher while limiting the effect on vascular Aβ, and hopefully limited VE or ARIA. Three monoclonal antibodies, gantenerumab (R-1450), crenezumab (MABT-5102A), and AAB-003, are currently being tested in Phase II trials.

10.2.3 Gamma-secretase Inhibitors and Modulators

γ-secretase, the enzyme responsible for the final step in Aβ generation, is one of the main complexes involved in intramembranous cleavage of several proteins, including APP and Notch receptor. Development of γ-secretase inhibitors is difficult because this enzyme has many substrates. γ-secretase inhibitors have had several significant side effects thought to be related to the impact on the Notch signaling pathway, such as hematological and gastrointestinal toxicity, skin reactions, and changes to hair color.

Several compounds have been or are being tested in patients with AD, such as tarenflurbil, semagacestat (LY-450139), MK-0752, E-2012, BMS-708163, PF-3084014, begacestat (GSI-953), ELND006, and NIC5-15.

Flurizan® (tarenflurbil) was the first of this class to be tested in Phase III. Tarenflurbil is not a direct inhibitor of γ-secretase, but belongs to a group of agents known as selective β-amyloid-lowering agents (SALAs). Tarenflurbil was tested in Phase III randomized clinical trials (RCTs) in patients with mild AD, but did not show clinical effects, possibly due to low γ-secretase modulator potency, poor CNS penetration, or inhibition of microglia-mediated Aβ clearance by residual non-steroidal anti-inflammatory drug (NSAID) activity.

Semagacestat is a direct inhibitor of γ-secretase, reduces Aβ concentrations in the plasma and Aβ production in the CNS. Phase III trials for the Notch-inhibiting drug, semagacestat, did not meet its primary endpoints. In fact, findings showed that semagacestat not only failed to slow disease progression, but was also associated with worsening of clinical measures of cognition and the ability to perform the activities of daily living, and a higher incidence of skin cancer in the treatment group than the placebo group.

Other more selective γ-secretase inhibitors and modulators have been developed and tested, such as BMS-708163 and PF-3084014, but those have also suffered from collateral side effects due to Notch. At least seven γ-secretase inhibitors have discontinued development.

10.2.4 β-secretase Inhibitors

β-secretase (also known as the β-site amyloid protein precursor (APP)-cleaving enzyme, BACE1) initiates the amyloidogenic pathway. This pathway is also challenging due to β-secretase affecting other substrates which may also cause collateral damage. Most of the work here has been focused on how to make these compounds more selective.

No Phase III programs with β-secretase inhibitors have started, but there are several programs now moving into Phase II, such as MK-8931 and LY2886721. The MK-8931 trial is an adaptive Phase II/III trial and aims to enroll more than 1,900 subjects.

10.2.5 Aβ Anti-Aggregants

Compounds that inhibit Aβ aggregation or destabilize Aβ oligomeric species can act by either binding to Aβ monomers, thereby preventing oligomerization and allowing Aβ elimination, or by reacting with Aβ oligomers, thereby neutralizing their toxicity and promoting their clearance.

Despite promising preclinical and Phase II studies, tramiprosate (homotaurine, Alzhemed; a small orally administered compound that binds preferentially to soluble $A\beta$, maintaining it in non-fibrillar form) did not show clinical efficacy in a North American Phase III RCT (Alphase study) in patients with mild to moderate AD.

Scyllo-inositol (ELND-005), an orally administered stereoisomer of inositol, crosses the blood–brain barrier using inositol transporters. Scyllo-inositol is thought to bind to $A\beta$, modulate its misfolding, inhibit its aggregation, and promote dissociation of aggregates. Scyllo-inositol failed to meet its endpoints in a Phase II RCT.

Clioquinol (PBT1), an inhibitor of $A\beta$ aggregation that works by interfering with interactions between copper and zinc, showed encouraging results in Phase II RCTs, but manufacturing problems (high concentrations of toxic di-iodo impurity) stalled further development. PBT2 is a second-generation inhibitor of metal-induced $A\beta$ aggregation that is orally administered and has a greater blood–brain barrier permeability than clioquinol does. It is currently in Phase II development.

Although there have been many recent failures in Phase II and Phase III AD programs (Table 10.3), the field is encouraged by new ways to diagnose patients, and new and improved ways of targeting $A\beta$ and other pathways. It will take a significant number of new trial centers and trial subjects to test all of these new therapies and ultimately get to an approved treatment.

TABLE 10.3   Major Phase III DMD AD Programs in the Past Eight Years

Compound	AB Strategy	Last Phase of Development	N (Subjects)	Number of Countries Utilized	Result
Tramisrosate	Anti-Aβ aggregation	3	~2000	12	Did not meet endpoints
Tarenflurbil	γ-secretase	3	~2500	12	Did not meet endpoints
Dimebon	NA	3	~1500	9	Did not meet endpoints
Semagacestat	γ-secretase	3	~2000	33	Did not meet endpoints
Bapineuzumab	Passive antibody	3	~4500	27	Did not meet endpoints
Solanezumab	Passive antibody	3	~2200	17	Did not meet endpoints
Number of subjects utilized			~14,000		

10.3 CHALLENGES AND OPPORTUNITIES SEEN WITH GLOBAL ALZHEIMER'S CLINICAL TRIALS

10.3.1 Variability with Diagnosis/Patient Selection

The data from recently completed clinical trials using bapineuzimab and solaneuzumab have raised an interesting point for consideration for future trials which utilize an amyloid-targeting product as a potential DMD. These trials showed that approximately one-third of subjects recruited into these trials tested negatively for amyloid when assessed using AV-45 (Amyvid®, Lilly) or PET-PIB. Thus, these subjects had signs and symptoms consistent with the diagnosis of mild to moderate AD, but did not appear to have an amyloid-based AD.

As a result, a significant number of new trials using potential DMDs are now requesting that potential subjects have demonstrable amyloid before they are progressed through to randomization, usually via a PET scan. This places further burden on both sites and subjects, as well as on the sponsor company, as up to one-third of subjects undergoing this procedure will fail at this stage—further increasing the costs to the sponsor.

In addition, this request could limit the number of available sites and countries that are able to participate in these next stages of global AD trials, due to lack of availability of a PET scanner or, more likely, due to the geographical locations of the distribution depots of the amyloid ligand being used. Some PET ligand manufacturers, e.g., GE (flutametamol), are willing to audit a site's GMP labeling facility to ensure that it is acceptable and then provide the cold ligand to the site for local labeling and quality control. They then provide support to the sites as needed. This approach would enable many sites in Eastern European countries to be further involved in DMD trials, as this is often the rate-limiting factor. The majority of countries do have access to a PET scanner.

10.3.2 Patient Endpoints: Symptomatic Therapies

The endpoints in mild to moderate AD trials are generally all similar, with the majority being changes on the Alzheimer's Disease Assessment Scale-cognitive portion (ADAS-Cog) and a functional or global scale, at various time points—and these range from 3 to 18 months in treatment duration.

If a trial is designed as a pure placebo-controlled trial (i.e., not as an add-on to another agent such as Aricept®), then, practically speaking, it should last three months or less, as it is unlikely to be approved for a longer period, and there will also be challenges in recruiting subjects. However, sponsors may be concerned with a short duration in case the trial endpoints are not met within this timeframe. Even a trial of only three months' duration may have limited country approvals. In addition, even if such a pure placebo trial is approved, then it is critical to select appropriate sites that will recruit subjects. At the majority of global sites, subjects have several trials to choose from and will typically select the one that ultimately presents them with the best opportunity for a measurable and prolonged response. Where possible in such situations, it is recommended that the trial be followed by an open-label extension, where those subjects who were assigned to the placebo arm have an opportunity for therapy—whether it is the investigational product or an approved AD medication.

Depending on the mechanism of action of the investigational product, it is becoming commonplace to see trials with symptomatic products being used in an "add-on" setting as additional therapy to stable AD therapy, most usually Aricept (donepezil) or other acetyl cholinesterase inhibitors. Such trials are easily accepted in a placebo-controlled setting, as the subject is still receiving "standard of care," compliance is usually good, and recruitment is fairly predictable. The protocol-mandated dose of donepezil is important—the majority of subjects with mild disease will be on a dose of 10 mg; however, as the disease progresses, it is commonplace to see the higher doses being prescribed, although to date only the US has the 23 mg Aricept dose approved.

Of note, in a number of countries in Eastern Europe, a subject might well have utilized their healthcare providers' limit for reimbursement of donepezil by the time their Mini Mental State Examination (MMSE) score decreases to below 20. At this stage, they would need to pay for additional treatment themselves and thus any trial-related request for stable background therapy could be a challenge for some subjects. Provision of the requested add-on therapy by the sponsoring company will expand the potential number of subjects available to the trial in this region.

The endpoints are scale assessments—we rarely see biomarkers involved—and there can be a range of scales used at varying time points over the lifespan of the trial.

10.3.3 Disease-Modifying Drugs

The aim of trials involving DMDs is to show a decrease in the rate of progression of the subjects' AD and thus there is often a more complex design applied to these trials. In addition, the costs of these trials to the sponsor company are usually significantly higher than for a trial utilizing a symptomatic therapy, due to the additional biomarker assessments required and the longer duration of the trials.

There are several specific challenges with these trials, in particular working with the subject and caregiver to ensure that the subject does not drop out of the trial due to a perceived "non-response;" due to the likely mode of action of these products, we do not expect to see an easily recognizable symptomatic response, but rather a slowing down of disease progression. This also leads to longer studies than for symptomatic agents, which must be explained to the caregiver and family so that they remain motivated to ensure that subjects remain in the trial. This is a critical factor for the successful retention of subjects, and time spent educating site staff appropriately will be reflected in better retention rates.

In addition, trials involving potential DMDs nearly always involve biomarker assessments as an integral part. Thus, it is critical to select those sites with proven high compliance with biomarkers, in particular, with the ever-increasing request for lumbar punctures (LPs). The "usual" biomarker assessments involve LPs, MRIs and PET imaging with some amyloid ligand or fluorodeoxyglucose (FDG). It is critical to ensure that these biomarker assessments are performed on an ongoing basis and that there are at least two measures per subject for each biomarker. In order to achieve this, it is imperative to select the sites carefully and ensure that the principal investigators fully appreciate the importance of compliance, and work with the subject and caregiver to achieve the highest level possible.

Use of a central imaging provider is almost always required for these trials in order to provide an unbiased and masked interpretation of the imaging data to the regulators. Contract research organizations (CROs) and pharmaceutical companies have successfully incorporated all countries in DMD trials to varying extents and these have been mostly limited by the availability of a PET scanner, or ligand, rather than an MRI scanner.

Of note, Hughes et al. [18] has observed that MRI compliance is higher when there is an on-site imaging facility. If subjects need to travel to an off-site imaging facility, then there is a lower compliance with this biomarker assessment.

10.3.4 Rater Training

For any AD trial or program to meet its goals, all study scales must be administered uniformly and consistently across all sites in all countries. Experience has shown three key factors that require special management on AD trials: robust and consistent training for raters and Clinical Research Associates (CRAs); completion of worksheets and case report form transcription; and staff turnover at sites. All of these factors can contribute to inconsistent rating. In addition, continuous "real time" (or as close to this as possible) monitoring of scale data throughout the lifespan of the clinical trial will help identify inconsistencies at an early stage and thus permit retraining as required.

Training includes rater training and assurance of inter-rater reliability. This training brings all raters closer to the "gold standard" norm, although it cannot guarantee 100% consistency. However, the objective is to identify those raters at either extreme of the curve. To succeed in these objectives, the following options should be considered:

- Rater training, testing, and/or certification on primary scales at investigator meetings
- Tapes sent by mail (to sites for rater test and/or from sites for expert evaluation)
- Visits to sites by expert consultants or trained professionals
- Follow-up rater skills assessment at predetermined intervals
- Web-based rater training methods
- On-site training/follow-up if there is rater turnover at the site.

Effective implementation of an inter-rater reliability training program involves the selection of a qualified expert in the desired assessment scale. Copyrights and/or usage fees associated with certain scales must also be understood and taken into account in planning. Principal investigators must also pre-select qualified raters from their existing staff members and verify their availability for the investigator meeting, as well as for the duration of the program. It is becoming more commonplace for a sponsor company to request that for a site to be qualified for trial participation they need two or more raters trained and available for the trial, placing an additional burden on the sites.

It is also critical that each CRA understands how to score properly, reviews the worksheets carefully for proper completion, and makes sure the scores are correctly transcribed to the Case Report Form (CRF). Thus, they will be trained in methods similar to the investigators on the rating scales to ensure consistency.

For rater training, local language training may aid comprehension and result in more consistent data. The majority of the scales are now available in many languages and have been fully validated and translated by their owners before being released to the sponsor company.

In terms of scale fatigue—either by the subject or the rater—we are not aware of objective data on the number of scales and duration of scale assessments that an AD subject can undertake and still provide a reliable, consistent and robust outcome. Neither have we seen objective data with regards to the "learning" effect of scale completion, although we are aware of such concerns.

We would always recommend that a subject completes the scale(s) that represent the primary outcome of the trial first, that the scales are administered in a set order and that imaging modalities—which may upset the subject—are performed after the scale assessments. It is often suggested that the LP procedure is performed on a separate day to the scale assessments, preferably afterwards, in order to not have any bias from any anxiety or distress from the LP itself, which could affect the completion of the scales.

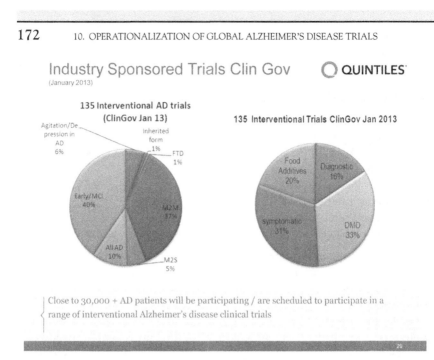

FIGURE 10.1   Planned AD subjects for all clinical trials.

10.3.5 Recruitment/Competition

The pie charts in Figure 10.1 show the split of interventional trials (as of January 2013, extrapolated from Clinicatrials.gov). The first chart shows the split between the various stages of AD, illustrating a shift towards earlier stage AD trials and then the mild to moderate stage. There are some 30,000 AD subjects targeted at this time for inclusion in interventional trials, the majority of who will have early-to-moderate AD. The second chart shows how the class of interventional product is distributed across this large cohort of subjects. There is approximately the same percentage of trials scheduled or ongoing using potential DMDs as there are symptomatic trials.

Thus, in order to achieve the interventional trial burden as shown above, it will be critical to ensure there are sufficient countries and sites available to conduct these concurrently. The high percentage of DMD trials will saturate available sites and countries that have easy access to the required biomarker equipment, i.e., PET scanners, and ready availability of the PET ligand and MRIs. In particular, if the trend of only recruiting subjects who are amyloid positive at screening continues, this will also limit a number of sites and countries in Eastern Europe and other regions due to the currently limited availability of some of the PET ligands in these regions. However, there are also significant numbers of planned and ongoing trials using symptomatic products, and these trials will rely on robust recruitment from other regions to achieve timelines. Thus, it is important to ensure that we continue to develop new and emerging sites and countries, as these are also the regions that are predicted to see the highest increase in AD subjects and thus caregiver and healthcare burden.

10.4 NEW CHALLENGES

As AD trials have become increasingly complicated, there are several logistical concerns that will need to be addressed. Due to the concern with patient selection, biomarkers are being used more frequently as selection criteria in clinical trials. For a therapy targeting beta-amyloid (Aβ), it makes a lot of sense to ensure that Aβ is present. Until recently, this was not possible in clinical trials. With the advent and increased use of the new radioligands, and increased use of cerebrospinal fluid (CSF), the reality of Aβ testing for patient selection is now being realized. While this should lead to more efficient use of trial subjects and less variable results, it poses significant hurdles to the operational management of trials.

To use amyloid PET as an inclusion/exclusion test, sponsors will have to select PET centers along with their primary clinical sites for participation in the trials. While the methods of selecting clinical sites for AD treatment trials are well established, this is not so clear for PET centers. There are a significant number of AD clinical investigators with years of AD trial experience, who are well known in the field and have developed a good staff of pharmacists, study coordinators, sub-investigators and raters. However, few of these centers have developed relationships (either working or contractually) with sophisticated PET centers. This requires that sponsors qualify PET centers to be used in concert with a given clinical center. The staff needed to qualify a PET center goes beyond the normal CRA role of ensuring trial experience, appropriate staff, good records, and good clinical practice (GCP) training. It requires technical experience with imaging, assessing PET scanners, and ensuring proper acquisition methods. In some areas, a PET center may service more than one clinical site. The PET centers often require their own contracts with the sponsor, as well as separate regulatory paperwork and sometimes separate institutional review boards (IRBs)/ethics committees (ECs). In other words, aligning a PET center with a clinical site takes additional resources and an additional level of knowledge and understanding.

Another challenge to using amyloid PET as an inclusion/exclusion test is ensuring that the radioligand is available in close proximity to the clinical site. For instance, C-11 PIB has a short half-life and must be produced on-site where it is administered. This requires use of a cyclotron, which are rather rare and generally found only at top university hospitals. There are also logistical challenges in manufacturing and delivering the radioligand to the patient in a short timeframe. F-18 radioligands, such as florbetapir and flutemetamol, have a longer half-life and can be manufactured off-site and transported to the clinic within a few hours. It is much easier to use these compounds in trials that require many subjects, as it is possible to reach more clinical sites. However, these manufacturing centers still need to be within a four hour drive of the clinical sites. The product could be flown, but is too cost-prohibitive.

Over the past couple of years, both flutemetamol and florbetapir have become widely available in the US and Western Europe, allowing trials using PET for inclusion/exclusion to be conducted there. However, the agents are less readily available in other regions and there have been no trials to date conducted outside of the US and Western Europe using amyloid PET as a selection test. Another concern for emerging markets is access to adequate PET scanners for the amyloid scan. As more compounds are tested for AD, and the need to enroll patients more selectively increases, the availability of such compounds and technology will need to expand greatly.

Some of the same concerns also relate to availability and qualification of MRI imaging facilities. MRIs are used at baseline in almost all AD trials in an attempt to exclude subjects with other comorbidities, such as stroke or other causes of cognitive decline. In trials using Aβ immunization, patients are being excluded if they have too many microhemorrhages or significant amounts of leaky blood vessels, in order to protect against possible effects of VE or ARIA. Volumetric MRIs may also be utilized for quantitative analysis of the effect of the agent on brain volume. The appropriate MRI technology is needed to ensure that the right subjects are being enrolled safely. In many cases, the MRI imaging facility is also a separate entity to the clinical site, and will need to be independently qualified and contracted. As with PET centers, this requires technical experience from the qualifier. In trials using MRI and PET, sometimes the MRI imaging facility, PET center and clinical site comprise three separate entities, and effective coordination is paramount. As with PET centers, there is a need for the expansion of MRI technology into emerging markets to more effectively expand the use of clinical sites and gain access to larger populations.

10.4.1 Treatment-Naïve Mild Cognitive Impairment/Early AD/ Prodromal AD patients

These trials are extremely challenging in terms of identifying suitable subjects for trial inclusion. Prodromal Alzheimer's disease (pAD)/mild cognitive impairment (MCI) symptoms are prevalent in the community, but patients do not self-identify with these conditions [18]. In surveys conducted to date by Quintiles via the on-line patient community, MediGuard.org., no patients have ever self-reported a diagnosis of pAD and only 5% have reported a diagnosis of MCI [18]. Rather, they seem to align with the symptoms they experience. Types of symptoms most commonly mentioned include: less interest in hobbies/activities (16%), daily problems with thinking/memory (12%), problems with judgment (e.g., making decisions) (10%), trouble remembering appointments (9%), repeating the same things (8%), trouble handling financial affairs (7%), trouble learning how to use a tool/gadget/appliance (7%), and forgetting the month/day/year (3%). Of the patients reporting at least one symptom, only 15% were being treated for cognitive functioning.

Only 30% of patients experiencing at least one symptom have visited a physician, suggesting a large available pool of community-based patients for a pAD/MCI study [18]. Due to the fact that these patients are not identified, even within a primary care physician's office, supplemental patient recruitment through digital outreach is critical to the successful enrolment of these studies.

In common with AD patients, the potential for LP and other procedures, as well as the study time commitment, are primary concerns in pAD/MCI patients. Across the pAD/MCI surveys conducted to date, around 40% of patients would not participate in a study requiring an LP, making this study element one of the highest of any non-physician-related factor ever tested by Quintiles. In general, the study time commitment is an issue as well, with 15–20% not interested in participating due to the study length (often three years), the number of visits, and the duration of the visit. Developing a patient study aid that clearly explains the potential benefit of the study medication, and the crucial role that the LPs and other procedures play in the drug development process will prove useful in educating patients. One patient put it this way: "I would explain in general terms about the [lumbar punctures] and how it will help people down the road."

This challenge is seen not only in sites in Western Europe and the US, but also across all sites globally that are involved in recruitment to pAD trials. The screen failure rate is extremely high—especially if subjects are required to have a positive amyloid burden at this stage—and the main source of subjects can be via digital outreach.

10.4.2 AD Trials are More Expensive than Ever

The costs of conducting a trial using a potential DMD product—including MRIs, PET imaging, LPs and scale administration—can be significantly higher than for a symptomatic trial, which utilizes scales as the primary endpoint and is usually of a shorter duration. The costs per patient can be up to four times higher for DMD trials [18] and thus it is critical to ensure that every subject recruited not only meets the required entry criteria but is also able to undergo all the necessary assessments and imaging modalities.

In addition, many sponsors are looking at other endpoints which require a significantly lower number of subjects in order to determine a response to treatment, e.g., changes in brain volume. However, until a sponsor undertakes such a trial—with the full support of the regulatory agencies—then it is up to the pharma company and CRO (as indicated) to work with the countries and sites to determine the best options for timely recruitment, quality subjects, confirmed diagnosis of subjects, and high quality data.

References

[1] Alzheimer's Association Alzheimer's disease facts and figures. Alzheimers Dement 2010;6(2):158–94.
[2] Wimo A, Prince P. World Alzheimer Report 2010: The global economic impact of dementia. Alzheimer's Disease International, London, 2010. London.
[3] Brookmeyer R, Johnson E, Ziegler-Graham K, Arrighi HM. Forecasting the global burden of Alzheimer's Disease. Johns Hopkins University, Department of Biostatistics Working Paper; January 2007. Available at: <http://biostats.bepress.com/jhubiostat/paper130/>.
[4] Fratiglioni L, De Ronchi D, Agüero-Torres H. Worldwide prevalence and incidence of dementia. Drugs Aging 1999;15(5):365–75.
[5] Ferri CP, Prince M, Brayne C, Brodaty H, Fratiglioni L, Ganguli, M, et al. Disease International Global prevalence of dementia: a Delphi consensus study. Lancet 2005;366(9503):2112–7. doi:10.1016/S0140-6736(05)67889-0.
[6] Hardy J, Selkoe DJ. The amyloid hypothesis of Alzheimer's disease: progress and problems on the road to therapeutics. Science 2002;297(5580):353–6.
[7] Nelson PT, Abner EL, Schmitt FA, Kryscio RJ, Jicha GA, Santacruz K, et al. Brains with medial temporal lobe neurofibrillary tangles but no neuritic amyloid plaques are a diagnostic dilemma but may have pathogenetic aspects distinct from Alzheimer disease. J Neuropathol Exp Neurol 2009;68(7):774–84.
[8] Querfurth HW, LaFerla FM. Mechanisms of disease: Alzheimer's disease. N Engl J Med 2010;362(4):329–44. Available at: <http://www.nejm.org/doi/full/10.1056/NEJMra0909142>.
[9] Hampel H, Shen Y, Walsh DM, Aisen P, Shaw LM, Zetterberg H, et al. Biological markers of amyloid beta-related mechanisms in Alzheimer's disease. Exp Neurol 2010;223(2):334–46.
[10] Gunn AP, Masters CL, Cherny RA. Pyroglutamate-Abeta: role in the natural history of Alzheimer's disease. Int J Biochem Cell Biol 2010;42(12):1915–8.
[11] Guntert A, Dobeli H, Bohrmann B. High sensitivity analysis of amyloid-beta peptide composition in amyloid deposits from human and PS2APP mouse brain. Neuroscience 2006;143(2):461–75.
[12] Meyer-Luehmann M, Mielke M, Spires-Jones TL, Stoothoff W, Jones P, Bacskai BJ, et al. A reporter of local dendritic translocation shows plaque-related loss of neural system function in APP-transgenic mice. J Neurosci 2009;29(40):12636–12640.

[13] Shankar GM, Li S, Mehta TH, Garcia-Munoz A, Shepardson NE, Smith I, et al. Amyloid-beta protein dimers isolated directly from Alzheimer's brains impair synaptic plasticity and memory. Nat Med 2008;14(8):837–42.

[14] McKhann G, Drachman D, Folstein M, Katzman R, Price D, Stadlan EM. Clinical diagnosis of Alzheimer's disease: report of the NINCDS-ADRDA work group under the auspices of the department of health and human services task force on Alzheimer's disease. Neurology 1984;34:939–44.

[15] Dubois B, Feldman HH, Jacova C, Dekosky ST, Barberger-Gateau P, Cummings J, et al. Research criteria for the diagnosis of Alzheimer's disease: revising the NINCDS-ADRDA criteria. Lancet Neurol 2007;6(8):734–46.

[16] Dubois B, Feldman HH, Jacova C, Cummings JL, Dekosky ST, Barberger-Gateau P, et al. Revising the definition of Alzheimer's disease: a new Lexicon. Lancet Neurol 2010;9:1118–27. [Epub 2010 October 9].

[17] CDR – Clinical Dementia Rating GDS – Global Deterioration Scale MMSE – Mini-Mental State Examination Neurology 2005;65(Suppl. 3):S10–7. Modified with permission from Reisberg B, et al. Alzheimer Dis Assoc Disord 1994;8(suppl. 1):5188–5205].

[18] Hughes L, Kalali A, Vanbelle C, Cascade E. Innovative Digital Patient Recruitment Strategies in Prodromal AD trials. Poster presentation of the fifth conference CTAD. 29–31 October, 2012, Monte Carlo.

Alzheimer's Disease Mortality and Patient Retention in Clinical Trials: The Impact of Alzheimer's Disease on Mortality

H. Michael Arrighi

Janssen Research & Development, South San Francisco, California, USA

Mortality in Alzheimer's disease (AD) is increased relative to the population of the same gender and age [1]. This risk is estimated to be around two times higher than a comparable population. Table 11.1 presents the relative risk for mortality from selected publications. Evans [4] observed a 1.4 relative rate in a cohort of 467 persons aged 65 years or more located in the Pennes region in France, while one of the highest relative rates reported, 3.2, was observed in the Helsinki Aging Study [5]. Perkins and colleagues [3] performed the identical study in two different geographic locations. Among Africans in Ibadan, Nigeria and African Americans in Indianapolis, Indiana, USA, the estimate of the increased mortality risk from AD was nearly identical with RR point estimates of 2.1 (95% confidence interval [CI] 0.7, 6.4) and 1.8 (95% CI 0.8, 3.7), respectively. This direct evidence indicates that the increased relative risk that AD confers on mortality may be independent of other factors contributing to mortality.

In a representative, population-based study in Northern Manhattan, New York, USA, an overall mortality rate of 10.7 per 100 person-years was observed in the AD population aged 65 years or more; Northern Manhattan is an ethnically/racially diverse area with the AD cases predominately comprised of Hispanics (55%), African Americans (33%), and non-Hispanic whites (11%) [6]. In a representative sample from

M. Bairu & M.W. Weiner (Eds):
Global Clinical Trials for Alzheimer's Disease.
DOI: http://dx.doi.org/10.1016/B978-0-12-411464-7.00011-0

TABLE 11.1   The Impact of AD on the Risk of Death

Reference	Country	N	Age Range	Point Estimate (95% CI)	Estimate Type
Eaker [2]	USA	811	not stated	1.9 (1.4, 2.6)	Hazard Ratio
Evans [4]	USA	467	65+	1.4 (1.1, 2.0)	Relative Rate
Ganguli [7]	USA	1,681	65+	1.4 (1.2, 1.8)	Hazard Ratio
Helmer [45]	France	3,675	65+	1.7 (1.3, 2.2)	Relative Rate
Jagger [46]	Great Britain	377	75+	1.5 (1.1, 2.2)	Relative Rate
Perkins [3]	Nigeria	2,487	65+	1.8 (0.8, 3.7)	Relative Rate
Perkins [3]	USA	2,212	65+	2.1 (0.7, 6.4)	Relative Rate
Qiu [47]	Sweden	1,296	75+	3.1 (1.8, 5.4)	Relative Rate
Tilvis [5]	Finland	550	75–85	3.2 (1.7, 6.2)	Relative Rate

TABLE 11.2   Mortality Rate for AD patients by Age and Gender [7]

Age at Death	Men Rate Per 1000 Person-Years	Women Rate Per 1000 Person-Years
65–74	38.2 (10.5,139.3)	39.5 (13.4–116.1)
75–84	102.8 (172.9, 280.9)	98.1 (76.6, 125.8)
85+	220.4 (172.9, 280.9)	182.5 (147.6, 225.7)
Total	142.7 (118.6, 171.6)	127.8 (108.9, 150.0)

south-west Pennsylvania, USA, a population that is predominately white and lower socio-economic status, among those with AD, an overall mortality rate of 13.4 per 100 person-years was observed [7]. From a health maintenance organization in the north-west USA, incidence patients were identified who were followed and a overall crude mortality rate of 10.2 per 100 person-years was observed [8].

In the general population, the underlying risk of death is related to both age and gender. As expected, the same pattern is observed in AD patients: The mortality rate increasing with increasing age and men generally have higher mortality rates than women. Table 11.2 presents typical observations [7]. Mortality rates for AD patients increase with increasing age and women generally have lower mortality rates than men.

While in the general population mortality rates for men are elevated compared with women, regardless of age [9], the published literature on the additional impact of AD on mortality indicated that there is little difference between men and women [6,7]. Among AD patients, the hazard ratio for male gender compared with females on AD mortality was 1.12 (95% CI 0.73, 1.72), adjusted for ethnicity, education, significant comorbidities, and stratified by age [6]. Ostbye [10] reported slightly higher point estimates for the mortality rate ratios among women compared with men but the confidence intervals were overlapping. Similarly, Aevarsson [11], among AD patients aged 85 years or more, reported a nearly identical MRR for women of 2.9 (95% CI 1.9, 4.3) and for men at 2.6 (95% CI 1.5, 4.7). To date, preponderance of evidence indicates that gender does not influence the differential impact of AD on mortality and the interpretation is that the impact of AD on mortality is independent of the impact from gender.

Among adults, the risk for mortality increases with age and by the age of 60 the relationship is nearly exponential with a doubling of the mortality risk for approximately every eight years in age [9]. While the underlying risk of death increases with age, the additional mortality risk conferred by AD exhibits an inverse relationship with age, when expressed as a ratio [1,10,12,13]. Ostbye [10] compared the mortality among persons with AD to the general Canadian population and reported age- and gender-specific mortality rate ratios of 6.5, 2.9 and 1.7, for women and 9.6, 4.1 and 19.0, for men, aged 65–74, 75–84, and 85 or more years, respectively. Similarly, Katzman [14] evaluated a cohort in China and compared the mortality rates among persons diagnosed with AD with persons without AD. A higher mortality rate ratio of 5.4 was observed among persons aged 65–74 years compared with the lower mortality rate ratio of 2.8 for persons aged 75 years or more. Thus, a younger person with AD has a higher relative mortality compared with contemporaries than an older person with AD.

Ratio measures are a common method used to compare rates, which incorporates a multiplicative scale. As the underlying mortality rate in the general population increases with increasing age and the relative increase in mortality risk due to AD has an inverse relationship, an additive structure may provide an improvement to characterize the relationship on mortality by AD and age, an additive structure which incorporates a constant increase in mortality risk across all ages. For example, in the general population, if the probability of death during a year is 0.06 for a person aged 80 years, a doubling of the risk would result in 0.12 and adding a risk increase of 0.06 would result in 0.12, a doubling of the risk. At the age of 60, the annual probability of death is 0.01 for the general population; a doubling of the risk for AD results in a annual probability of 0.02, while adding 0.06 results in an annual probability of 0.07 or a 7-fold increase. Similarly, for the population aged 90 years and over, a doubling of the general population's annual risk results in 0.30 for those with AD and adding 0.06 results in a risk of 0.21 or a 1.4 relative increase over the general population's risk of 0.15.

Johnson and colleagues [13] evaluated an additive, two-stage model to estimate the impact of AD. A two-stage model allows for the incremental impact of AD on mortality to differ by whether the person is in early or late stage AD. The additive incremental increase incorporates the assumption that the additional risk conferred by AD is similar within a stage and essentially "constant" across age. The two-stage, additive model was observed to fit the empirical data from the Baltimore Longitudinal Study of Aging (BLSA) more closely than a one-stage, multiplicative model. Subsequently, a two-stage, multiplicative model was used to estimate the prevalence of AD [15]. The model allows for the estimation of age- and gender-specific median survival times. The challenge is that a two-stage model requires the specification of more parameters than a one-stage model; the latter incorporates more assumptions with fewer parameters to specify.

An alternative way to express mortality is to observe the life expectancy of an AD patient. As with mortality rate, comparison across different studies is generally not possible due to the variations in study design. A Korean-based study reported a median survival time of 12.6 years (95% CI 11.7, 13.4) from the time of symptom onset and 9.3 years (95% CI 8.7, 9.9) from diagnosis [16]. In a US-based study, Helzner [6] reported median survival times after diagnosis of 3.7 years (95% CI 1.5, 5.9) among non-Hispanic whites, 4.8 years (95% CI 4.0, 5.7) among African Americans, and 7.6 years (95% CI 6.4, 8.7) among Hispanics. The Korean-based study had a mean age of AD onset of 71 years [16] and of 83 years for the US-based study. The BLSA, a study of a predominately white population based in the USA, reported a median survival from diagnosis of 4.4 and 3.8 years, for men and women, respectively.

An intriguing finding was reported by Helzner [6] who observed that non-Hispanic white AD patients had reduced survival compared with Hispanics and African Americans. The study is based on a representative sample of Medicare recipients, aged 65 years or over, in Northern Manhattan, New York. The AD cohort was restricted to incident cases and the analysis was adjusted for demographics and significant comorbidities. Similar findings were reported by Mehta et al.[17] using data from the National Alzheimer's Coordinating Center (NACC). African Americans and Latino Americans had lower mortality hazard ratios when compared with white Americans, of 0.85 (95% CI 0.74, 0.96) and 0.57 (95% CI 0.46, 0.69), respectively. These differences persist across all sub-group analyses, by age, gender, and Mini-Mental Status Examination (MMSE) score.

Apart from age, the apolipoprotein E (ApoE) ε4 allele is perhaps the strongest risk factor for AD [18], with one copy of the ε4 allele doubling one's risk and two copies increasing the risk 4- to 8-fold. However, the impact of the allele on mortality after the onset of AD has not been extensively studied. Among persons with AD, Helzner [6] observed a modest

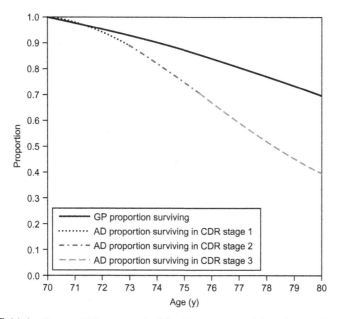

FIGURE 11.1 Expected 10-year survival for AD patients and the US general population aged 70 years [22].

increase in risk due to the presence of one or two ApoE ε4 alleles with a hazard ratio of 1.27, but the 95% CI was wide (0.81, 1.99).

The severity of the stage of AD contributes to mortality risk, with increasing severity associated with increasing mortality across different measures of severity, MMSE [8], CDR-global score [19], and verbal fluency [20]. Additionally, the rate of prior change is an additional component [8,21]. Thus, two patients observed to have the same stage of AD will have different mortality risks if they differed on the prior rate of progression.

Considering all the factors, Figure 11.1 shows the projected survival for a person aged 70 years with new onset AD [22]. With onset at age 70, the median survival is approximately eight years. Additionally, the rate of mortality accelerates as the patient progresses into more severe stages. Over a 10-year interval, the expected survival duration is three years at CDR stage 1, three years at CDR stage 3, and four years at CDR stage 4. By age 80 the overall expected survival is 39%, substantially lower than the general US population at 70%; notably the US general population includes people with AD.

An alternative approach is to present mortality as years of life expectancy. The literature presents varying estimates but requires consideration of the age, gender, current severity, and whether survival is from

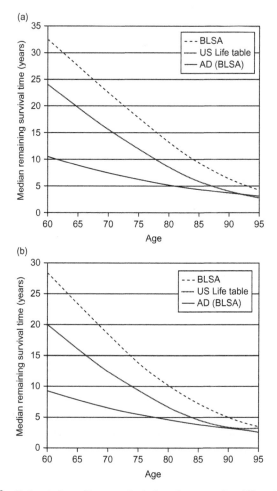

FIGURE 11.2   Estimated median survival time in years for AD patients compared with BLSA participants and United States 1998 Life Tables: a. women; b: men, *adapted from Brookmeyer [23].*

AD diagnosis or onset. Figure 11.2 shows the expected median remaining years of life expectancy from the diagnosis of AD for women (Figure 11.2a) and men (Figure 11.2b) by age [23]. Estimates were based on a Weibull model using data from the BLSA from the age at diagnosis, with separate models for women and men. For comparison, the median survival time for all BLSA participants was estimated using a similar model and the United States population from 1998 life tables. Estimated life expectancy decreases with increasing age; for example, a woman diagnosed at age 65 had 8.9 years of life expectancy while if diagnosed at age 85 she would have 4.4 years. The corresponding expected life expectancies for a man diagnosed with AD were estimated at 7.8 and 3.8, respectively. Across all ages, a women diagnosed with AD has a slightly longer life expectancy than a man, which is substantially lower than all BLSA participants. The later in life one is diagnosed with AD, the proportion of life lost due to AD is substantially reduced; a woman in the BLSA diagnosed at age 60 with AD has less than a third of life expectancy compared with a similar woman without an AD diagnosis; diagnosed with AD at age 90, a woman would retain more than 60% of life expectancy compared with a woman of a similar age without AD.

When evaluating the literature on mortality in AD, substantial variation in the results exists. Differences in risk estimates are anticipated due to the variations across study designs. Substantial differences across studies include the number of persons enrolled, age range, and duration of observation, all of which may influence the observed mortality rates. Additionally, different analysis methods were used, in particular the selection of which covariates to adjust for in the models. Whether survival is based on disease onset or diagnosis will contribute to variations in risk estimates and survival times. However, the factor that may contribute the most in variation across studies is how participants are identified and then diagnosed with AD; in a review of AD prevalence studies, heterogeneity in identification and diagnostic criteria were identified as the factors contributing the most to the variation across prevalence estimates for AD [24,25]. Overall, AD mortality rates provide a strategic view of the burden in that community. However, overall mortality rates should not be compared across studies unless they are adjusted to the same population characteristics.

11.1 ALZHEIMER'S DISEASE MORTALITY RISK DURING CLINICAL TRIALS

Estimating the mortality rate from clinical trials is generally not possible as clinical trials generally report the number of events out of the total number enrolled and who met the ITT (Intent-to-Treat) or mITT (modified-ITT) criteria. Thus, the clinical trial literature reports the risk or cumulative incidence—a proportion as opposed to a rate. Comparing risk, i.e., proportions, across different studies is further challenged by the varying duration of the studies and the different number of participants who withdraw and no longer contribute to the at risk population. Additionally, adverse events, including deaths, are generally reported within a specified number of half-lives of therapy. The CIOMS VI recommendation is "at least an additional five half-lives" (p. 96,[26]). Using a half-life interval relative to last exposure further complicates the ability to estimate the person-time at risk based on the published literature, as this interval is generally not described in the manuscript's method section. For therapies, such as monoclonal antibodies that may have a half-life of several weeks [27], the time when adverse events may be reported may extend substantially beyond the date of the last study visit. The potential for differential reporting among sub-groups, such as receiving active therapy or placebo, cannot be excluded.

As an example, in a Phase II trial of bapineuzumab, 234 patients were randomized and included in the safety evaluation [27]. One hundred and fifty-eight, 67.5%, completed the trial and received all infusions and the week 78 safety assessment. Three deaths were reported. The population evaluated for safety included all patients who were randomized and received at least one dose of treatment, which differs from the mITT. The mITT is a subset of the safety population, n = 229, as an additional requirement is imposed as having at least one post baseline, evaluation for efficacy. Even though, overall, approximately 72% of both those assigned placebo and active therapy completed the trial, the authors reported differential study completion rates among subjects who were ApoE ε4 carriers compared with those who were not. Completion rates were observed to vary by assigned dose, ranging from 89% to 54%. Thus, comparing three deaths in 229 patients from this study with other clinical trials is likely to be non-comparable. Another clinical trial of mild to moderated AD had a safety population sample size of 394 [27]. However, the definition of mild to moderate AD from Peskind [28] differs from Salloway [2009], the former had an MMSE at baseline from 22 to 10 and the latter from 26 to 16. A total of 332 completed the 24 week trial, or 82%, with two deaths reported. Ignoring random error, attempting to infer similarity or difference in mortality across these two studies is not possible due to differences in the operational definition of disease severity, duration of study, and proportion of patients who discontinued.

11.2 HEALTHY VOLUNTEER EFFECT

Participants who volunteer for clinical trials and non-interventional studies differ from the general patient population. Empirical evidence for this is seen from the BLSA and shown in Figure 11.2. BLSA participants have substantially lower mortality rates than the corresponding US general population [23]. The eligibility criteria are one source of this difference, particularly for clinical trials. The criteria to enroll may be quite restrictive, excluding individuals with mixed dementia types, restricting the age range, restricting the severity of AD to a narrow range, and excluding comorbidities common in the AD patient population. The substantive impact of study participation is that AD patients who volunteer will tend to be healthier than the general AD patient population, which may result in lower mortality rates than expected when based on AD patients in general, even when adjusting for age, gender, ethnicity/race, and disease severity.

The healthy volunteer effect creates another consideration during the course of a study. Over time, participants' health status may change and they may experience events that increase their mortality risk, either acutely or chronically. Thus, even when considering changes in age, demographics, and AD severity, the mortality rate may be increased later during the study. The impact may be to give the impression that there is an increasing mortality rate over time, which may be more substantial and more difficult to interpret during an open-label extension (OLE) study, when there is no contemporaneous comparison group. An implication is that an OLE study may manifest slightly higher mortality rates than during the parent study, even when appropriately correcting for age, gender, and AD severity. The optimal comparison is to maintain a contemporaneous comparison group, particularly when transitioning into OLE studies.

11.3 PLANNING MORTALITY PROJECTIONS FOR CLINICAL TRIALS

When planning a clinical trial, particularly one with a long duration for both enrollment and patient participation, estimating mortality prior to the beginning of the study assists with interpreting deaths that occur early in the study. Given the caveats stated above regarding factors that may influence mortality rates for AD patients in general and those who participate in clinical trials, estimating the expected mortality rate is not a trivial task and variation around the estimate is warranted to provide additional context for interpretation.

For estimating the number of deaths in a clinical trial, a potential source of expected rates is using the placebo arm from studies of similar design, particularly with respect to eligibility criteria. One data source is the CAMD (Coalition Against Major Diseases) (www.c-path.org) initiative to combine the placebo data from AD clinical trials and the C-Path Online Data Repository (CODR). Information on CODR and an application can be found online at http://www.c-path.org/CAMDcodr.cfm. Additionally, other publically available data may be utilized such as the ADNI (the Alzheimer's Disease Neuroimaging Initiative) (http://www.adni-info.org/) or the CERAD (Consortium to Establish a Registry in Alzheimer's Disease) (http://cerad.mc.duke.edu/). Given that a particular study is unlikely to be exactly duplicated using other sources, the generation of expected mortality rates should not result in a single number but should consider a potential range of estimates.

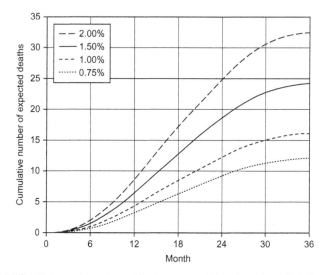

FIGURE 11.3   Estimated number of deaths among AD patients in a clinical study with a total n = 1,000; a duration of 24 months; an enrollment period of 12 months; and an annual withdrawal rate of 20%, under varying annual mortality rates of 0.75, 1, 1.5, and 2 deaths per 100 person-years.

To estimate the number of expected deaths before the trial begins, some of the information needed includes the estimated rate of enrollment or the time estimated to complete enrollment, the maximum study duration for participation, the rate of discontinuation, and the basic demographics of the study population. The demographics need to include, at a minimum, an estimate of the gender distribution and the expected mean age. From the basic demographics, the expected mortality rate may be generated from other sources of data. Using the basic trial parameters and the expected mortality rate, a cumulative plot of the total number of events may be created.

An example of such is shown in Figure 11.3. The curves in Figure 11.3 are based on the number of expected deaths in a study of 1,000 patients, with participant duration of two years and with enrollment expected to take one year. An annual withdrawal rate of 20% was assumed and the withdrawal rate includes deaths. Four expected mortality rates are assumed— 0.75, 1.00, 1.50, and 2.00 per 100 person-years, or % per year. Six months after the study was initiated, one to two deaths are expected, specifically 0.75, 1.00, 1.51, and 2.02, respectively for the 0.75%, 1.0%, 1.5%, and 2.0% annual mortality rates. This information may assist the safety monitoring committee (SMC) in an interpretation of the observed number of deaths at the six-month interval. Given the small number of expected events, the likelihood that all would occur in one treatment arm is probable. Even one year into the study, the expected number of deaths is less than 10, or 3.19, 4.26, 6.41, and 8.57, respectively, for the four mortality rates 0.75%, 1.0%, 1.5%, and 2.0%.

Additionally, during the course of the study, the number of expected deaths may be refined by periodically generating the person-time on the study by a combination of age, say in five-year categories, and gender. Providing an estimate of the person-time at period intervals assists to more accurately estimate the number of expected deaths by more closely matching person-time at risk to age- and gender-specific mortality rates.

11.4 MORTALITY AND STUDY DISCONTINUATION

As previously mentioned, a complicating factor for clinical trials is that adverse events, including deaths, are reported related to a pre-specified number of half-lives. CIOMS VI guidance recommends five times the half-life [26]. Some therapies, such as the monoclonal antibodies, have a half-life that is measured in weeks and the potential interval for which adverse events, including death, may be reported will be extended considerably after the patient's last visit. Some adverse events in AD clinical trials of amyloid modifying therapy are considered to be related to the therapy, for example, ARIA (Amyloid-Related Imaging Abnormalities), and are generally considered mild [29]; thus, a patient may continue in the study. Over a study of long duration, an ARIA, or similar event, increases the likelihood of unblinding the investigator and if the safety reporting interval extends beyond the last patient visit, due to a long half-life, the likelihood of introducing a false positive safety event is increased. Thus, patients in active therapy may have more deaths reported during this post-study window.

A recommendation is to include a formal post-study assessment of vital status, at the end of the therapy's interval for safety assessment. This follow-up applies to all participants, regardless of therapeutic assignment and the individuals undertaking the assessment should be blinded to the patient's assigned therapy and any other adverse events. For example, if the last study visit is at 12 months, with the last treatment at 11 months and an assessment for safety events is 3 months after the last therapy session then all patients' vital status would be assessed at 14 months.

Another implication of the differential interval for efficacy and safety is its potential impact on the evaluation of the benefit-risk ratio for which more quantitative methods are being utilized [30–32]. The implication is that the risk interval and safety population differ from the efficacy population and period in which efficacy is assessed. To perform a balanced benefit–risk assessment both aspects—benefit and risk—should be assessed in the same population and observed with equal propensity during the same interval; to do otherwise, may introduce bias.

11.5 PATIENT RETENTION

AD is a complicated disease with impacts on both the patient and the patient's caregiver, which is partly attributable to the high rates of morbidity and mortality and partly due to the complexity of care and demands imposed by the disease itself. Thus, annualized withdrawal rates of 20% are not uncommon in clinical trials with AD patients and the number of patients enrolled needs to consider the discontinuation rate to ensure the level of statistical precision desired is achieved. Given the complexity of the trial, the number of sites will have to increase and the number of patients screened, with a significant dedication of resources to achieve the required number of patients. As study duration of 18 months and more is becoming the norm for AD clinical trials, participant withdrawal has the potential to introduce a significant source of bias.

Patient retention is of significant concern for AD trials [33,44]. Even in studies as short as six months, 20–30% of the population may withdraw [34]. After reviewing the literature on retention in AD clinical trials, Grill and Karlawish [34] concluded that study duration had little impact on retention rates, although larger trials tended to have lower retention rates and small trials had higher retention rates. Commercial trial sites as opposed to academic trial sites were observed to have half the retention rate compared with those AD research centers funded by the National Institute on Aging [35].

The conventional notion is that withdrawal would tend to attenuate the effects of treatment, under the assumption that persons who discontinue from placebo are more likely to be those who exhibit a greater rate of progression, i.e., patients assigned placebo who progress slowly may believe that treatment is working and stay in the trial. Additionally, subjects on active treatment may discontinue due to potential adverse effects, although some adverse effects may be potential markers of treatment efficacy; thus, those with potentially the largest treatment effect may discontinue. The implication is that either factor alone would tend to attenuate the observed efficacy of a treatment, even if the overall withdrawal rates were identical across the groups assigned to placebo and to active therapy. Additionally, under these same assumptions, the implication is that a bias toward false positive safety events may occur; that is, an event is interpreted as a safety event when it is not. However, high withdrawal rates may artificially mask treatment efficacy or erringly introduce a false safety signal, either of which may stop the use of a potentially beneficial therapy. Thus, strategies that improve patient retention should be adopted and additional efforts to identify ways to improve retention are encouraged [36,37].

11.5.1 Strategies to Improve Patient Retention

Prior to starting the study, attention should be given to the potential to improve patient retention [38,39]. Pre-study focus groups are useful for talking with patients and caregivers prior to starting the study about what would assist their ability to maintain study participation. Additionally, during the study periodic focus groups about what may be modified to assist retention are useful. Focus groups are preferred over questionnaires or checklists, as a difficulty is anticipating the response.

A community-level involvement adds a level of support and accountability to the participants [16]. The community may have local or cultural-specific issues that may be directly addressed. Consider using alternative means for assessment, using the telephone, or home-based visits [36,40]. Reduce the number of visits, which is a balance between having interim measures for those who discontinue early and having as few measures as possible to improve retention. The selection of study sites and personnel should be undertaken so as to have centers with a motivated, caring, and knowledgeable study personnel. Study personnel are a resource, particularly for longer trials; they are able to provide insight and ongoing assessment of issues and challenges. As study personnel are the "face" of the trial, they are in a position to identify patients at high-risk of discontinuation, and can attempt an intervention strategy. Infrastructure and continuity of care, coordinating care with other providers, should be considered, particularly for large trials of long duration. As AD patients are complex and may still be seen by other healthcare providers, assistance to the caregiver and the patient to coordinate activities in the least burdensome way would lead to improved patient retention. Improving the caregiver's experience is another aspect to consider. Would the caregiver be interested in attending a support group while the patient is in the clinic? Is the caregiver's area in the clinic comfortable and relaxing? Does it create a welcoming and comfortable environment, as the clinic visits often last several hours.

Maintain the current participant's information, their current living situation and contact information, caregiver, and consider including an alternative contact person [36,40,41]. Use visit reminders and prompts to improve adherence to scheduled visits, particularly for studies that may have several weeks between visits. Utilize alternative means of contact that are suitable for the patient/caregiver, such as e-mail and text messages, to update them on upcoming visits and other status information. Create a project identity; the identity should link to the reason and objectives of the research, i.e., that the study has benefits and will help the community. Use multiple forms of media to maintain contact both to and from the patient/caregiver, including toll free numbers, hot lines, help lines, and websites. In the VIOXX study, the first listed reason for retention was the 24-hour availability of a nurse [42].

AD patients have particular challenges that impact retention. Transportation is a challenge for the AD patient/caregiver dyad. Finding ways to reduce travel, such as by home visits, telephone interviews, or reducing the number of visits, is of critical importance. Consider providing assistance in transportation, beyond just monetary vouchers. When the caregiver is not related to the AD patient, the risk for discontinuation increases and increasing caregiver burden is an additional risk factor [43].

Constant monitoring for significant life events, chronic lateness, and missed appointments are cues to issues related to retention. When problems begin to emerge, reach out to re-engage the patient/caregiver in order to identify the sources of the problems and determine ways to adapt the trial to their current demands, where possible; for example by modifying dates of clinic visits, and combining or splitting visits. Providing a supportive and caring environment is essential for retention, regardless of whether the issue is something that the study is able to address. A recovery and re-contact process should be planned as part of the original study and be in place prior to the enrollment of the first patient.

11.6 SUMMARY AND CONCLUSION

Mortality in AD patients is elevated and has the potential to impact on clinical trials particularly with respect to introducing a bias against therapy. Pre-planning with regard to the number of expected events will assist in placing into context deaths that occur early in the study, when there are relatively few events and an imbalance among treatment groups may occur by chance. To reduce ascertainment bias, plan a vital status assessment at the end of study for all subjects that includes the safety interval based on the therapy's half-life.

AD patients withdraw from clinical trials at rates that have the potential to introduce significant bias, which may mitigate efficacy or misleadingly label an event as increased among those receiving active therapy. Thus pre-planning, periodic evaluation and assessment, and incorporating strategies to both increase retention rates and identify and improve such techniques, should be part of the study process.

References

[1] Guehne U, Reidel-Heller S, Angermeyer MC. Mortality in dementia: a systematic review. Neuroepidemiology 2005;25:153–62.
[2] Eaker ED, Vierkant RA, Mickel SF. Predictors of nursing home admission and/or death in incident Alzheimer's disease and other dementia cases compared to controls: a population-based study. J Clin Epidemiol 2002;55:462–8.

[3] Perkins AJ, Hui SL, Ogunniyi A, Gureje O, Baiyewu O, Unverzagt FW, et al. Risk of mortality for dementia in a developing country: the Yoruba in Nigeria. Int Geriatr Psychiatry 2002;17:566–73.

[4] Evans DA, Smith LA, Scherr PA, Albert MS, Funkenstein HH, Hebert LE. Risk of death from Alzheimer's disease in a community population of older persons. Am J Epidemiol 1991;134:403–12.

[5] Tilvis RS, Strandberg TE, Juva K. Apolipoprotein E phenotypes, dementia and mortality in a prospective population sample. J Am Geriatr Soc 1998;46:712–5.

[6] Helzner EP, Scarmeas N, Cosentino S, Tang MX, Schupf N, Stern Y. Survival in Alzheimer's disease: a multiethnic, population-based study of incident cases. Neurol 2008;71:1489–95.

[7] Ganguli M, Dodge H, Shen C, Pandav RS, Dekosky ST. Alzheimer's disease mortality: a 15-year epidemiological study. Arch Neurol 2005;62:779–84.

[8] Bowen JD, Malter AD, Sheppard L, Kukull WA, McCormick WC, Teri L, et al. Predictors of mortality in patients diagnosed with probable Alzheimer's disease. Neurol 1996;47:433–9.

[9] Arias E, Rostron BL, Tejada-Vera B. United States life tables, 2005. National vital statistics reports; vol 58 no 10. Hyattsville: National Center for Health Statistics; 2010.

[10] Ostbye T, Hill G, Steenhuis R. Mortality in elderly Canadians with and without dementia: a 5-year follow-up. Neurology 1999;53:521–6.

[11] Aevarsson O, Svanborg A, Skoog I. Seven-year survival rate after age 85 years: relation to Alzheimer's disease and vascular dementia. Arch Neurol 1998;55: 1226–32.

[12] Tschanz JT, Corocran C, Skoog I, Khachaturian AS, Herrick J, et al.The Cache County Study Group Dementia: the leading predictor of death in a defined elderly population: The cache county study. Neurol 2004;62:1156.

[13] Johnson E, Brookmeyer R, Ziegler-Graham K. Modeling the effect of Alzheimer's disease on mortality. Int J Biostat 2007;13(1):a13.

[14] Katzman R, Hill LR, Yu ES, Wang ZY, Booth A, Salmon DP, et al. The malignancy of dementia: predictors of mortality in clinically diagnosed dementia in a population survey of Shanghi, China. Arch Neurol 1994;51:1120–5.

[15] Brookmeyer R, Johnson E, Zeigler-Graham K, Arrighi HM. Forecasting the global burden of Alzheimer's disease. Alzheimers Dement 2007;3(3):186–91.

[16] Go SM, Lee KS, Seo SW, Chin J, Kang SJ, Moon SY, et al. Survival of Alzheimer's disease patients in Korea. Dement Geriatr Cogn Disord 2013;35:219–28.

[17] Mehta KM, Yaffe K, Pérez-Stable EJ, Stewart A, Barnes D, Kurland BF, et al. Race/ethnic differences in AD survival in US Alzheimer's disease centers. Neurol 2008;70:1163–70.

[18] Devanand DP, Pelton GH, Zamora D, Liu X, Tabert MH, Goodkind M, et al. Predictive utility of apolipoprotein E genotype for Alzheimer's disease in outpatients with mild cognitive impairment. Arch Neurol 2005;62(6):975–80.

[19] Neumann PJ, Araki SM, Arcelus SM, Longo A, Papadopouls G, Kosik KS, et al. Measuring Alzheimer's disease transition probabilities: estimates from CERAD. Neurol 2001;57:957–64.

[20] Cosentino S, Scarmeas N, Albert SM, Stern Y. Verbal fluency predicts mortality in Alzheimer's disease. Cog Behav Neurol 2006;19:123–9.

[21] Van Sanden S, Diels J, Gaudig M, Spencer M, Thompson G, Arrighi HM. Faster cognitive decline is associated with decreased survival in patients with Alzheimer's disease. (Abstract) Value Health 2012;15:A277.

[22] Arrighi HM, Neumann PJ, Lieberburg IM, Townsend RJ. Lethality of Alzheime's disease and its impact on nursing home admission. Alzheimer Dis Assoc Disord 2010;24:90–5.

VI. OPERATIONALIZATION OF GLOBAL ALZHEIMER'S DISEASE TRIALS

[23] Brookmeyer R, Corrada MM, Curriero FC, Kawas C. Survival following a diagnosis of Alzheimer's disease. Arch Neuro 2002;59(11):1764–7.

[24] Corrada M, Brookmeyer R, Kawas C. Sources of variability in prevalence rates of Alzheimer's disease. Int J Epidemiol 1995;24:1000–5.

[25] Brookmeyer R, Evans DA, Hebert L, Langa KM, Heeringa SG, Plassman BL, et al. National estimates of prevalence of Alzheimer's disease in the United States. Alzheimer Dement 2011;7:61–73.

[26] Report of CIOMS Working Group VI. Management of Safety Information from Clinical Trials. Council for International Organizations of Medical Sciences, Geneva, 2005.

[27] Salloway S, Sperling R, Gilman S, Fox NC, Blennow K, Raskind M, et al. A phase 2 multiple ascending dose trial of bapineuzumab in mild to moderate Alzheimer disease. Neurology 2009;73(24):2061–70.

[28] Peskind ER, Potkin S, Pomara N, Ott B, Graham S, McDonald S, et al. Memantine treatment in mild to moderate Alzheimer disease: a 24-week randomized clinical trial for the Memantine MEM-MD-10 Study Group. Am J Geriatr Psychiatry 2006;14(8):704–15.

[29] Sperling RA, Jack CR, Black SE, Frosch MP, Greenberg SM, Hyman BT, et al. Amyloid-related imaging abnormalities in amyloid-modifying therapeutic trials. Recommendations from the Alzheimer's Association Research Roundtable workgroup. Alzheimer Dement 2011;7:367–85.

[30] European Medicines Agency Benefit-Risk Methodology Project, EMA/213482/2010. Available at: <http://www.ema.europa.eu/ema/index.jsp?curl=pages/special_topics/document_listing/document_listing_000314.jsp&mid=WC0b01ac0580223ed6&murl=menus/special_topics/special_topics.jsp&jsenabled=true>; 2010. (Cited 30 March 2013).

[31] Coplan PM, Noel RA, Levitan BS, Ferguson J, Mussen F. Development of a framework for enhancing the transparency, reproducibility and communication of the benefit–risk balance in medicines. Clin Pharmacol Ther 2011;89:312–5.

[32] Yuan Z, Levitan B, Berlin JA. Benefit–risk assessment: to quantify or not to quantify, that is the question. Pharmacoepidemiol Drug Safety 2011;20:653–6.

[33] Vella B, Pesce A, Robert PH, Aisen PS, Ancoli-Israel S, Andrieu S, et al. AMPA workshop on challenges faced by investigators conducting Alzheimer's disease clinical trials. Alzheimer Dement 2011;7:e109–17.

[34] Grill JD, Karlawish J. Addressing the challenges to successful recruitment and retention in Alzheimer's disease clinical trials. Alzheimer Res Thera 2010;2:34. Available at: <http://alzres.com/content/2/6/34>.

[35] Edland SD, Edmond JA, Aisen PS, Petersen RC. NIA-funded Alzheimer centers are more efficient than commercial clinical recruitment sites for conducting secondary prevention trials of dementia. Alzheimer Dis Assoc Disord 2010;24:159–64.

[36] Shumaker SA, Dugan E, Bowen DJ. Enhancing adherence in randomized controlled clinical trials. Control Clin Trial 2000;21:226S–32S.

[37] Olin JT, Dagerman KS, Fox LS, Bowers B, Schneider LS. Increasing ethnic minority participation in Alzheimer disease research. Alzheimer Dis Assoc Disord 2002;16(Suppl. 2):S82–9.

[38] Areán PA, Alvidrez J, Nery R, Estes C, Linkins K. Recruitment and retention of older minorities in mental health services research. Gerontol 2003;34:36–44.

[39] Mody L, Miller DK, McGloin JM, Freeman M, Marcantonio ER, Magazineer J, et al. Recruitment and retention of older adults in aging research. J Am Geriatr Soc 2008;56:2340–8.

[40] DeKosky ST. Maintaining adherence and retention in dementia prevention trials. Neurol 2006;67(Suppl. 3):S14–6.

[41] Blanton S, Morris DM, Prettyman MG, McCulloch K, Redmond S, Light KE, et al. Phys Ther 2006;86:1533.

[42] Mor M, Niv G, Niv Y. Patient retention in a clinical trial: a lesson from the rofecoxib (VIOXX) study. Dig Dis Sci 2006;51:1175–8.

[43] Coley N, Gaurdette V, Toulza O, Gillette-Guyonnet S, Cantet C, Nourhashemi Predictive factors of attrition in a cohort of Alzheimer's disease patients. The REAL.FR study. Neuroepidemiol 2008;31:69–79.

[44] Cohen-Mansfield J. Recruitment rates in gerontological research: the situation for drug trials in dementia may be worse than previously reported. Alzheimer Dis Assoc Disord 2002;16:279–82.

[45] Helmer C, Joly P, Letenneur L, Commenges D, Dartigues JF. Mortality with dementia: results from a French prospective community-based cohort. Am J Epidemiol 2001;154:642–8.

[46] Jagger C, Clarke M, Stone M. Predictors of survival with Alzheimer's disease: a community-based study. Psychol Med 1995;25:171–7.

[47] Qiu C, Backman L, Winblad B, Aguero-Torres H, Fratiglioni L. The influence of education on clinically diagnosed dementia incidence and mortality data from the Kungsholmen Project. Arch Neurol 2001;58:2034–9.

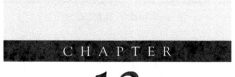

CHAPTER

12

Minimizing Trial Costs by Accelerating and Improving Enrollment and Retention

Debbie N. Cote

Debbie Cote Associates, USA

In recent decades, clinical trials have seen rising costs, complexity, and workloads, declining productivity, and stagnant volunteer participation. Biopharmaceutical companies are driving efficiency and controlling costs by outsourcing partnerships with contract research organizations, moving clinical trials to developing countries; they're reducing trial costs and enhancing productivity by forecasting—a process of translating the strategic objectives of the trial into operational elements to project the cost and use of resources. The budgeting process is built on the forecast model and the final clinical protocol. The final budget consists of both internal resources and external costs. The planning and execution of clinical trials involve stakeholders in different organizations conducting numerous activities across different stages of the trial. Project management involves planning, coordinating, and tracking key tasks, including the timeline, budget, risk, and contingency planning. Overall, the clinical trial business is complex; it involves many players and stakeholders, all of whom are ultimately dependent upon the investigative site to perform.

12.1 UNDERSTANDING THE PATIENT RECRUITMENT MARKET

Clinical trials account for 40% of the US pharma/biotech research budget, totaling US$ 7 billion per year. The estimated cost of patient

M. Bairu & M.W. Weiner (Eds):
Global Clinical Trials for Alzheimer's Disease.
DOI: http://dx.doi.org/10.1016/B978-0-12-411464-7.00012-2

197

BOX 12.1 STATISTICS OF VOLUNTEER DEMOGRAPHICS

- Nearly 80% of all clinical studies fail to finish on time, and 20% of those delayed are for six months or more.
- 85% of clinical trials fail to retain enough patients.
- The average dropout rate across all clinical trials is around 30%.
- Over two-thirds of sites fail to meet original patient enrollment for a given trial.
- Up to 50% of sites enroll one or no patients in their studies.

recruitment is 4% of the total budget, or US$ 1.89 billion. Patient recruitment is a weak link in the development pipeline and one would expect there to be a vetted plan that seeks to accelerate the time to market and consequently deliver the medicine to the patient and profitability to the shareholders in a more efficient manner.

Volunteer demographics are very important; to anticipate the challenges of optimizing recruitment, it is necessary to become aware of the statistics [1] (Box 12.1).

Data from an ECRI Evidence Report, which reviewed 11 studies investigating the reasons for participating and not participating in clinical trials, revealed no consistent findings; however, by using random-effects calculations to combine results from all the studies, the researchers were able to estimate the typical percentages of patients who cited reasons for participation in three general categories: potential health benefits (45%), physician influence (27%), and potential benefit to others (18%).

Studies have shown that while 44% of people find out about studies through the media, 14% gain the information from their physicians. An overwhelming majority of people (77%) say that they would consider getting involved in an appropriate clinical research study if asked; however, 10% of those eligible to participate in clinical trials do so in the United States [2].

Minority physicians have been shown to have a positive impact on minorities' involvement in clinical trials. At the time of writing, only about 7% of all physicians in the United States belong to a minority group and a very small percentage are actively involved in clinical research. Several medical societies and associations are now looking for ways to encourage minority physician involvement in clinical trials [3].

In 2007, a survey conducted on 717 adults (in the USA) found high levels of public distrust in clinical research staff. The breakdown showed that this level of distrust was significantly higher in minority adults, as 73% said they were "very likely" or "likely" to be treated as guinea pigs without their consent, whereas 49% of Caucasians responded this way [4].

12.2 PERSPECTIVES ON PATIENT RECRUITMENT: FIGHTING FEARS WITH FACTS

Currently, there are online conversations about clinical trials, indicating that patients are uneasy about clinical trials. From such discussion, most of the fear and misunderstanding seems to be due to a lack of understanding and education. In the 1980s, research was predominantly in the domain of the larger academic medical centers, where recruiting patients required communication about the trial to colleagues who had access to these types of patients. When a particular patient was identified by the clinic to be a "potential study candidate," the principal investigator (PI) or research nurse would be paged to the clinic to inform a patient about the trial. Most of the time, consent was obtained and screening procedures initiated; this is due in part to the PI or study nurse completing a proper "informed consenting process" as per International Conference on Harmonization/Good Clinical Practices (ICH/GCP) requirements.

There has been a dramatic shift in study participation since the evolution of the information age. In 1995, only one third of the several hundred patients were self-referrals; nearly two thirds had their physician or nurse refer them to trials. In 2004, 50% were self-referrals while 34% came from physician referrals. In a survey among several thousand health consumers, 60% said they would be willing to participate in an appropriate trial despite 74% of them acknowledging that they knew little—if anything—about what was expected of them. A poll of 5,348 adults conducted in May 2003 found that 77% of consumers would consider participating in trials if their physicians asked it of them [5].

Study volunteers are uniquely motivated to find medical information on the research process; many people have become empowered—and, in turn integrate the knowledge they acquired by approaching their health more proactively. Of the three million people who participate in clinical trials in the United States annually, it is estimated that 40% receive their healthcare from a health management organization (HMO). More than 70% of the US population receive their primary care through a managed care network [5]. Metrics have demonstrated that study volunteers are empowered to step outside their healthcare network—often without the permission of their primary care physician. This may show to be true based on a survey conducted in 2000 among 1,000 people: 70% said they have never spoken with their physician or nurse [6].

It's necessary to consider clinical trials from the patient and caregiver perspective and to investigate the reasons why an individual may or may not participate in a research trial; factoring in the difficulties of dealing with Alzheimer's disease (AD) makes committing to trials more complex and challenging.

Not much is written as to why people choose not to take part in consenting AD patients and their caregivers into clinical trials: in most cases, it's no longer a one-patient disease, but requires a caregiver and possibly a legal authorized representative (LAR). Many times, LARs would say "no" to taking part in a research trial: Common responses were that caregivers didn't have the time; some people didn't want their loved one to be a "guinea pig"—especially if the risks outweighed the unknown benefits; or, in some cases, travel to and from the study site was too risky for the caregiver to comfortably travel alone with a confused elderly person. Their plates are very full, leaving little time to spend additional hours at a study site.

The reality is that Memory Disorder Centers train their staff on how to care for this specialized population who are predominantly over the age of 65, and they have little if any prior medical or psychological experience to take care of a person with AD. Caregivers typically do not focus their time on themselves but with education through advocacy groups: By educating the general public and healthcare professionals in the value, risks, and benefits of clinical research participation, groups have started to connect patients and medical professionals together.

12.3 PUBLIC PERCEPTION AND THE STIGMA OF AD

Society's attitude toward AD—in some instances—is not very nice. The impact of stigma around symptoms, recognition, and diagnosis plays front and center in the minds of patients, their families, and close friends. People report a hesitation in admitting they had AD for fear of negative public perception about the disease and its potential for causing social isolation. Keeping the diagnosis a secret is very common—denial helps for the first few years: The risk of this debilitating disease is so far in the future that it's easy to be convinced it's not real. A potential study participant (or spouse) may not consider participating if they are embarrassed by their medical condition, or if frequent visits to the physician's office might be a painful reminder they are living with a devastating disease.

AD is often a "rule out" diagnosis; significant cognitive deficits are often noticed by family and close friends, prior to the diagnostic criteria of the disease being met. There are many incorrect assumptions about the disease, and some are held by the people that have it. Due to the perception that early symptoms are part of normal aging or the negative stigma associated with the disease, patients with AD often delay seeking treatment for their symptoms. The diagnostic process is challenging and accepting one's condition is difficult; but once the process is complete, people tend to report many benefits—and they even go on to encourage others to seek diagnosis.

12.4 THE SIGNIFICANCE OF THE CAREGIVER'S ROLE AND IMPACT ON AD TRIALS

Wikipedia's definition of *caregiver* (US, Canadian and Chinese usage) and *carer* (UK, NZ, Australian usage) are words normally used to refer to unpaid relatives or friends of a disabled individual [7] who help that individual with his or her activities of daily living (ADLs) [8,9]. As per the Alzheimer's Association 2013 Facts and Figures Report, more than 15 million Americans provide unpaid care for people with AD and other dementias. There is ethnical and racial diversity in caregiving among caregivers of people with AD and other dementias [10] (Box 12.2).

The care provided to people with AD and other dementias is wide-ranging, and, in some instances, all-encompassing. The types of dementia care provided are shown in Box 12.3 [11].

In addition to assisting with ADLs, 64% of caregivers advocate for their care recipient with government agencies and service providers; nearly half (46%) arrange and supervise paid caregivers from community agencies; 43% of people with AD and other dementias provide care for one to four years; and 32% of dementia caregivers provide care for over five years [12].

BOX 12.2 ETHNICAL AND RACIAL DIVERSITY IN CAREGIVING

- More white caregivers assist a parent than caregivers of individuals from other racial/ethnic groups (54% vs 38%).
- On average, Hispanic and African American caregivers spend more time caregiving (approximately 30 hours per week) than non-Hispanic white caregivers (20 hours per week) and Asian American caregivers (16 hours per week).
- Hispanic (45%) and African American caregivers (57%) have a higher probability to experience a higher burden from caregiving, than whites and Asian-Americans.

BOX 12.3 DEMENTIA CAREGIVING TASKS (2013 DATA) [13]

- Help with instrumental activities of daily living (IADLs), such as household chores, shopping, preparing meals, providing transportation, arranging for doctor's appointments, managing finances and legal affairs and answering the telephone.
- Helping the person take medications correctly, either via reminders or direct administration of medications.
- Helping the person adhere to treatment recommendations for dementia or other medical conditions.
- Assisting with personal ADLs such as bathing, dressing, grooming, feeding and helping the person walk, transfer from bed to chair, using the toilet and managing incontinence.
- Managing behavioral symptoms of the disease such as aggressive behavior, wandering, depressive mood, agitation, anxiety, repetitive activity and nighttime disturbances.
- Finding and using support services such as support groups and adult day service programs.
- Making arrangements for paid in-home, nursing home or assisted living care.
- Hiring and supervising others who provide care.
- Assuming additional responsibilities that are not necessarily specific tasks, such as:
  - Providing overall management of getting through the day.
  - Addressing family issues related to caring for a relative with AD, including communication with other family members about care plans, decision-making and arrangements for respite for the main caregiver.

12.5 FACILITATING BEST PRACTICES TO SUCCEED AS AN INVESTIGATIVE AD TRIAL SITE

Despite the myriad of challenges associated with successfully executing trials, sound clinical trial forecasting and execution practices can meaningfully reduce trial costs while enhancing productivity. Best practices are proven methods and processes employed by companies to maximize strategic, operational, and financial advantage [14]. It's these important drivers that enable a study site to succeed and achieve results by using standardized and consistent methodologies to demonstrate effectiveness.

By developing best practices, sites can reassert the essential roles study staff and healthcare professionals play in recruiting and retaining patients for AD trials.

Personal relationships with study staff influence many AD patients and families in their decision to volunteer, and in their willingness to complete participation. There is an overwhelming majority of participants that praise the "support system" of study staff—including physicians, nurses, and study coordinators—as highly skilled, personable, and accessible. For some, the study staff offers a friendly face, an open ear, and a level of concern that might have been lacking in their previous medical encounters.

Personal relationships develop with physicians and study coordinators who tend to go out of their way to accommodate trial patients and their families. Practical steps to help patients feel valued need not be expensive: instead, if sites treat all patients as if they were "special research patients"—meaning most have 24 hour direct access to a study coordinator or investigator for safety reporting, travel assistance using a debit card system, dedicated waiting rooms with internet access and snacks, and access to geriatric care professionals. The sites that implement some or all of these services receive patient loyalty which goes a long way towards retention.

The workload for investigators and site study staff has increased significantly, posing additional challenges for clinical trial execution. Regulations governing clinical research activities have become more complex, increasing the work burden on investigators in terms of additional needs for compliance, documentation, and training. A recent study showed that the work burden for clinical researchers increased by 67% from 1999 to 2005 [15].

Additionally, the AD landscape is changing in the way trials are designed: They are no longer recruiting from the general AD population, but instead are targeting specific sub-populations. Some of these are derived from ApoE allele, MMSE, NPI, and Alzheimer's Disease Assessment Scale-cognitive portion (ADAS-Cog) psychometric scores for entrance into the trial. Sites that are affiliated with PET centers—and have the ability to perform lumbar punctures—may more easily qualify as a study site than those without access to these specialized diagnostic (biomarker) procedures.

12.6 RECRUITING AD PATIENTS AND CAREGIVERS INTO CLINICAL TRIALS

In our country, patients are the most underutilized resource, and they have the most at stake. They want to be involved and they can be involved. Their participation will lead to better medical outcomes at lower costs with dramatically higher patient and customer satisfaction.

Charles Safran, MD President, American Informatics Association Testimony before
the Subcommittee on Health of the House Committee on Ways and Means [16].

Effective patient engagement can improve clinical trial participation
with heightened transparency, intense competition, and tighter budgets; sponsors cannot afford to let their communications with study participants operate inefficiently. Patient engagement tools must efficiently
communicate complex and unfamiliar information [17]. Sponsors, sites,
and communication teams need to be sensitive to "adopt" patient and
caregiver perspectives as they work to understand how they feel: How
are these conditions affecting them? How will the trial work from their
perspective? Trial communication should be in "user-friendly terms"—
convenient and understandable to patients and sensitive to their
preferences.

There is a mounting need for sponsors to effectively engage professional sites as real assets in the clinical trial process. Potential engagement tactics might include: educational and communication efforts
targeting healthcare professionals in specific communities prior to trial
initiation; involvement of study staff during project initiation; and
general and targeted communication that positions study staff as partners in the recruitment process. Right now, recruitment and retention
strategies tend to marginalize the role of the study staff and trusted
healthcare professionals, whereas they need to work in conjunction
with the staff to enhance the trial experience and facilitate a timely
outcome.

12.7 THE CHALLENGES OF THE INFORMED CONSENT PROCESS

Often the first interaction with the patient and the trial is at the
recruitment visit. If the patient is interested and eligible, the informed
consent process is initiated. This is the process that formally opens the
door to the screening process. This process, to be effective, must engage
and educate: Often times, the informed consent is seen as a legal document filled with medical terms that are unfamiliar to most people.
Traditionally, it has been paper based, and investigators typically viewed
consents as an instrument needed to meet regulations rather than an
educational opportunity; this is due in part to the length of consent
documents and the typical complexities as trial protocols evolve. (The
informed consent form (ICF) for the bapineuzumab Phase III trial was
24 pages, in 2009).

The challenge for any study site is to improve the recruitment success
rate at the largest segment of the funnel: the internal patient population.

Having the investigator explain the study in the most non-threatening way, with standardized delivery of consent information, brings a higher yield of enrollment—thus reducing the overall workload of the research staff.

During the consenting discussion, it's beneficial to ask what patients were most worried about, and what motivated them to join the trial. The responses will help keep the patient and caregiver engaged, and circumvent a situation that could lead to early terminations of the trial.

It's also important to allow time for questions to be asked: This alleviates fear and concerns in some people, and it might make a person ineligible for the trial, thereby reducing the cost of screen failures. An MRI scan, for example, involves lying in a narrow tube—an experience that may cause intense claustrophobia for some. Such people are advised not to volunteer. Also, many people fear that a lumbar puncture will cause an intense headache and could lead to spinal cord damage and may refuse to participate.

12.7.1 Alzheimer's Disease Patient and Securing a Legalized Authorized Representative (LAR)

The consenting process is the first most important task when considering enrolling in a clinical trial; but, knowing the mental capabilities of your audience (AD patient and caregiver) is extremely important to ensure the consenting process was followed as per GCP/ICH Guidelines [15].

The institutional review boards (IRBs) have approved the use of LARs for patients with a wide range of chronic and acute psychological and neurological impairments. Prior to identifying a LAR, the PI or designee determines if a potential study patient has the capacity to make a decision and voluntarily give informed consent. Patients with dementia related to AD may be cognizant of their surroundings at the time of screening, but they might become impaired a few months later as the disease state declines: This can make it difficult and unethical to consent a person who does not have the mental capacity to make an informed decision.

The National Institutes of Health (NIH) states, "It is important to take prospective subjects' abilities, impairments, and needs into account when considering whether to invite them to participate in research [17]".

When a patient has dementia of the AD type, and they do not have the mental capacity to give informed consent for themselves, then a LAR may give informed consent (or "permission") on their behalf. The LAR's "right" to consent is an extension of the patient's right. Using "substituted judgment" based on "the best knowledge of the LAR," the LAR makes a decision and acts in the "best interests" of the study subjects to determine whether or not consent to participate in a clinical trial is appropriate.

Obtaining informed consent from an LAR is just the same as obtaining it from the study subject with the following additional steps:

- Modify the informed consent form to allow consent by the LAR.
- Obtain IRB app roval for the use of LARs in the study by explaining the need for LARs and demonstrating safeguards to protect potential subjects.
- Determine that potential subjects do not have the decision-making capacity to give informed consent [18,19].

It is important to identify the LAR-provided state law, which allows for LARs involvement with clinical research. The AD patient can designate his or her LAR prior to the advancement of the disease; however, if an impaired person has not already designated an LAR and the state has a statutory hierarchy of people who can serve as LARs, the site can identify the LAR for the person according to the hierarchy. By participating in clinical studies, they can also help improve the quality of care for future patients.

12.8 TRIAL FORECASTING AND RECRUITMENT TACTICS

The forecasting exercise starts with study concept. Each trial is designed to achieve specific study objectives and approaches; these items vary accordingly from a dose escalating design to placebo-controlled, double-blind parallel arms. The subject population is defined, and specific inclusion and exclusion criteria are identified to further refine the target population. Endpoints are designed to achieve the desired safety, efficacy, pharmacokinetics, and testing regimen modeled according to the drug's mechanism of action and preliminary profile. The study size is determined based on statistical calculations and key assumptions such as treatment effect and variability.

Traditionally, patient recruitment was modeled based on the sponsor's continual reliance on investigators who had successfully recruited a number of study subjects from within their referral network and practices. In the mid 1990s, the clinical research industry became a multicenter global enterprise: Trials were more complex, requiring additional tests for exploratory analysis and demanding many more volunteers, which made it ever more difficult for investigative sites to fulfill their commitment of enrolling patients from their private practices.

Nowadays, federal regulations require sponsors to select investigators who are qualified according to their training and experience with a new investigational drug. It's challenging when the same investigator has limited experience launching a successful recruitment campaign.

Training staff on the protocol and procedures, achieving consensus on recruitment initiatives, obtaining commitment on scheduling and follow up visits, and supplying staff with literature to read about the condition being studied helps to prioritize the focus; these items improve employee morale, boost the interest in wanting to do a good job, and alleviate the overwhelming feelings held by study coordinators who do not really understand their responsibilities when they undergo a rushed training session (Box 12.4).

To optimize accrual, clinical operational planning should take into account a more focused approach in setting recruitment goals and timelines.

Study execution should focus on the following:

- Unstructured attempts at recruitment have been replaced by carefully researched plans, which pinpoint AD investigators and sites that are best suited for a particular trial. Patient enrollment is an extremely labor intensive aspect of the clinical trial process, and it is the leading cause of trial delays (behind contract and budget delays), which can take up to 30% of the clinical timeline.
- Improving patient recruitment rates offers pharmaceutical companies one of the biggest opportunities to accelerate the pace of clinical

---

BOX 12.4 TIPS ON BEST RECRUITMENT PRACTICES

- Identify recruitment challenges: protocol design, inclusion/exclusion criteria, specific procedures.
- Isolate motivators and public perceptions impacting the disease or clinical trial participation.
- Design an effective intake form to assess site resources and enrollment projections.
- Develop customized recruitment and retention plans that educate and inform, leading to a call for action on the part of the AD patient and their family.
- Prioritize multiple recruitment strategies with staggered roll-out.
- Develop a concept and brand the name for the trial for recognition and effective advertising through posters, flyers and brochures, and online social media campaign.
- Identify ethical cultural and regulatory considerations that impact recruitment and retention.
- Evaluate the effectiveness of recruitment and retention programs.

trials—making it possible to reduce time to market [20]. As the number of AD patients needed for clinical trials rises—as safety and regulatory issues trend toward larger and longer trials—the demand for patient recruitment services has grown exponentially.

- Having a line item in the budget for recruitment services encourages planning and execution of the program during start-up planning. Successful factors resulting in enhanced recruitment are directly impacted when study teams and sites focus on "how to" locate and communicate with patients and families of AD patients.

12.9 DETERMINING A RECRUITMENT FUNNEL

Experienced recruitment providers have long acknowledged that scientific and artistic skill sets are needed to develop successful recruitment campaigns. The science is locating the right study sites based on databases and metrics. There are also intangible components that require an artistic flare to help develop the messaging and the appropriate material. Mapping across regions, countries, and study sites may give a false sense of confidence that the evidence-based recruitment initiative will identify the right audience. Yet, despite this degree of specificity, without the right message a recruitment campaign may not be successful.

Branding the trial to appreciate the needs, interests, and motivations of the target audience is the most effective route: The message needs to be understandable, interesting, eye-catching, and ear-catching with an emotional appeal that creates a call to action without crossing the threshold into material needing the approval of an IRB.

If the right message reaches the intended audience, there will be many people aligning their trial experience, as stated by caregiver Becky Teel: "The comfort I got from working with a team of people who were sympathetic, empathetic, and driven to help was enormous. They were like another family to me, and they put us at the cutting edge of research [21]". See also Box 12.5.

12.9.1 Recruitment Effort Launch "All Systems in Place"

Early planning is a technique that is followed as sites are being selected, rather than after sites are initiated. The investigator meeting may be an excellent opportunity to be proactive and solicit input from the investigators on the best way to recruit.

Relationship building is becoming more mainstream as protocols become more complex: Providers need to collaborate to amass the full range of services if sponsors wish to launch a successful campaign. The materials listed in Box 12.6 are essential to an effective campaign.

BOX 12.5 GOALS OF THE DRUG INFORMATION ASSOCIATION (DIA) PATIENT RECRUITMENT SUBCOMMITTEE

- Define metrics for measuring progress.
- Use data-driven analysis to identify and share best practices among participants.
- Develop and implement educational programs and communication tools.
- Interface and provide input to advocacy organizations regarding ethical issues associated with the enrollment of participants into clinical trials.
- Develop a site-specific questionnaire that cites complete detailing enrollment challenges and offers options to develop a custom recruitment campaign.
- Develop and implement patient-focused communications regarding the risks and benefits of volunteering for clinical trials.

BOX 12.6 EDUCATIONAL RECRUITMENT MATERIALS

- Educational brochures to raise awareness of the trial (local site contact information).
- Posters, wall boards with pull- off flyers.
- Pre-screening tool tri fold containing key entry criteria.
- Advertisement—print and TV.
- Referral letters—PI to doctor, and doctor to patient.
- Study-branded website may include pre-screening ability, location site finder.

The IRB must review all direct advertising for research subjects: that is to say advertising intended to be seen or heard by prospective subjects to solicit their preparation in the study [22,23]. Communications that are educational or provide general information, such as postings or podcasts describing symptoms or an underlying disease, do not need to be submitted to the IRB.

The term "social media" refers to Internet-based modes of communication that allow users to interact with the medium (typically a website) or other users. The term includes social networking websites (such as Facebook, LinkedIn, and Twitter), and social photo and video sharing websites (such as Instagram, Pinterest, and YouTube). Social media can also include blogs, podcasts, and text messages. Social media outlets are revolutionizing the ability of study sponsors and researchers to conduct clinical trials, but the Food and Drug Administration (FDA) and the Office of Human Research Protection (OHRP) have provided little guidance on their use [24]. The FDA held hearings on the use of social media in clinical research in late 2009 and has promised to issue guidance specific to this topic, but no guidance has been issued to date [25].

Social media presents an incredible opportunity to connect with trial participants on a level never seen before—"Patients engage" regularly with each other in online health communities. In a recent pilot test, a PR firm—with a specialized social media focus—sought to facilitate a patient recruitment campaign alongside a large-scale AD study. In the three months that the group was actively engaging with the community, one million digital impressions were proof of the widespread exposure to the group's effort. They had generated traffic to an AD-specific web asset, contributing to the dialogue surrounding the disease in the social sphere, and consequently harnessed a group of around 300 unique users (including large AD support groups) who interacted with the account on a daily basis. In a matter of 90 days, the PR firm had gotten a foothold on the digital AD discussion and had showed how a social media campaign can play a highly effective part in patient recruitment.

These community-oriented conversations offer patients and families information with a personal spin, and foster potent patient-to-patient relationships [26]. As social media campaigns are designed to raise awareness, they strive to become influencers within the virtual AD community by developing content to be shared throughout all the social spheres. As the campaign builds momentum, and followers take note, the audience is expanded—thus driving interested followers to priority web assets. The content on the website is educational, disease focused, and an intake prescreener questionnaire directs visitors to a site locator to identify the closest study site without exposing study-specific information. It is recommended that all North American trial websites post one central number to collate all data points into one central place. For sites outside NA, European Union regulatory authorities do not accept pre-screening potential patients via call centers. List investigator site and contact information on the study website, Clinical Trials.gov or Trial Match (Alz.org AD trial site) so that prospective patients can follow up directly with the investigative site.

The use of centralized call centers fosters the rapid processing of large volumes of data across multiple sites, protocols, and various social marketing campaigns. They have been used to identify trends in recruitment and retention challenges, and they are often referred to as aggregators and distributors of data. Recent data point to an upswing in spending on central call centers with annual growth reaching an estimated US$120 million in 2003 [27]. IRBs review and approve call scripts and HIPAA compliance statements, along with existing standard procedures for the protection of patient privacy being made available from call centers that are considering providing recruitment and retention services to the industry. So often people are interested in finding out more about clinical research and may prefer the option of speaking to a person outside the study site to understand more about clinical research trials prior to being "transferred" to the trial site.

One of the many benefits of having a dedicated call center is having a live and trained professional responding to potential study participants: They ask a series of questions to determine if candidates are eligible based on subsets of questions. If the caller meets certain criteria they are asked if they would like to "opt in" and be transferred to the closest study site. The call center has a direct line to the study site and transfers the caller directly to a site staff member; if the caller passes the pre-screener questions and meets basic study entry requirements, an appointment is made to meet with the investigator to determine eligibility. This is a great alternative to sites that do not have the resources to respond to callers until after hours.

As efficacy is measured, recruitment strategies becomes more scientific and evidence-based relying on informatic tools such as disease incidence databases, insurance claims databases, prescribing databases, and investigator databases to pinpoint the right sites and investigators. Along with media campaigns, multiple strategies using several tactics will most likely achieve the best outcome. As trials progress, the efforts of the recruitment campaign are measured on a continual basis of allowing the metrics to be developed and fine-tuned, leading to completion of enrollment on time.

12.10 BUDGETING THE STUDY

Costing out procedures of an AD clinical trial requires a thorough analysis of the specific protocol tasks, and appropriate knowledge of and familiarity with institutional and standalone research site resources; delineation of standard-of-care from research events and procedures to understanding CPT coding and billing; familiarity with relevant federal and state laws governing trials; estimating a reasonable, average number of cycles or days each patient will be in the study; and a clear understanding of the study completion timeline and requirements triggering payments as stated in the clinical trial agreement.

Tips for successful budgeting include looking at a flow chart that breaks down the protocol into specific paths for each patient with sections divided by service provider; this will create a master timeline that plots each participant's usage of critical resources over time, such as MRI test space available weekly, or infusion center for delivery of investigational product.

How patients are accrued onto a protocol will often determine the overtaxing of clinical research resources: Create a worst-case scenario timeline and one according to plan. Create a billing grid—usually derived from the study calendar—to monitor the cost of the trial during the early phase when one-third of the sites are active and enrollment is just starting; and then midway through recruitment, at the height of activity and site participation, and at the end of the study's finalizing queries, close out visits, etc.

Another tip for successful budgeting is to understand the patient population and be realistic as to where patients will be recruited (either from clinic databases or the general community) to accurately estimate the accrual rate. An assessment of study metrics identifying screen failure trends may require amending the protocol instead of adjusting the recruitment campaign.

The general rule of thumb to factor in for site labor costs is to allow 4–10 hours per visit (or 1–2 hours per time point for clinical research center (CRC) labor), 1–3 hours per visit for faculty labor, and 2–3 hours per visit for psychometric and clinical rater; if applicable, a 30% screen failure rate is considered to be fair.

Hold firm on the time required to chart screenings and logs that can consume enormous amounts of time. Perform a workload analysis by tracking all trial activities in monthly reports to document the amount of work done within a certain timeframe. This will help create benchmarks for your institution or group.

Common mistakes such as overestimating the ease of obtaining subjects, underestimating the time required for regulatory affairs, under budgeting for the unexpected, and overestimation of research staff efficiency and expertise may delay regulatory filing.

12.11 THE REALITY OF PATIENT ENROLLMENT AND RETENTION

According to a 2011 *New York Times* report, industry-wide research and development spending has increased to more than US$ 45 billion annually, more than doubling since 2000 [28]. Among these and other figures seen in the pharmaceutical and healthcare industry—e.g., annual national health expenditures to expand to US$ 4.6 trillion in 2020, according to the US Department of Health and Human Services [22]—seldom considered is the value these dollars have against the trial participants.

These subjects represent an invaluable population to the sponsor, CRO, and investigative site; therefore, metrics-driven approaches are

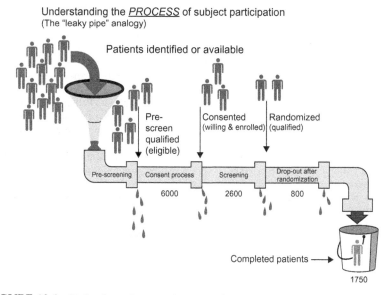

FIGURE 12.1   Defined metrics to evaluate recruitment success.

necessary to determine a complete tracking at all stages including: pre-screening, first screening visit/signed consent, dosed/randomized and enrolled, discontinued/early termination, completers/evaluable. Through close oversight and continuous measurement of the actions, linking to referral sources and outcomes at the study site will show significant information.

The "leaky pipe" analogy provides a visual display of where along the recruitment and retention continuum the majority of patients are lost. The diagram in Figure 12.1 closely resembles the metrics from a large multinational Alzheimer trial, which consisted of approximately 240 sites; 6,000 participants' signed consent, 2,650 were randomized/dosed, and 1,715 subjects completed the trial.

Enrollment forecasting was predicted to be 18 months, instead it took three years to complete; this was due in part to having to cast a much wider net then originally predicted, due to a 41% screen failure rate and a drop-out rate of 30%. The "leaky pipe" analogy may divulge a reasonable or expected patient loss through the pre-screening or screening process; but, if the informed consent process is not successful, this may dictate an alternative intervention. Monitoring the flow of patients through the pipeline—and focusing on the "leaks"—may diminish the response to specific interventions. While sponsors, sites, and recruitment specialists work to refine their metrics, tracking and reporting systems, the process of subject participation may significantly improve the rate of return for recruitment and retention in future trials.

References

[1] Getz K. Guide to Making Informed Decisions About Volunteering for a Clinical Trial. Jerian Publishing; 2007. p. 42.

[2] Center for Information and Study on Clinical Research Participation. Public Attitudes and Perceptions—Generation Information About Clinical Trials [Internet]. Available at: <http://www.ciscrp.org/professional/facts_pat.html>.

[3] ECRI Health Technology Assessment Information Services. Patients' Reasons for Participation in Clinical Trials and Effect of Trial Participation on Patient Outcomes. April 2002. Issue No. 74, 3. Available at: <https://www.ecri.org/Documents/Clinical_Trials_Patient_Guide_Evidence_Report.pdf>.

[4] Getz K. Public Confidence and Trust Today. Measuring Trust in Clinical Trials, The ACRP Monitor September, 2008, 18–19. Available from: <http://www.ciscrp.org/downloads/articles/Getz_publicopinion.pdf>.

[5] Getz K. "Improving Recruitment and Retention in Industry—Sponsored Clinical Trials." Drug Information Association meeting, April, 2003.

[6] Woolley M, Prospst S. Poll Data on Attitudes Towards Medical Research. Research! America. In: Visions of a Healthier Future: Annual Report. Presented at the Institute of Medicine's Clinical Roundtable, Washington DC, September 25, 2000. JAMA 2005;294:1380–1384.

[7] Definition: Disability. WikiPedia.org. May 2013. Available from: <http://en.wikipedia.org/wiki/Disablility>.

[8] Definition: Activities Of Daily Living. Wikipedia.org, April 2013. Available from: <http://en.wikipedia.org/wiki/Activities_of_daily_living>.

[9] Alzheimer's Disease Facts And Figures. Alzheimer's & Dementia, Ethical and Racial Diversity in Caregiving, Volume 8, Issue 2, 2013, 31. Available from: <http://www.alz.org/cacentral/documents/facts_and_figures_2013.pdf>.

[10] Alzheimer's Association. Alzheimer's Disease Facts And Figures. Alzheimer's & Dementia, Caregiving Tasks, Volume 8, Issue 2, 2013, 32. Available from: <http://www.alz.org/cacentral/documents/facts_and_figures_2013.pdf>.

[11] Best Practices Studies: What Is An APQC Best Practices Study? American Productivity and Quality Center (APQC). Available from: <http://www.apqc.org/best-practices-studies>.

[12] Tufts Center for the Study of Drug Development. Growing Protocol Design Complexity Stresses Investigators. Tufts CSDD Impact Report, Volume 10, No.1. Jan/Feb 2008. Available at: <http://csdd.tufts.edu/reports/description/impact_reports>.

[13] Alzheimer Association. 2013. *Alzheimer Dementia* 9(2), Slide 32, Table 5.

[14] Greenwald, M. Caregiving in the US. National Alliance for Caregiving in collaboration with AARP. Funded by MetLife Foundation, November 2009. Available from: <http://www.caregiving.org/data/Caregiving_in_the_US_2009_full_report.pdf>.

[15] Food and Drug Administration. Guidance for Industry E6 Good Clinical Practice: Consolidated Guidance. FDA. April 1996. Available from: <http://www.fda.gov/downloads/Drugs/Guidances/ucm073122.pdf>.

[16] Safran, C. Hearing Before the Subcommittee on Health of the Committee on Ways and Means, US Congress, J une 17, 2004. Available from: <www.waysandmeans.house.gov/media/transcript/9897.html>.

[17] National Institutes of Health Research Involving Individuals with Questionable Capacity to Consent: Points to Consider. November 2009 [cited 2011 Jan 1]. Available from: <http://grants.nih.gov/grants/policy/questionablecapacity.htm#_ftn11>.

[18] National Institutes of Health "Research Involving Individuals with Questionable Capacity to Consent: Points to Consider". Nov 2007. Available from: <http://grants.nih.gov/Grants/policy/questionablecapacity.htm>.

[19] Katzen J. Legally authorized representatives in clinical trials. J Clin Res Best Pract 2011;7(3) Available from: <http://firstclinical.com/journal/2011/1103_LAR.pdf>.

[20] Anderson DLA. Guide to patient recruitment and retention: the artistic side of patient recruitment. CenterWatch Weekly 2004:107.

[21] Teel B. Center for information and study on clinical research participants. Patient Perspectives, 2009.

[22] US Department of Health and Human Services, Office for Human Research Protections. September 20, 2005. Guidance on Institutional Review Board Review of Clinical Trials Websites. Available from: <www.fda.gov/RegulatoryInformation/Guidances/ucm126428.htm>.

[23] US Food and Drug Administration. 2010. Recruiting Study Subjects—Information Sheet. Available at: <www.fda.gov/RegulatoryInformation/Guidances/ucm126428.htm>.

[24] Gearhart C. JD IRB Review of the Use of Social Media in Research. The Monitor, Issue 7/Volume 26, 2012, 39–42.

[25] Redfearn, S. First FDA Draft Guidance on social media leaves clinical trials industry waiting for more CenterWatch Weekly, January 9 2012, p. 1.

[26] Dolan, AP. Patient-leaders of online health communities discuss patient-to-patient conversations on clinical trials. The Monitor. Volume 26, Issue 2, 2012, 58–63.

[27] Anderson DL. Applied Clinical Trials on line. Improving Recruitment and Retention Practices Based on Input from Public and Patients. CenterWatch, Boston, MA, 2003.

[28] Wilson, D. Drug Firms Face Billions in Losses in '11 as Patents End. NY Times, March 6, 2011. Available from: <http://www.nytimes.com/2011/03/07/business/07drug.html?pagewanted=all.&_r=0>.

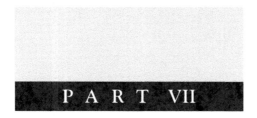

PART VII

ENHANCING LOW AND MIDDLE INCOME COUNTRIES' CAPACITY AND CAPABILITY TO CONDUCT ALZHEIMER'S DISEASE TRIALS

CHAPTER

13

South America's AD Clinical Trials Experience: Lessons Learned from Argentina and Brazil

Ricardo F. Allegri[1], Pablo Bagnati[1], Sonia Brucki[2] and Ricardo Nitrini[2]

[1]Memory and Aging Center, Instituto De Investigaciones Neurologicas "Raúl Carrea" (FLENI), Buenos Aires, Argentina
[2]Hospital das Clínicas, Department of Neurology, University of São Paulo School of Medicine, São Paulo, Brazil

13.1 INTRODUCTION

The world's population is aging. Improvements in healthcare in the past century have contributed to people living longer and healthier. However, this has also resulted in an increase in the number of people with age-related diseases like dementia. The growth of dementia in the next 20 years will be much more acute in those countries with low and medium incomes, in comparison with those nations with high incomes [1].

In 2012, the World Health Organization and Alzheimer's Disease International wrote a report which makes a major contribution to our understanding of dementia and its impact on individuals, family and society around the world; the report calls on all governments, policymakers, and stakeholders to define dementia as a public health priority [2].

Clinical trials are growing as a result of considering dementia as an epidemic disease in the coming years. ClinicalTrials.gov showed that 363 Alzheimer's disease (AD) studies were open worldwide but only 1.1% are ongoing in South America [3].

M. Bairu & M.W. Weiner (Eds):
Global Clinical Trials for Alzheimer's Disease.
DOI: http://dx.doi.org/10.1016/B978-0-12-411464-7.00013-4

Dementia clinical trials have been progressively more difficult to undertake and need to enrol high numbers of patients to meet the requirements of the regulatory agencies (Food and Drug Administration (FDA) and European Medicines Agency (EMEA)). South America has larger urban populations than other emerging regions and could provide treatment-naïve patients for clinical trials [4].

The aims of this chapter will be to discuss the advantages and disadvantages of AD clinical trials in South America, starting with the lessons learned from Argentina and Brazil.

13.2 GEOGRAPHY, DEMOGRAPHY, AND ECONOMY

The South American region is one of the top emerging markets, together with Southeast Asia and Eastern Europe. The region includes several countries, but the two most important are Brazil and Argentina. Both cover 12.3 million square kilometers, with a population estimated at over 240 million. Portuguese is the language in Brazil whereas Spanish is the language in Argentina and the other countries in South America. Brazil is the largest South American country both in area (8.5 million square kilometres) and in population (around 200 million). Argentina is the second largest in area (3.8 million square kilometers) with 40 million inhabitants. There are large urban sections in both, such as São Paulo (11 million residents) and Buenos Aires (3 million residents) [5].

Between 2010 and 2015, life expectancy worldwide will be 78 years for men and 82 years for women and in South America it will 80 years for men and 83 years for women, which is similar to Europe [5].

The population in South America shows great diversity. At the beginning of the sixteenth century, Portugal and Spain began to colonize the region. Brazil had an African immigration, which began with slavery in the seventeenth century and continued into the nineteenth century, with a huge amount of interracial marriages and descendants. During the nineteenth century, the region saw a large migration of Italians, Jews, Japanese, Germans, Lebanese, Syrians, Arabs, Russians, and Polish, and from oriental Europe in the twentieth century during the World War II period. The predominant religion is Roman Catholic.

South America is an important emerging market; Argentina is ranked in 24th position in the world economy and Brazil, which is the largest Latin American economy, in 7th position [6]. Social disparity remains a significant problem in Latin America; in almost half of the countries, half or more of the population live below the poverty line. The human development index is considered in a very high level in Argentina, coming 45th out of 187 countries, and Brazil is in 84th position, with a high level [7].

Educational level in Argentina is around nine years, with a literacy rate of 97.7%, and in Brazil this rate is 90.4% with a mean of seven years of education. This is an important issue, since dementia has a higher rate, and probably an earlier onset, in low educated individuals, due to their low cognitive reserve [8].

A pooled data of prevalence of dementia surveys from six Latin American countries showed that the dementia rate among illiterates was 15.67% whereas in literate individuals it was 7.16% [9].

13.3 HEALTHCARE INFRASTRUCTURE

Resources and healthcare infrastructure are well suited for enabling global clinical trials [4]. In fact, compilation of data from 2006 to 2010 shows that Argentina had 30 physicians per 10,000 population, more than the USA, which has 24, while the number was 17 in Brazil. Argentina had 45 hospital beds per 10,000 populations, more than the USA, which has 30, while the number was 24 in Brazil. In 2009, total expenditure on health as a percentage of gross domestic product was 9.5 in Argentina and 8.8 in Brazil compared with 17.6 in the USA [1].

Healthcare in Argentina is shared between the public and private sector. The public sector provides care to low and middle income populations, mainly in public hospitals, whereas the private sector tends to provide care to middle and high income populations, including home assistance [10]. Unfortunately, this distribution is unequal: More than 17 million people (43% of the population) have access only to the public health system, which receives only 28% of the total health resources [11]. On the other hand, most elderly people (91% of people aged 65 and over) receive medical care from Social Security Support, in an optimal inclusive model, but the economic instability in the country through the years makes its efficacy fluctuate to cover the disease's demands. Despite this, in the last five years the system has shown a slight improvement [12].

In Brazil, healthcare is provided in most cases by the government and public healthcare—the Unified Health System (SUS). There is a medication program, which is responsible for the free distribution of basic medications (arterial hypertension, diabetes, for example) and special treatments (atypical antipsychotics, anticancer drugs, for example). In 2007, the Brazilian government spent R$ 1,956,332,705.60 (about US$ 980 million) on medications [13]. Distribution of the three available cholinesterase inhibitors (donepezil, rivastigmine and galantamine) is free. There are centers in many cities that regulate this distribution, making a validation of diagnosis and drug necessity. Drugs are available only for

AD; patients with other dementias, like Lewy body dementia or vascular dementia, do not receive these medications on this program.

13.4 REGULATORY INFORMATION

South American regulatory authorities increasingly employ good clinical practice (GCP) terminology and have adopted features of GCP within regulations and guidelines; however, no country is a signatory of International Conference on Harmonization (ICH)–GCP guidelines. Each country in the region has different local regulatory requirements. On the whole, procedures, regulations, and processes are not harmonized within the region [4].

The Pan American Health Organization has developed a document called *Documento de las Americas* (*Document of the Americas*). The objective was to propose guidelines for good clinical practice that can serve as a foundation for regulatory agencies, as well as for investigators, ethics committees, universities, and businesses. It was developed with representation of the regulatory agencies from Argentina, Brazil, Chile, Costa Rica, the Caribbean Community (CARICOM), Cuba, Mexico, the USA, and Venezuela.

Each country has its own regulatory agency that, as a part of the Ministry of Health or in association with it, regulates clinical trials conducted in the country. Ethics review is typically an important component, but the details vary among the countries.

When the clinical trials program includes a placebo control, there are restrictions in Brazil and Argentina, where the National Ethics Committee and Federal Council of Medicine prohibit the conduct of clinical trials in which a placebo is administered as the sole treatment when an approved treatment is available for use as a comparator.

In Brazil and Argentina, there are additional restrictions on clinical trials related to post-study access to the drug. If the study doctor considers the study drug to be the best treatment option for a participant, the patient must be assured of continued access to the drug. In both countries, the ethics committees prohibit payment for the patient's participation in clinical trials.

Additional challenges include ensuring that site facilities are adequate and that staff members have appropriate levels of experience, and ensuring provision of the study drug, comparators, and background medication required for the conduct of the clinical trial. Sponsors must also often supply insurance as well as written assurance that treatment for injuries related to the study will be provided.

13.5 EPIDEMIOLOGY OF AD

The total number of people with dementia worldwide in 2010 was estimated at 35.6 million and is projected to nearly double every 20 years, to 65.7 million in 2030 and 115.4 million in 2050. The total number of new cases of dementia each year worldwide is nearly 7.7 million, implying one new case every four seconds [2]. The growth of dementia in the next 20 years will be much more acute in those countries with low and medium incomes, compared with those nations with high incomes [2].

The total estimated worldwide costs of dementia were US$ 604 billion in 2010. In high income countries, informal care (45%) and formal social care (40%) account for the majority of costs, while the proportionate contribution of direct medical costs (15%) is much lower. In low income and lower middle income countries (LMIC), direct social care costs are small and informal care costs (i.e., unpaid care provided by the family) predominate. Changing population demographics in many LMIC may lead to a decline in the ready availability of extended family members in the coming decades [2].

In Argentina, there are no complete epidemiological works with the required information for an efficient planning of health strategies in the prevention and assistance of dementia. A recent initiative in Argentina by the National Health Department has become the model of the first centralized Registry of Cognitive Pathologies in Argentina (ReDeCAr, Registro de DeterioroCognitivo en Argentina), which appears as an epidemiological initial kick-off, unpublished in the country at the time of writing. The hope is that this work will be transformed in the short term into a platform for a whole national plan to tackle dementia [14]. ReDeCAr is an observable prospective study carried out in hospitals and health centers throughout the country, using software at a national level, which includes systems of epidemiological watch, connected to the National Health Department [14].

In this context, the prevalent dementia rate in Argentina is estimated as 12.18% of people over 65 years old [15]. An epidemiological study in Cañuelas (a city in the Buenos Aires province) found that 23% of people over 60 years old had cognitive impairment [16]. According to these numbers, it can be inferred that there are approximately 1,000,000 people with cognitive impairment and 480,000 with dementia in the country [17].

Dementia creates an important economic, social, and personal burden. In this respect, local investigations were conducted to find out the costs of dementia in Argentina. The study carried out by Allegri et al. [18] showed that the annual costs were US$ 3420,40 in mild Alzheimer's dementia and up to US$ 9657,60 in severe forms, adding up to US$ 14,447,68 including care paid by the patient's family. A recent study conducted in our country shows that the different types of dementia (AD, vascular and frontotemporal dementia) have different costs. Vascular dementia is slightly more expensive, probably because of the presence of behavioural symptoms and functional level impairment [19].

Population-based studies in Brazil have observed rates from 5.1 to 19% of dementia; AD is responsible for 55–60% of the cases [20–24]. We can observe heterogeneous rates among countries, probably due to educational levels, and different diagnostic criteria. In the pooled data of epidemiology of dementia surveys from six Latin American countries, the overall prevalence rate of dementia was 7.1% for subjects aged 65 or more [9]. In that study, AD was the most frequent cause of dementia in all included countries, ranging from 49.9% in Maracaibo, Venezuela, to 84.5% in Concepcion, Chile. Vascular dementia was the second most prevalent disease causing dementia, ranging from 8.7% in Lima, Peru, to 26.5% in Maracaibo,Venezuela [9]. Prevalence of dementia could be different according to different criteria; it was shown by Rodriguez et al. [25] that the prevalence of dementia was underestimated when using the Diagnostic and Statistical Manual of Mental Disorders (DSM)-IV criterion compared with the 10/66 dementia algorithm, mainly in rural and less-developed sites.

13.6 HEALTHCARE INFRASTRUCTURE IN DEMENTIA CARE

As in general healthcare, as described above, dementia care in Argentina and Brazil is shared between the public and private sector. In the assessment, diagnosis and treatment of dementia, Argentina presents an unequal distribution of specialists (neurologists, psychiatrists and geriatricians), with most of them located in large cities, while there is a shortage of specialists in small towns and rural areas. The facilities needed for accurate diagnosis are scarce around the country, except in Buenos Aires and a few other large provincial cities. There are few specialists trained in geriatric neuropsychiatry [26].

In Brazil, in a survey of dementia specialists who care for dementia patients in their region, we observed that depending on region there is a different distribution of specialists taking care of these patients: 50–70% of the neurologists see patients with dementia, 10–20% of psychiatrists, and 10–40% of the geriatricians.

In the last 10 years the so-called memory clinics, or dementia clinics, have been playing an important role in Argentina. Most of these memory clinics are based on private initiatives. In a recent questionnaire, 20 directors of the most relevant memory clinics were interviewed [27]. Among its main findings, this questionnaire showed that 70% of these memory clinics only assist private clients; 60% are directed by neurologists. However, every clinic had at least one psychiatrist among their staff. Only 35% of the centers perform clinical trials and only 20% of the groups present original papers or studies at meetings. Interestingly, 60% of the centers have day care services, 35% of the clinics provide training courses for caregivers, and 80% of the memory clinics offer counselling for spouses and caregivers [27].

Private care in Brazil is undertaken by physicians in their private offices, but is not common in specialized memory or dementia clinics. This last type of care is given in universities, with a multidisciplinary approach. All centers have a research clinic independent from assistance places. These memory clinics in the universities usually see from 15 to 80 Alzheimer's patients per month; with around 4–10 patients per month being new cases.

We know how useful information related to dementia care can be. More than two-thirds of people with dementia live at home and the majority are cared for by family members [28]. Argentina has a similar profile [29,30]: Most senior citizens live at home with their families and approximately 15% are institutionalized in nursing homes [31]. Family and nonfamily caregivers need information and counselling about dementia care. In our country, these resources are improving. ALMA (Asociación de Lucha contra el Mal de Alzheimer—Association against AD) is the main local entity (an Alzheimer's Disease International member) fighting against the disease; it works locally, to promote and offer care and support for people with dementia and their carers. It has more than 20 associations around the country [32].

Our group wrote the first book in the country about dementia family care in 2003, re-edited in 2010 [33]. More books and publications have been written to help families in the early detection and treatment of dementia in Argentina [34,35].

In Brazil we have ABRAz (Associação Brasileira de Alzheimer—Alzheimer's Brazilian Association) that supports caregivers, giving juridical assistance and advice on how to cope better with patients with dementia. It is an organization created by families of demented people.

The very early dementia diagnosis in Argentina is another current challenge. It may be possible to improve the predictive validity of the prodromal risk indicators based upon cognitive decline and subjective impairment. One widely advocated approach is the incorporation of disease biomarkers that may indirectly represent the extent of underlying neuropathology: structural neuroimaging (medial temporal lobe or hippocampal volume), functional neuroimaging ($A\beta$ ligands, to visualize amyloid plaques in vivo), and cerebrospinal fluid (CSF) [36]. In this regard, in February 2011 in Buenos Aires, Argentina, FLENI [37] became part of ADNI (Alzheimer's Disease Neuroimaging Initiative) [38,39],

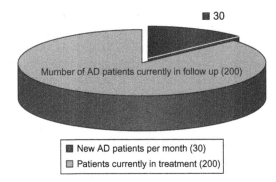

FIGURE 13.1   Number of AD patients recruited each month and number of patients in follow-up treatment. *(Survey: AD Research Sites in Argentina, 2012)*

a public sector–industry partnership founded in 2004 to develop biomarkers to predict the progression from normal aging or mild cognitive impairment to the dementia phase of AD. The study requires volumetric magnetic resonance imaging (MRI) and positron emission tomography (PET) with fluorine-18-labeled deoxyglucose scans and Aβ ligands (PiB and AV45), cognitive and neurological evaluations, and analysis of CSF biomarkers (Aβ42, tau and f-tau). In addition, FLENI houses one of the brain banks in South America [37]. We carried out a survey of 10 important investigation sites in Argentina, which showed a high per site recruitment (30 new AD patients per month) and a significant number of patients who continued with treatment (mean 200) (Figure 13.1).

The Brazilian Aging Brain Study Group has a brain bank at the University of São Paulo which consists of a large number of brains of elderly people, including non-demented subjects, and a large spectrum of pathologies related to aging brain processes. The subjects are selected from the São Paulo Autopsy Service, with a comprehensive interview with relatives about the deceased, including a Clinical Dementia Rating (CDR) interview and a functional questionnaire. Brain parts are frozen and fixated. CSF, carotids, kidneys, heart and blood are also collected, and DNA is extracted. During the first 21 months, 1,602 samples were collected and were classified by CDR as CDR0: 65.7%; CDR0.5:12.6%, CDR1:8.2%, CDR2:5.4%, and CDR3:8.1% [40].

Thirteen centers are developing protocols to follow up on 480 subjects divided into subjective memory complainers, mild cognitive impairment and AD (senile and presenile onset) for three years, with ADNI protocol and their own adaptations. Patients will be submitted to clinical, neurological, and neuropsychological evaluations; all of them will include an MRI scan, a PET-FDG scan, CSF biomarkers, and genetic analysis. Patients with familial disease will be tested for presenilin 1 and 2.

Among these centers, all have MRIs with 1.5 or 3 tesla, eight have PET-FDG, and 10 will be able to perform spinal fluid biomarkers. PET scans with amyloid markers have not been available until now, but will probably become available in 2013.

13.7 INVESTIGATOR PROFILE

Most principal investigators and sub-investigators in South America have completed their medical training in the USA or Europe, often including exposure to clinical trial participation. As a result, to qualify to conduct clinical trials these investigators generally only need training in GCPs and consultation to ensure that facilities are appropriate [4].

Within the medical community, awareness and adoption of GCPs and ICH guidance are widespread. Principal investigators must comply with certain requirements (e.g., licenses and training) before receiving authorization to act as a principal investigator.

In Argentina, several private (e.g., Universidad Austral) and public (e.g., Universidad de Buenos Aires) universities, as well as non-profit organizations such as SAMEFA (Argentinean Medical Association of the Pharmaceutical Industry, www.samefa.org.ar) and FECICLA (Foundation for Clinical Research's Ethics and Quality, www.fecicla.org.ar), offer clinical trial training programs for site staff, clinical research associates, and ethics committees.

In Brazil, the SBMF (Brazilian Medical Society of Pharmaceutical Medicine, www.sbmf.org.br) as well as some other non-profit organizations like the SBPPC (Brazilian Society of Clinical Research Professionals, www.sbppc.org.br) and the newly created SOBEPEC (Brazilian Society of Clinical Research Nurses, www.sobepec.com.br) play significant roles in training activities. Sites must establish that they have the facilities required to conduct a specific trial, as specified in ANVISA's norm number 4 (local regulation). Local ethics committees must be registered and approved in CONEP (Comissão Nacional de Ética em Pesquisa); all universities have their own local ethics committee and the time necessary to analyze protocols is around 60 to 90 days. Our centers have being participating in clinical trials in II, III and IV phases.

13.8 PATIENT PROFILE

Strong local ties in the population and the availability of large hospitals mean that patients often receive treatment at the same hospital or institutions throughout their lives. Clinical investigators and site staff usually work within a network of referrals, allowing outside patient populations to be enrolled through referrals from physicians who, though not acting as investigators, recognize that trial participation may offer the chance of better treatment. Patient retention is excellent in South American investigative sites because of the ongoing relationships between physicians and patients.

13.9 CLINICAL TRIALS

Nowadays, of the 715 closed interventional studies worldwide, 34 included South America (Chile 20, Argentina 17, Brazil 8, Peru 4, Colombia 1, and Venezuela 1). Three hundred and sixty-three AD drug studies worldwide were open and only two are taking place in South America: Studies of gantenerumab in patients with prodromal AD from Roche are ongoing in Brazil, Argentina and Chile, and studies of solanezumab in AD patients are ongoing in Brazil and Argentina [3].

Clinical trials worldwide are growing as a result of considering dementia as an epidemic disease in the coming years; South America has larger urban populations than other emerging regions and could provide treatment-naïve patient populations for clinical trials. These population characteristics enable accelerated enrolment, high persistent recruitment levels, high patient retention rates, and simplified patient follow-up. These factors can make a dramatic difference in trial efficiency, in an environment of tighter timelines and funds [4].

13.10 CHALLENGE AND OPPORTUNITIES

South America, especially Argentina and Brazil, has suitable conditions for conducting and developing clinical trials, incorporating particularities of our cultures and necessities. There is a great market for drugs to control and reverse dementia, mainly AD; developing countries will be the main source of aging people in the future. Trials are becoming more complex and clinical trial designs are changing: there are greater demands to meet the requirements of the FDA and EMEA. At the same time, the new paradigm of prodromic AD has increased the inclusion of biomarkers (CSF Abeta42 and Tau, FDG PET, MRI hippocampal volume) in the majority of the trials, which can limit the number of places that use that technology. Our countries have large urban populations and high recruitment levels per site. There are well-equipped centers, memory clinics, and a great number of specialists in dementia, which has been proven by an increasing number of publications. Together with an emerging financial evolution in our countries, we will remain important points of future research.

References

[1] World Health Organization. World Health Statistics [cited Mar 2013]. Available from: <http://www.who.int/healthinfo/EN_WHS2012_Full.pdf>; 2012.

[2] World Health Organization. Dementia: A Public Health Priority. [cited Mar 2013]. Available from: <http://www.who.int>; 2012.

[3] ClinicalTrials.gov. A service of the US National Institute of Health (USA). [cited 2013 Jan 2]. Available from: <http://www.clinicaltrials.gov/ct2/results?term=Alzheimer& recr=Open>; 2013.

[4] Ukuwu H, Parma M, Guimaraes A, Fernando de Oliveira CF, Mas AP, Villeponteaux E. Clinical trials in latin America, Chin R, Bairu M, editors. Global Clinical Trials; 2011 pp. 271–308.

[5] United Nations. Population Aging. [cited Jan 2013]. Available from: <http://www.un.org/esa/population/publications/2012WorldPopAgeingDev_Chart/2012PopAgeingandDev_WallChart.pdf>; 2012.

[6] World Economic League. [cited 2013 Feb 2]. Available from: <http://www.cebr.com/wp-content/uploads/WELT-press-release-EMBARGOED-00.05-GMT-26-Dec-2012.pdf>; 2013.

[7] United Nations of Development Programs. 2011. Summary Human Development Report.

[8] Nitrini R. Dementia incidence in middle-income countries. Lancet 2012;380:1470.

[9] Nitrini R, Bottino CMC, Albala C, Capunay NSC, Ketzoian C, Rodriguez JJL, et al. Prevalence of dementia in Latin America: a collaborative study of population-based cohorts. Int Psychogeriatr 2009;21:622–30.

[10] Ritchie CW, Ames D, Burke J, Bustin J, Connely P, Laczo J, et al. An International perspective on advanced neuroimaging: come the hour or ivory tower? Int Psychogeriatr 2011(Suppl. 558–564):23.

[11] World Health Organization. World Health Statistics. Geneva: World Health Organization. <http://www.who.int/whosis/whostat/EN_WHS08_Full.pdf>; 2008 [Accessed Oct 2012].

[12] PAMI. National Institute of Social Services for Retired People and Pensioners (INSSJP/ PAMI). <http://www.pami.org.ar>; 2011 [Accessed Sept 2013].

[13] Vieira FS. Ministry of Health's spending drugs: program trends from 2002 to 2007. Rev Saude Publica 2007;43:674–81.

[14] Melcon CM, Bartoloni L, Katz M, Del Mónaco R, Mangone C, Melcon MO, et al. Propuesta de un Registro centralizado de casos con Deterioro Cognitivo en Argentina (ReDeCAr) basado en el Sistema Nacional de Vigilancia Epidemiológica. [Cognitive Impairment Centralized Case Registry in Argentina (ReDeCAr) based on Epidemiological Surveillance Model] Neurol Argent 2010;2(3):161–6.

[15] Pages Larraya F, Grasso L, Mari G. Prevalencia de las demencias de tipo Alzheimer, demencias vasculares y otras demencias en la República Argentina. [Prevalence of Alzheimer's dementia, vascular dementia and other dementias in Argentina] Rev Neurol Argent 2004;29:148–53.

[16] Arizaga RL, Gogorza RE, Allegri RF, Barman D, Morales MC, Harris P, et al. Deterioro cognitivo en mayores de 60 años en Cañuelas (Argentina). Resultados del Piloto del Estudio Ceibo (Estudio Epidemiológico Poblacional de Demencia). [Cognitive impairment in aging peoples in Cañuelas (Argentina) Pilot Study "Ceibo Study"] Rev Neurol Argent 2005;30(2):83–90.

[17] Allegri RF. Primer Registro Centralizado de Patologías Cognitivas en Argentina (ReDeCAr). Resultados del Estudio Piloto. [First Centralized Register of cognitive disease in Argentina (ReDeCAr), Results from the pilot study] Publicación del Ministerio de Salud 2011;5:7–9.

[18] Allegri RF, Butman J, Arizaga RL, Machnick G, Serrano C, Taragano FE, et al. Economic impact of dementia in developing countries: an evaluation of costs of Alzheimer-type dementia in Argentina. Int Psychogeriatr 2006;18:1–14.

[19] Galeno R, Bartoloni L, Dillon C, Serrano C, Iturry M, Allegri RF. Clinical and economic characteristics associated with direct costs of Alzheimer's, frontotemporal and vascular dementia in Argentina. Int Psychogeriatr 2011;23(4):554–61.

[20] Herrera Jr. E, Caramelli P, Barreiros AS, Nitrini R. Epidemiologic survey of dementia in a community-dwelling Brazilian population. Alzheimer Dis Assoc Disord 2002;16:103–8.

[21] Lebrão ML, Duarte YAO. O projeto SABE no município de São Paulo: uma abordagem inicial. [SABE project in San Pablo: an initial assessment] Brasília: Organização Pan-Americana da Saúde 2003.

[22] Lopes MA, Hototian SR, Bustamante SE, Azevedo D, Tatsch M, Bazzarella MC, et al. Prevalence of cognitive and functional impairment in a community sample in Ribeirão Preto, Brazil. Int J Geriatr Psychiatry 2007;22(8):770–6.

[23] Bottino CMC, Azevedo Jr. D, Tatsch M, Hototian SR, Moscoso MA, Folquitto J. Estimate of dementia prevalence in a community sample from São Paulo, Brazil. Dement Geriatr Cogn Disord 2008;26:291–9.

[24] Scazufca M, Menezes PR, Vallada HP, Crepaldi AL, Pastor-Valero M, Coutinho LM, et al. High prevalence of dementia among older adults from poor socioeconomic backgrounds in São Paulo, Brazil. Int Psychogeriatr 2008;20:394–405.

[25] Llibre Rodriguez JJ, Ferri CP, Acosta D, Guerra M, Huang Y, Jacob KS, 10/66 Dementia Research Group Prevalence of dementia in Latin America, India, and China: a population-based cross-sectional survey. Lancet 2008;372:464–74.

[26] Sarasola D, Taragano F, Allegri R, Arizaga R, Bagnati P, Serrano C, et al. Geriatric neuropsychiatry in argentina. IPA Bull 2006 pp. 10 and 19.

[27] Kremer J. Memory Clinics in Argentina. Questionnaire. [cited Feb 2012]. Available from: <http://www.institutokremer.com.ar>; Córdoba, Argentina 2011.

[28] Rabins P, Lyketsos CG, Steele CD. Pract Dent Care 1999;7:111.

[29] Taragano FE. Síntomas neuropsiquiátricos en la Enfermedad de Alzheimer. [Neuropsychiatric Symptoms in Alzheimer's disease] Revista de ALMA (Asoc Lucha Mal de Alzheimer) 2011:10–11.

[30] Pollero A, Gimenez M, Allegri RF, Taragano FE. Síntomas neuropsiquiátricos en pacientes con enfermedad de Alzheimer. [Neuropsychiatric symptoms in patients with Alzheimer's disease] Vertex 2004;15(55):5–9.

[31] Taragano F, Mangone C, Comesaña Diaz E. Prevalence of neuropsychiatric disorders in nursing homes. Revista de la Asociación Argentina de Establecimientos Geriátricos 1995

[32] ALMA (Asociacion de Lucha contra el mal de Alzheimer, Argentina). <http://www.alma-alzheimer.org.ar>; 2013 [Accessed Feb 2013].

[33] Bagnati PM, Allegri RF, Kremer JL, Taragano FE. Enfermedad de Alzheimer y otras demencias. Manual para la familia. [Alzheimer's disease and other dementias. Handbook for the family] Buenos Aires, Argentina: Editorial Polemos; 2010.

[34] Manes F. Convivir con personas con EA u otras demencias. [Living with people with AD and other dementias] Buenos Aires, Argentina: D. Palais Ediciones; 2005.

[35] González Salvia M. Manual para familiares y cuidadores de personas con Enfermedad de Alzheimer [Handbook for the family and caregivers with Alzheimer's disease]. Editorial del Hospital Italiano:. Argentina: Buenos Aires; 2006.

[36] Alzheimer Disease International (ADI). World Alzheimer Report, London. 2011. p. 12.

[37] Memory and Aging Center, Institute of Neurology, FLENI, Buenos Aires, Argentina. [cited 2012 Feb 9] Available from: <http://www.fleni.org.ar>.

[38] ADNI (Alzheimer Disease Neuroimaging Initiative) FLENI partnership. [cited Feb 2012] Available from: <http://www.alz.org/research/funding/partnerships>; 2011.

[39] Burton A. Big science for a big problem: ADNI enters its second phase. Lancet 2011;10:206–7.

[40] Grinberg LT, Ferretti RE, Farfel JM, Leite R, Pasqualucci CA, Rosemberg S, Brazilian Aging Brain Study Group Brain bank of the Brazilian aging brain study group–a milestone reached and more than 1,600 collected brains. Cell Tissue Bank 2007;8(2):151–62.

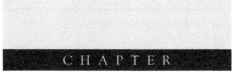

CHAPTER
14

Dementia Clinical Research in India

Tal Burt[1], Lynne Hughes[2], Amir Kalali[3] and P. Murali Doraiswamy[4]

[1]Duke Global Proof-of-Concept (POC) Research Network, Duke Clinical Research Unit (DCRU) & Duke Clinical Research Institute (DCRI), Department of Psychiatry and Behavioral Sciences, Duke University, Durham, NC, USA [2]Quintles, Reading UK [3]Quintles, San Diego, USA [4]Departments of Psychiatry and Medicine, and the Duke Institute for Brain Sciences, Duke University, Durham, NC, USA

14.1 MOTIVATION FOR GLOBAL AND INDIAN ALZHEIMER'S DISEASE CLINICAL RESEARCH

India has powerful drivers and attractive features favoring dementia research. Rapid increase in life expectancy globally and in India is likely to increase the prevalence of individuals suffering from all types of dementia including Alzheimer's disease (AD) [1,2]. Such increase in prevalence is not yet matched by the provisions of the healthcare system or indigenous medical research. The aspirations of this rapidly emerging market, on track to becoming the world's second-largest economy by 2050, are indeed to be self-sufficient in providing care to its growing population of elderly people and basing such care on home-grown research. This chapter begins with a description of the environment in India, its characteristics and potential for dementia research, then proceeds to describe current dementia research and associated challenges, and concludes with suggestions for future researchers and policymakers seeking global equity of the India dementia research ecosystem.

In addition to the growing need and demand there are unique features favoring India as a location for dementia research. Ethnic differences in a genetically heterogeneously population may affect the presentation

M. Bairu & M.W. Weiner (Eds):
Global Clinical Trials for Alzheimer's Disease.
DOI: http://dx.doi.org/10.1016/B978-0-12-411464-7.00014-6

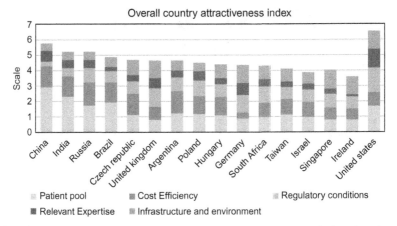

FIGURE 14.1 Most attractive global locations for the conduct of all clinical trials outside the USA, 2006. *Adapted from [7]*.

and outcome of interventions, making generalizations from studies done elsewhere difficult and making a strong case for indigenous dementia research [2–6]. India offers many operational advantages likely to appeal to multinational drug developers and contract research organizations (CROs) seeking to improve feasibility of their global trials. A study in 2006 by A.T. Kearney found India second only to China on the "Country Attractiveness Index for Clinical Trials" (Figure 14.1) [7]. Modest effect sizes in dementia pharmacological trials call for large sample sizes and rapidly recruiting sites. Large healthcare center catchment areas and a treatment-naïve population offer such advantages in most Indian urban areas. Cost advantage (40–60% when compared with Western sites) is an additional advantage. The presence of an English-speaking environment facilitates communication with patients and their families, though attention has to be given to dominance of local languages and dialects. Finally, harmonization of clinical research guidelines and regulations, and availability of Western-trained and English-speaking investigators, also represent valuable advantages for clinical research operators, though not without their challenges (discussed below) [8].

14.2 SCOPE OF DEMENTIA IN INDIA

In an aging world, dementia prevalence is increasing, especially in places with the steepest increase in life expectancy, i.e., low and middle income countries [1]. In 2010, 35.6 million people were estimated to live with AD worldwide, the number increasing to 115.4 million in 2050 [1]. In India, recent surveys have found dementia prevalence rates ranging between 3.3% (in an urban population in South India) and 4.8% in a systematic review of dementia epidemiological studies from Southeast Asia, results consistent with prevalence rates from Western countries [1,9]. However, another study found AD incidence rates from Ballabgarh in North India to be 4.7 per 1000 person-years and considerably lower than rates of 17.5 per 1000 person-years from a corresponding site in the USA [10]. Amongst those aged 65 and older, dementia rates (standardized for age sex and education) were 8.2% in urban India and 8.7% in rural India using the 10/66 dementia algorithm [11]. Rates of dementia in India are forecast to increase by more than 300% between 2000 and 2040 [1,12].

The various dementia subtypes have implications for diagnosis, pathophysiology, and response to treatment, and consequently, implications for study conduct and interpretation of results. Although considerable variability exists in India in prevalence of dementia (possibly in part due to diverging study methodologies), its subtypes and associated ApoE4, the relative prevalence of the various dementia subtypes and association with ApoE4 are more consistent [6,13–15]. Prevalence of dementia subtypes in a sample of 347 patients from a specialist clinic in India were 38.3% for AD, 25.4% for vascular dementia, 18.7% for Frontotemporal, and 8.9% for Lewy Body subtypes [16]. Mean age at presentation was 66.3 years, nearly a decade younger than in developed countries. The proportion of patients with early-onset dementia was high (49.9%). Similar findings were reported by Shaji et al. [9].

India's population ethnicity, race, and languages exhibit considerable diversity most prominent along a north–south divide. In dementia populations in India, associations with ApoE4 polymorphism were identified in AD and vascular dementia subtypes in both north and south India, and urban and rural populations, which is similar to the risk in Caucasians [14,15,17–19]. AD-related pathological findings were similar in aging populations from Mumbai and New York [20].

14.3 TREATMENT OF DEMENTIA IN INDIA

Rapid demographic changes are finding the Indian healthcare system, patients, their families and caregivers unprepared, and their needs unmet [21]. Formal care for the elderly is lacking and specialist healthcare providers are in short supply [21–23]. A recent study from Goa, a relatively prosperous region of India, found that only 5% of subjects with dementia received adequate care and access to modern diagnostic tools, and pharmacotherapy is limited [24]. Nevertheless, in a recent report from Mumbai [25], the use of research criteria to diagnose and manage patients with dementia has been demonstrated to be beneficial and feasible in public hospital memory clinics.

There is a concerted effort being made to diagnose and treat AD and it is primarily neurologists and psychiatrists who diagnose and treat these patients, not general practitioners. There are approximately 1,000 neurologists, 3,500 psychiatrists, 350 psychiatric social workers, and 40 neurology institutes/departments that are now associated with the management of AD [26]. Memory clinics or dementia clinics have recently been set up in many general/private tertiary care hospitals in India. These clinics are jointly run by departments of neurology and psychiatry and focus on the comprehensive management of AD patients, along with providing information and education for families and emotional support to caregivers.

It is these clinics that provide a substantial opportunity for the conduct of clinical trials as they have a huge catchment area, are managed by well-trained and motivated clinical staff, have access to a number of imaging modalities, and have the appropriately trained people to apply the rating scales.

14.4 CLINICAL RESEARCH REGULATORY ENVIRONMENT IN INDIA

The clinical research regulatory environment has come under sustained attack by patient and public advocates, and subsequently by the Indian Supreme Court for perceived unethical practices in the conduct of clinical trials [27]. A report by the Indian Parliament then identified deficiencies in enforcing regulations and claims of exploitation of Indian citizens by foreign pharmaceutical companies [28]. The report identified understaffed and under-resourced Central Drugs Standard Control Organization (CDSCO) as the main reasons for clinical research operations' non-compliance with regulations. Multiplicity and overlapping regulatory guidelines and sometimes ambiguous wording present additional challenges for the enforcement of guidelines. Lengthy turnaround times for clinical trial approvals have dissuaded both local and foreign sponsors from conducting clinical trials in India and have likely contributed to the reduction in the number of clinical trials in India since 2010 (Figure 14.2). Regulatory approvals relevant to dementia treatments manufactured by Indian companies include the Food and Drug Administration's approval of Dr. Reddy's generic galantamine in 2008 and Ranbaxy's generic donepezil in 2010.

However, there has been a recent change to the regulatory environment in India that is likely to discourage further placement of clinical trials in India until there is further clarification or another amendment. On January 30, 2013, The Ministry of Health and Family Welfare for

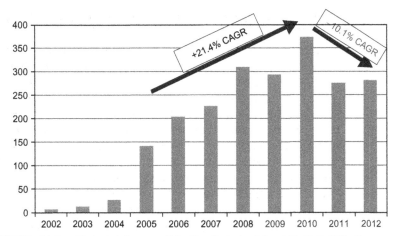

FIGURE 14.2   Clinicaltrials.gov: all-India clinical trials 2002–2012 [52]. Data were obtained from Clinicaltrial.gov on February 16, 2013. Methods: "Advanced Search" option was used; "India" entered in "Country' field." "First Received" field was used to include dates "From '01/01/...' To '12/31/...," for each year from 2002 through 2012. The following Compound Annual Growth Rate (CAGR) was used for the periods 2005–2010 and 2010–2012 (years prior to 2005 were deemed to contain data that was not meaningful):

$$\text{CAGR}\,(t_0, t_n) = \left(\frac{V(t_n)}{V(t_0)}\right)^{\frac{1}{t_n - t_0}} - 1;$$

$V(t_0); Start\ Value;\ V(t_n) : Finish\ Value;\ t_n - t_0 : Number\ of\ Years$

India issued an amendment to the Drugs and Cosmetics Act 1940 [29]. The Ministry of Law in India issued a final set of guidelines on patient compensation that now includes, once again, some of the very contentious clauses that many (in the industry) had lobbied hard to have removed by the Ministry of Health. Possibly the most contentious of these is the need to pay compensation should an experimental drug fail to show therapeutic benefit. These guidelines issued in January 2013 are in effect for all new and ongoing trials [29]. Companies are all currently working with the Indian Society for Clinical Research (ISCR), the Indian Pharmaceutical Association (IPA), and the Indian biotechnology companies' representative body to look at legal means to apply a hold to this implementation. These amendments have placed increased liability on clinical trial sponsors and CROs to provide medical management and compensation for research participants' injuries, including any study-related injuries or deaths from the use of a placebo in a placebo-controlled trial.

14.5 DEMENTIA CLINICAL RESEARCH IN INDIA

Of 1,202 dementia studies ever entered into the Clinicaltrials.gov database, only 5 (0.4%) have been conducted in India, a country that is home to 17% of the world's population. Although India clinical research activity was predicted to grow at an accelerated rate [8], there has been a decline since 2010 in the overall number of clinical trials (Figure 14.2). However, this is in contrast to the report by Kearney et al., which shows how India was deemed an attractive global location for clinical trials in 2006 (in third place after the USA and China) due mainly to a large patient population (Figure 14.1) [7]. However, trial sponsors are still not prepared to utilize this vast country's potential at the current time due to a variety of reasons as mentioned above.

Table 14.1 lists six AD/Dementia studies from Clinicaltrials.gov database. While the majority (4) are sponsored by international pharmaceutical companies, the list also includes a community-based non-pharmacological intervention and a government-sponsored testing of a herbal remedy (Curcumin) for AD.

14.5.1 Phase I AD/Dementia Trials in India

India has explicit language in the laws governing clinical trials prohibiting testing on Indians of compounds developed outside of India without prior presentation of Phase I data [30]. Furthermore, recent reports of unethical conduct in clinical research (some in AD trials) by non-Indian multinational companies has led to increased restrictions on conduct, report, and indemnification in clinical trials [28,29,31–33]. Of 240 Phase I AD trials ever entered into the Clinicaltrials.gov database, only one has been conducted in India. Figure 14.3 provides data from the Clinicaltrials.gov database on all Phase I clinical trials conducted in India between 2004 and 2012. The methodology is similar to the one used for Figure 14.2. No CAGR was calculated since no clear pattern was identified. In 2012 there appears to be an increase in the total number of Phase I trials, but of the 83 trials registered for the year, 65 (78%) were bioequivalence studies of generic drugs rather than Phase I of new drugs in development.

Early-phase clinical trials appear to be less represented than later-phase trials in the Asia-Pacific region [34]. Early-phase methodological sophistication, operational complexity, greater ethical sensitivities, and the lack of track record of Asia-Pacific sites and investigators may drive industry sponsors of such studies to conduct them elsewhere [35]. The experience of Duke University in Asia-Pacific early-phase collaborations with the National University of Singapore (NUS) in Singapore and Medanta the Medicity in India has been that East–West collaborations

TABLE 14.1 India Alzheimer's Disease/Dementia Studies (from Clinicaltrials.gov)

Name	Clinicaltrials.gov ID	Drug	Year Started	Year Completed	Sponsor	Phase	N	Population	Site
European Study of HF0220 in Mild to Moderate AD Patients	NCT00357357	HF0220	2006	2008	Hunter-Fleming Ltd	II	40	Mild to Moderate Alzheimer's	Multinational Study (three countries)
Effect of LY450139 on the Long-Term Progression of Alzheimer's Disease	NCT00594568	LY450139	2008	2011	Eli Lilly	III	164	Long-Term Progression Alzheimer's	Multinational (19 countries)
Rosiglitazone (Extended Release Tablets) as Adjunctive Therapy for Subjects with Mild to Moderate Alzheimer's Disease (REFLECT-2)	NCT00348309	Rosiglitazone XR	2006	2009	GSK	III	1496	Mild to Moderate Alzheimer's	Multinational (17 countries)
A Study of the Effect of Concomitant Administration of Rifampin on the Pharmacokinetics of BMS-708163 in Healthy Subjects	NCT01002079	BMS-708163	2010	2010	BMS	I (DDI)*	20	PK in Healthy Volunteers	India only
Efficacy and Safety of Curcumin Formulation in Alzheimer's Disease	NCT01001637	Curcumin	2009	Unknown	Jaslok Hospital and Research Centre	II	26	General Alzheimer's	India only
Evaluating the Effectiveness of a Community Based Intervention for Persons with Dementia and Their Caregivers in a Developing Country [23]	NCT00479271	Community-Based Intervention	2003	2005	London School of Hygiene and Tropical Medicine	N/A	81	Dementia Patients and Caregivers	India only

*DDI: Drug–Drug Interaction

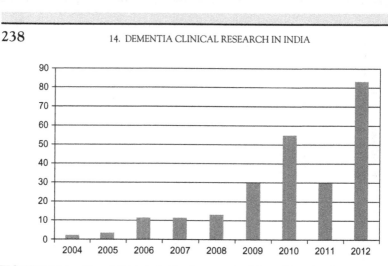

FIGURE 14.3   Phase I Trials in India. Data obtained from Clinicaltrials.gov on February 3, 2013. Methods: see Figure 14.2. CAGR was not calculated as no clear pattern was identified.

bringing together local clinical expertise with Western methodological and operational know-how foster sponsor confidence.

14.6 CULTURAL FACTORS RELATED TO DEMENTIA IN INDIA

A country as vast and heterogeneous as India can introduce ethnic and cultural variability as well as divergent local characteristics with the potential to impact on dementia research [36–39]. These can be grouped under manifestations and course of illness, clinical research environment, and study conduct.

14.6.1 Manifestation and Course of Illness

Ethnic physiological differences (body mass, pharmacokinetic differences) and pathophysiological differences (e.g., prevalence of ApoE4, speed of cognitive decline, cardiovascular risk factors, and pharmacodynamic differences) may impact disease manifestation, progression, and response to treatment [16]. Genetic differences amongst the various Indian ethnic groups and between Indians and the rest of the world may manifest in variability in disease manifestations and response to treatment including pharmacogenomic effects on parameters of drug response, both pharmacokinetic and pharmacodynamic (efficacy and safety parameters) [6,16]. Environmental factors such as diet and use of herbal medications may impact drug pharmacokinetics, including absorption, metabolism, and drug–drug interactions. Antioxidants in diet may reduce oxidative injury. Culture-specific behavioral changes (e.g., attitudes towards apathy as a pathological behavioral manifestation) and difficulties in assessing changes in activities of daily living (ADLs) where domestic help is widely available may impact the assessment of behavioral and psychological signs and symptoms of dementia [37]. Educational and occupational factors may confound diagnosis of dementia since lower education and professional attainment was found to be associated with slower progression of disease [40]. Societal influences include the extent to which extended families play a role in disease-management decision making [37] and attitudes about cognitive decline [16]. In rural communities a cognitively undemanding environment within a supportive extended family and societal network may mask AD's manifestations [10].

14.6.2 Clinical Research Environment

Public, patient, and caregiver education and attitudes about illness in old age and aging in general, and attitudes towards clinical trials, can all impact recruitment, adherence and support of dementia clinical trials. Paternalistic attitudes towards physicians as clinical research investigators may drive patients to put decisions of participation in clinical trials in the hands of their physician-investigators, thus compromising the validity of the informed consent process.

Local standard of care (e.g., availability of Western-type diagnostics and treatments) and practitioner experience and training are important considerations in the assessment of a clinical research environment and vary widely among regions and institutions in India [21]. Clinical trial guidelines in India include restrictions on studies conducted by non-Indian companies and in vulnerable populations, however, the enforcement of regulations and ethical principles is still far from optimal [30,35,36,41]. At least one AD study sponsored by a foreign pharmaceutical company made international news with claims that participants were not informed about receiving experimental treatment, and has triggered activist group protests [31]. There are also import/export restrictions on supply line and biological samples; however, they can usually be handled by submitting special permits to the appropriate regulatory authority. Institutional support (e.g., emergency services, ethics committees, and appropriate insurance and indemnification policies) is an important component of the clinical research environment, especially when conducting trials in the physically fragile and socially vulnerable populations of dementia research.

14.6.3 Study Conduct

Choice of diagnostic approaches is critical in dementia clinical trials, as is the applicability of Western criteria and assessment tools in India (e.g., Diagnostic and Statistical Manual of Mental Disorders (DSM)-IV vs 10/66 diagnostic criteria, translation of Alzheimer's Disease Assessment Scale-cognitive portion (ADAS-Cog) recall items) [36,38,39,42]. Clinical presentation of patients may be affected by demographics, risk factors, and attitudes. DSM-IV diagnosis may underestimate dementia prevalence (18% in rural India when compared with Europe) and may be an order of magnitude different from other dementia diagnostic algorithms (e.g., the 10/66) [11]. The experience of investigators and raters with dementia diagnosis, and their ability to distinguish dementia subtypes, is essential as is their assessment and inter-rater reliability when using Western assessment tools. Such experience and expertise are limited in India [2,16]. Therapeutic area expertise is crucial for the standardization of assessment [42]. Variability in study conduct can be introduced by many factors (e.g., rigor of the informed consent process, following of standard operating procedures, processing of biological samples, degree of training of research staff) [2]. Additional sources of variability amongst India research sites that can impact study conduct are the

TABLE 14.2 Impact of Ethnic and Cultural Variability and Local Characteristics on Illness and Dementia Research

A. Manifestation and course of illness
    1. Physiological differences (e.g., body mass)
    2. Pathophysiological differences (e.g., ApoE4, risk factors)
    3. Environmental (e.g., diet, climate)
    4. Behavioral (e.g., ADL)
    5. Educational and occupational
    6. Social (e.g., attitudes towards dementia, presence of support network).
B. Clinical research environment
    1. Attitudes towards research and physician-investigators
    2. Investigator competence
    3. Standard of care
    4. Regulatory environment
    5. Activist counter-research environment
    6. Institutional support.
C. Study conduct
    1. Diagnostic criteria and outcome measurements
    2. Staff experience and training in dementia research
    3. Informed consent process
    4. Site infrastructure
    5. Language barriers.

quality and maintenance of site infrastructures (e.g., availability of a steady power supply). Finally, language barriers (including availability of translation services) could impact comprehension of study objectives and compliance with study procedures. Table 14.2 shows the impact of ethnic and cultural variability and local characteristics on illness and dementia research.

14.7 DIAGNOSIS AND OUTCOME MEASURES USED FOR DEMENTIA TRIALS IN INDIA

Harmonization of screening, diagnosis, and outcome assessments is crucial to effective study methodologies and interpretation of their results [42–44]. Diagnosis of dementia made using DSM-IV criteria was found to have poor sensitivity to mild to moderate cases in low and middle income countries (LAMIC) including India [11,45,46]. An alternative scale, the 10/66 Dementia Research Group's cross-culturally validated diagnosis, appears more sensitive and consistent across different cultures [11,46]. Dementia under-diagnosis in resource-poor areas may be due to lack of access to healthcare facilities, isolation by relatives, stigma, high tolerance of health problems in elderly individuals, and high costs of diagnostic tests [47]. A comparison of the Hindi version of the Mini Mental State Examination (MMSE) (HMSE) with the original MMSE has identified inconsistencies, most prominent in the assessment of potential cognitive decline in illiterate populations [48]. An 11-item ADL scale was developed and validated for use in the elderly, rural, illiterate Indian population [49].

14.8 RECOMMENDATIONS FOR OPTIMAL ALZHEIMER'S / DEMENTIA CLINICAL RESEARCH ENVIRONMENT

Recommendations for an optimal outcome in dementia research are divided into short- and long-term recommendations and apply to industry and academic sponsors and operators of clinical research as well as government agencies and regulators (Table 14.3).

14.8.1 Short-term Considerations

Approach your potential trial sites well in advance and conduct comprehensive on-site feasibility. Feasibility should include general

TABLE 14.3   Recommendations for Optimal AD/Dementia Clinical Research Environment

---

A. Short-term considerations:
  1. Early site contact
  2. Comprehensive site feasibility assessment
  3. Collaborations with established, reliable research institutions
  4. Engagement of regulatory authorities
  5. Cultural and ethnic impact
  6. Diagnostic and assessment validity confirmation
  7. Sample size.
B. Long-term approaches:
  1. Long-term relationships with sites
  2. Dementia-supporting practice guidelines, regulations, and legislation
  3. Dementia healthcare infrastructure
  4. Dementia public awareness, advocacy, and self-help
  5. Government and academia promotion of dementia research.

---

infrastructure considerations (e.g., availability of imaging capabilities [including use of phantoms for image standardization], lab standards, human participant protection, and emergency power supplies) as well as competence and familiarity of the research team with clinical research procedures, local and globally harmonized regulations. It is especially important that site research teams be familiar in treating and conducting research in patients with dementia due to their social vulnerability and demanding healthcare management.

Research collaborators in India should be in established healthcare institutions, preferably with clinical research infrastructure including an approved ethics committee, regulatory expertise, insurance and indemnification policies, access to modern diagnostic and treatment tools, emergency services, and the appropriate research education and training programs [50]. Regulatory authorities and local ethics committees should be contacted early and requirements specific to protocol under considerations explained and implications to study conduct clarified. Cultural and ethnic impacts should be considered on study methodology and conduct (e.g., clinical presentation, interaction with caregivers, recruitment, and comprehension of informed consent, assessment tools, and study instructions) [38,39]. Such assessment should also include consideration of the impact of ethnic factors on test drugs (e.g., potential for being a pro-drug, genomic impact on linearity of pharmacokinetics, P450 enzymes) [38,39].

Careful attention should be given to diagnostic and assessment issues. Each investigator and rater should perform the rating at least five times, at each disease severity level [51]. Sample size in Indian sites should constitute a meaningful fraction (at least 20%) of the total study population to allow for valid ethnic-related analyses and meaningful generalizations and conclusions to be made [44]. Each site should have recruited enough patients (i.e., more than 5–8) to ensure data collected are not primarily from a site's "learning-curve" period. Recruitment feasibility should ensure studies are not conducted over long periods of sparse recruitment and high staff turnover as these could negatively impact familiarity with study procedures and reduce diagnosis and rating validity.

In local AD trials conducted in India, with a group of some 62 neurologists, the average recruitment rate, for subjects recruited in the mild–moderate MMSE range was 1–2 patients/site/month (psm) [26]. In addition, there was robust recruitment for subjects with a more advanced AD, and the sites consistently recruited at a rate above 1.5 psm. However, these were locally sponsored trials and not used for pivotal registration submissions.

14.8.2 Long-term Recommendations

Industry sponsors and CROs should establish long-term relationships with clinical research operators, preferably with established tertiary care facilities and/or academic centers with advanced diagnostic and treatment capabilities and clinical research experience and expertise, preferably in the dementia field. Government authorities and regulators of medical research should consider establishing legislation and regulations supporting dementia healthcare and research ensuring protection of rights of patients and caregivers, allocating the necessary resources. Together with academic experts and community leaders they should work to establish an adequate dementia healthcare infrastructure including community support networks, education and training of specialist care providers, and establishment of practice guidelines addressing the special needs of patients with dementia [24]. Such efforts should include the promotion and support of dementia advocacy and self-help organizations, and educate patients, families, caregivers, and the public at large about dementia and its management, including fighting stigma and supporting dementia research [21,24]. Other recommendations are given in Table 14.3.

14.9 SUMMARY

There is considerable interest, both nationally and internationally, in conducting dementia research in India. Motivated by a rapid increase in the aging population and a desire for indigenous, self-sufficient healthcare and medical research, dementia research in India is on course for rapid growth in the coming years. Several challenges will have to be overcome along the way. A solid and general clinical research culture and a supportive healthcare system, both tailored to the specific needs of the dementia field and its vulnerable patient population, will have to be established through careful guidance of government regulators and collaborations with academic, industry and public stakeholders both in and outside India.

Disclosures

Tal Burt has no conflicts of interest to disclose. Lynne Hughes and Amir Kalali are employees and stock holders in Quintiles. P. Murali Doraiswamy has received research grants and advisory or speaking fees from several companies in this field. He owns stock in Sonexa and AdverseEvents Inc. whose products are not discussed in this article.

References

[1] ADI. (2009). World Alzheimer Report, 2009.
[2] Cummings J, Reynders R, Zhong K. Globalization of Alzheimer's disease clinical trials. Alzheimers Res Ther 2011;3:24.
[3] Salloway S, Mintzer J, Cummings JL, Geldmacher D, Sun Y, Yardley J, et al. Subgroup analysis of US and non-US patients in a global study of high-dose donepezil (23 mg) in moderate and severe Alzheimer's disease. Am J Alzheimers Dis Other Demen 2012;27:421–32.
[4] Liu CC, Kanekiyo T, Xu H, Bu G. Apolipoprotein E and Alzheimer disease: risk, mechanisms and therapy. Nat Rev Neurol, 2013.;9:106–18.
[5] Farrer LA, Cupples LA, Haines JL, Hyman B, Kukull WA, Mayeux R, Myers RH, Pericak-Vance MA, Risch N, van Duijn CM. Effects of age, sex, and ethnicity on the association between apolipoprotein E genotype and Alzheimer disease. A meta-analysis. APOE and Alzheimer Disease Meta Analysis Consortium. JAMA 1997;278:1349–56.
[6] Singh PP, Singh M, Mastana SS. APOE distribution in world populations with new data from India and the UK. Ann Hum Biol 2006;33:279–308.
[7] Kearney AT. Make your move: taking clinical trials to the best location. Exec Agenda 2006:56–64.
[8] Gupta YK, Padhy BM. India's growing participation in global clinical trials. Trends Pharmacol Sci 2011;32:327–9.
[9] Shaji S, Bose S, Verghese A. Prevalence of dementia in an urban population in Kerala, India. Br J Psychiatry 2005;186:136–40.
[10] Chandra V, Pandav R, Dodge HH, Johnston JM, Belle SH, DeKosky ST, et al. Incidence of Alzheimer's disease in a rural community in India: the Indo-US study. Neurology 2001;57:985–9.
[11] Llibre Rodriguez JJ, Ferri CP, Acosta D, Guerra M, Huang Y, Jacob KS, et al. Prevalence of dementia in Latin America, India, and China: a population-based cross-sectional survey. Lancet 2008;372:464–74.
[12] Ferri CP, Prince M, Brayne C, Brodaty H, Fratiglioni L, Ganguli M, et al. Global prevalence of dementia: a Delphi consensus study. Lancet 2005;366:2112–7.

[13] Mastana SS, Calderon R, Pena J, Reddy PH, Papiha SS. Anthropology of the apoplipo-protein E (apo E) gene: low frequency of apo E4 allele in Basques and in tribal (Baiga) populations of India. Ann Hum Biol 1998;25:137–43.

[14] Ganguli M, Chandra V, Kamboh MI, Johnston JM, Dodge HH, Thelma BK, et al. Apolipoprotein E polymorphism and Alzheimer's disease: The Indo-US Cross-National Dementia Study. Arch Neurol 2000;57:824–30.

[15] Luthra K, Tripathi M, Grover R, Dwivedi M, Kumar A, Dey AB. Apolipoprotein E gene polymorphism in Indian patients with Alzheimer's disease and vascular dementia. Dement Geriatr Cogn Disord 2004;17:132–5.

[16] Alladi S, Mekala S, Chadalawada SK, Jala S, Mridula R, Kaul S. Subtypes of dementia: a study from a memory clinic in India. Dement Geriatr Cogn Disord 2011;32:32–8.

[17] Bharath S, Purushottam M, Mukherjee O, Bagepally BS, Prakash O, Kota L, et al. Apolipoprotein E polymorphism and dementia: a hospital-based study from southern India. Dement Geriatr Cogn Disord 2010;30:455–60.

[18] Mansoori N, Tripathi M, Alam R, Luthra K, Ramakrishnan L, Parveen S, et al. IL-6-174G/C and ApoE gene polymorphisms in Alzheimer's and vascular dementia patients attending the cognitive disorder clinic of the All India Institute of Medical Sciences, New Delhi. Dement Geriatr Cogn Disord 2010;30:461–8.

[19] Kota LN, Shankarappa BM, Shivakumar P, Sadanand S, Bagepally BS, Krishnappa SB, et al. Dementia and diabetes mellitus: association with apolipoprotein e4 polymor-phism from a hospital in southern India. Int J Alzheimers Dis 2012;2012:1–4.

[20] Purohit DP, Batheja NO, Sano M, Jashnani KD, Kalaria RN, Karunamurthy A, et al. Profiles of Alzheimer's disease-related pathology in an aging urban population sam-ple in India. J Alzheimers Dis 2011;24:187–96.

[21] Dias A, Patel V. Closing the treatment gap for dementia in India. Indian J Psychiatry 2009;51(**Suppl. 1**):S93–7.

[22] Varghese MPV. The Graying of India Agarwal SG, Salhan D, Ichhpujani R, Shrivastava R, editors. Mental Health: an Indian perspective 1946–2000. New Delhi: Elsevier; 2004. pp. 240–48.

[23] Das SK, Pal S, Ghosal MK. Dementia: Indian scenario. Neurol India 2012;60:618–24.

[24] Dias A, Dewey ME, D'Souza J, Dhume R, Motghare DD, Shaji KS, et al. The effec-tiveness of a home care program for supporting caregivers of persons with demen-tia in developing countries: a randomised controlled trial from Goa, India. PLoS One 2008;3:e2333.

[25] Nair G, Van Dyk K, Shah U, Purohit DP, Pinto C, Shah AB, et al. Characterizing cogni-tive deficits and dementia in an aging urban population in India. Int J Alzheimers Dis 2012;2012:1–8.

[26] Quintiles. From an internal, proprietary database using illustrative, de-identified data. Data on File, 2013.

[27] Srinivasan S. Ethical concerns in clinical trials in India: an investigation. Mumbai: Centre for Studies in Ethics and Rights; 2009.

[28] Rajya Sabha POI. Fifty-Ninth Report on the Functioning of the Central Drugs Standard Control Organization (CDSCO) Rajya Subha Secretariat, New Delhi, India 2012.

[29] Ministry of Health and Family Welfare. Drugs and Cosmetics (First Amendment) Rules, India, 2013.

[30] Government of India. Schedule Y. Requirements and Guidelines for Permission to Import and/or Manufacture New Drugs for Sale or to Undertake Clinical Trials. Drugs and Cosmetics Rules, 1945, India. 2003.

[31] Lakshmi R. India's drug trials fuel consent controversy. The Washington Post online, 1 January 2012.

[32] Shetty P. Vaccine trial's ethics criticized. Nature 2011;474:427–8.

[33] Srinivasan S. Patient protection in clinical trials in India: some concerns. Perspect Clin Res 2010;1:101–3.
[34] Louisa M, Takeuchi M, Setiabudy R, Nafrialdi, Takeuchi M. Current status of phase I clinical trials in Asia: an academic perspectives. Acta Med Indones 2012;44:71–7.
[35] Glickman SW, McHutchison JG, Peterson ED, Cairns CB, Harrington RA, Califf RM, et al. Ethical and scientific implications of the globalization of clinical research. N Engl J Med 2009;360:816–23.
[36] Schindler RJ. Study design considerations: conducting global clinical trials in early Alzheimer's disease. J Nutr Health Aging 2010;14:312–4.
[37] Chiu HF, Lam LC. Relevance of outcome measures in different cultural groups—does one size fit all? Int Psychogeriatr 2007;19:457–66.
[38] ICH. E5 Ethnic Factors in the Acceptability of Foreign Clinical Data 1998.
[39] ICH Expert Working Group. E5 Implementation Working Group Questions & Answers. International Conference on Harmonization, 2006.
[40] Stern Y, Albert S, Tang MX, Tsai WY. Rate of memory decline in AD is related to education and occupation: cognitive reserve? Neurology 1999;53:1942–7.
[41] Department of Health and Human Services Office of the Inspector General USA (2003). The globalization of clinical trials: a growing challenge in protecting human subjects: executive summary (2001). J Int Bioethique 14, 165–9.
[42] Diaz PR, Gil Gregorio S, Manuel Ribera Casado P, Reynish J, Jean Ousset E, Vellas P, et al. The need for a consensus in the use of assessment tools for Alzheimer's disease: the Feasibility Study (assessment tools for dementia in Alzheimer Centres across Europe), a European Alzheimer's Disease Consortium's (EADC) survey. Int J Geriatr Psychiatry 2005;20:744–8.
[43] Kalaria RN, Maestre GE, Arizaga R, Friedland RP, Galasko D, Hall K, et al. Alzheimer's disease and vascular dementia in developing countries: prevalence, management, and risk factors. Lancet Neurol 2008;7:812–26.
[44] Tsou HH, Chow SC, Lan KK, Liu JP, Wang M, Chern HD, et al. Proposals of statistical consideration to evaluation of results for a specific region in multi-regional trials—Asian perspective. Pharm Stat 2010;9:201–6.
[45] Jotheeswaran AT, Williams JD, Prince MJ. The predictive validity of the 10/66 dementia diagnosis in Chennai, India: a 3-year follow-up study of cases identified at baseline Alzheimer Dis Assoc Disord 2010;24:296–302.
[46] Prince M, Acosta D, Ferri CP, Guerra M, Huang Y, Llibre Rodriguez JJ, et al. Dementia incidence and mortality in middle-income countries, and associations with indicators of cognitive reserve: a 10/66 Dementia Research Group population-based cohort study. Lancet 2012;380:50–8.
[47] Maestre GE. Assessing dementia in resource-poor regions. Curr Neurol Neurosci Rep 2012;12:511–9.
[48] Tiwari SC, Tripathi RK, Kumar A. Applicability of the Mini-mental State Examination (MMSE) and the Hindi Mental State Examination (HMSE) to the urban elderly in India: a pilot study. Int Psychogeriatr 2009;21:123–8.
[49] Fillenbaum GG, Chandra V, Ganguli M, Pandav R, Gilby JE, Seaberg EC, et al. Development of an activities of daily living scale to screen for dementia in an illiterate rural older population in India. Age Ageing 1999;28:161–8.
[50] Burt T, Sharma P, Mittal S. Research question, study design and continuous research education and training exercises (CREATE) program. J Clin Prev Card 2012;1:35–43.
[51] Tractenberg RE, Yumoto F, Jin S, Morris JC. Sample size requirements for training to a kappa agreement criterion on clinical dementia ratings. Alzheimer Dis Assoc Disord 2010;24:264–8.
[52] Burt T, Dhillon S, Sharma P, Khan D, Deepa MV, Alam S, et al. PARTAKE survey of public knowledge and perceptions of clinical research in india. PLoS One 2013;8(7):e68666.

15

Alzheimer's Disease Clinical Trials in China

James (Dachao) Fan[1], Huafang Li[2] and Jing Yin[1]
[1]Medical and Safety Services, ICON Clinical Research Pte Ltd, Singapore,
[2]Shanghai Mental Health Center, Shanghai, China

15.1 PREVALENCE OF ALZHEIMER'S DISEASE IN CHINA

Alzheimer's disease (AD) and other dementias have become a burgeoning public health challenge in the aging world, including in China. Since the implementation of the one-child policy in 1979, the birth rate in China has been decreasing and the number and proportion of elderly people continues to increase. The percentage of people aged 65 years and over increased from 4.9% in 1982 to 9.1% in 2011, and the old-age dependency ratio (the ratio of older dependents to the working age population) increased from 8.0% in 1982 to 12.3% in 2011 [1]. The population of people aged 65 years and over reached 122.88 million in 2011 [1]. A few epidemiology studies have been conducted on the prevalence of dementia in some regions of China; however, given the large population and the diversity of race, culture and economy in different regions, the quality and quantity of these studies is not sufficient and further studies are required to provide a consistent overview and national figures.

In one large population-based prevalence study of four major regional cities of China (n = 34,807), the prevalence of dementia in people over the age of 65 was 4.8% for AD and 1.1% for vascular dementia (VD), results similar to the prevalence of dementia subtypes in developed countries. The study also showed that the prevalence of AD doubled every five years in people between the ages of 65 and 85 years [2]. A World Health Organization (WHO) report estimated that there were 35.6 million people with dementia worldwide in 2010, with 5.4 million living in China [3]. It is undisputed that China is the country with the largest

M. Bairu & M.W. Weiner (Eds):
Global Clinical Trials for Alzheimer's Disease.
DOI: http://dx.doi.org/10.1016/B978-0-12-411464-7.00015-8

number of people with dementia, and the rate of increase in China is projected to be more rapid (117%) than that of developed countries (40–89%) [3]. AD may therefore impose a heavier social and economic burden on China and there is a huge market for the drugs that can prevent or treat the disease. However, currently no treatment is available to cure AD, and only a few drugs have been approved to relieve the symptoms. Therefore, China has high demand for the development of effective interventions for AD, including the conduct of AD clinical trials.

15.2 HISTORY AND CURRENT STATUS OF AD CLINICAL TRIALS IN CHINA

The history and development of AD clinical trials in China is heralded by two important milestones—the first AD clinical trial, which adapted Food and Drug Administration (FDA) and European Medicines Agency (EMEA) guidelines in 1999 and the release of "Technical Guidance on Clinical Trials of Medicinal Products for the Treatment of Alzheimer's Disease" in 2007 [4].

Table 15.1 summarizes a selection of important AD clinical trials that were started before 1999 or in early 1999 [5–8]. During this period, AD trials in China had no systematic assessment of therapeutic efficacy. These clinical trials all targeted mild and moderate AD. Utilization of assessment instruments to evaluate the efficacy of experimental drugs was limited to the Mini-Mental State Examination (MMSE), Clinical Dementia Rating (CDR) and other relatively insensitive instruments for mild to moderate AD. Sample size of the clinical trials was small (between 68 and 124 among the selected trials). Treatment period in the clinical trials was short: 12 weeks in the donepezil trial, [5] and 16 weeks in the rivastigmine [7] and the memantine trials [8]. There was no follow-up period to demonstrate long-term safety. Most studies were either open-label or single-blinded [8]. Hence the ability to draw robust conclusions from these early clinical trials is limited.

In 1999, Peking Union Medical College Hospital initiated the use of the Alzheimer's Disease Assessment Scale (ADAS) and standardized AD clinical trial protocols by adapting FDA and EMEA guidelines [4]. The standards for conducting AD clinical trials in China slowly improved. Table 15.2 summarizes a selection of influential AD clinical trials started between 1999 and 2007 [9–11]. The sample size of the clinical trials increased (between 202 and 258 among the selected trials). In accordance with the requirement by the Chinese State Food and Drug Administration (SFDA) Regulations for Implementation of the Drug Administration Law of the People's Republic of China (2002), to obtain registration of imported drugs which have been approved in other countries, randomized clinical trials must be conducted in at least 100 pairs

TABLE 15.1 Selected AD Clinical Trials Started before 1999 in China

Year Started	Drug	Design	Enrollment	Diagnostic Criteria	Outcome Measure	Results
1996 [5]	Tacrine	Multicenter, randomized, double-blind, placebo-controlled, 24-week treatment period	68 mild and moderate AD patients from 7 sites, randomized into treatment group and placebo group	NINCDS-ADRDA, DSM-III-R	MMSE, ADL, ADS, CGI, C-CGIC	Compared with the placebo group, the tacrine group has significant improvement in MMSE, ADL, CGI and CGIC, no significant improvement in ADS, significant increase in the AE rate of some gastrointestinal disorders. ALT increase (14%) was observed more frequently in tacrine group, but was not statistically significant.
1998 [6]	Donepezil	Multicenter, randomized, single-blind, placebo-controlled, 12-week treatment period	89 mild and moderate AD patients from 15 sites, randomized into treatment group and placebo group	NINCDS-ADRDA, DSM-IV	MMSE, CDR, ADL	Compared with the placebo group, the donepezil group had >3 points increase in MMSE, and significantly lower CDR and ADL. No significant difference in AE rate (4.7% in treatment group).
Early 1999 [7]	Rivastigmine vs. donepezil	multicenter, randomized, open-labeled, controlled, 16-week treatment period	124 mild and moderate AD patients from 10 sites, randomized into rivastigmine group and donepezil group	NINCDS-ADRDA, DSM-IV	MMSE, Blessed-Roth Dementia Scale, GDS	Both groups had significant improvement of MMSE, Blessed-Roth and GDS compared with baseline. Rivastigmine could improve the activity of daily life but donepezil could not. No other significant difference between the two groups. AE rate was 12.9–28.8% in two groups, mainly gastrointestinal disorders.

(Continued)

TABLE 15.1 (Continued)

Year Started	Drug	Design	Enrollment	Diagnostic Criteria	Outcome Measure	Results
1999 [8]	Memantine vs donepezil	Multicenter, randomized, single-blind(?)*, controlled, 16-week treatment period	100 mild and moderate AD patients from 6 sites, randomized into memantine group and donepezil group	NINCDS-ADRDA, DSM-IV-R	MMSE, Blessed-Roth Dementia Scale, GDS	Both groups had significant improvement of MMSE, Blessed-Roth and GDS compared with baseline. No significant difference between the two groups. AEs were mild and transient in both groups.

AD: Alzheimer's Disease; ADL: Activities of Daily Living; ADS: Alzheimer Deficit Scale; AE: Adverse Events; C-CGIC: Caregiver Clinical Global Impression of Change; CDR: Clinical Dementia Rating; CGI: Clinical Global Impression; DSM-III-R: Diagnostic and Statistical Manual of Mental Disorders, Third Edition, Revised; DSM-IV: Diagnostic and Statistical Manual of Mental Disorders, Fourth Edition; DSM-IV-R: Diagnostic and Statistical Manual of Mental Disorders, Fourth Edition, Revised; GDS: Global Deterioration Scale; MMSE: Mini-Mental State Examination; NINCDS-ADRDA: National Institute of Neurological and Communicative Disorders and Stroke and the Alzheimer's Disease and Related Disorders Association.

*Binding method of this study was not specified in the publication. It was only stated that the study was not double-blind.

TABLE 15.2 Selected AD Clinical Trials Started between 1999 and 2007 in China

Year Started	Drug	Design	Enrollment	Diagnostic Criteria	Outcome Measure	Results
1999 [9]	Huperzine A	Multicenter, randomized, double-blind, placebo-controlled, 12-week treatment period	202 mild and moderate AD patients from 15 sites, randomized into huperzine A and placebo group	NINCDS-ADRDA, DSM-IV	ADAS-Cog, MMSE, ADL, ADAS-non-Cog, CIBIC-plus	Compared with baseline, the huperzine A group had significant improvement in MMSE (2.7 points), ADAS-Cog (4.6 points), ADAS-non-Cog (1.5 points), and ADL (2.4 points). There was also significant improvement compared with the placebo group. Main AEs were gastrointestinal disorders, and there was no significant difference in AE rate between two groups (3%).
1999 [10]	Galanthamin vs. donepezil	Multicenter, randomized, double-blind, controlled, 16-week treatment period	223 mild and moderate AD patients from 9 sites, randomized into galanthamin group and donepezil group	NINCDS-ADRDA	ADAS-Cog, ADCS-ADL, NPI	Significant improvement in all three assessments in the two groups compared with baseline. Galanthamin group had more improvement in ADAS-Cog compared with donepezil. AEs (rate = 44%) were mainly transient gastrointestinal disorders and neurological disorders.
2004 [11]	Memantine	Multicenter, randomized, double-blind, placebo-controlled, 16-week treatment period	258 moderate and severe AD patients from 8 sites, randomized into memantine group and placebo group	NINCDS-ADRDA, DSM-IV-R	SIB, ADCS-ADL₁₉, NPI, MMSE	SIB in both groups increased mildly compared with baseline, though not statistically significant. Excluding deviation factors, post-hoc analysis showed significant improvement in the memantine group SIB (2.17 points), MMSE (0.97 points) and no decrease in ADL. AE rate (8%) was similar to the placebo group.

AD: Alzheimer's Disease; ADAS-Cog: Alzheimer's Disease Assessment Scale-Cognitive Behavior Section; ADAS-non-Cog: Alzheimer's Disease Assessment Scale-Non-Cognitive Section; ADCS-ADL: Alzheimer's Disease Cooperative Study Activities of Daily Living Inventory Scale; ADL: Activities of Daily Living; AE: Adverse Events; CIBIC-plus: Clinician's Interview-Based Impression of Change-Plus Caregiver Input; DSM-IV: Diagnostic and Statistical Manual of Mental Disorders, Fourth Edition; DSM-IV-R: Diagnostic and Statistical Manual of Mental Disorders, Fourth Edition, Revised; MMSE: Mini-Mental State Examination; NINCDS-ADRDA: National Institute of Neurological and Communicative Disorders and Stroke and the Alzheimer's Disease and Related Disorders Association; NPI, Neuropsychiatric Inventory; SIB: Severe Impairment Battery.

of patients. Most studies adopted a double-blind masking design. The memantine study [11] was the first clinical trial in China targeting moderate and severe AD patients.

Another important trial during this period was the huperzine A trial. This was the first AD clinical trial in China that strictly followed evidence-based medicine principles [4,9]. Huperzine A was the first compound that was originated and developed in China for the treatment of AD. It is an alkaloid compound extracted from the Chinese herb *Huperzia serrata*, and acts as a potent, highly selective and reversible acetylcholinesterase (AChE) inhibitor (similar to donepezil, rivastigmine and galantamine) and an N-methyl-D-aspartate receptor antagonist (similar to memantine). Early small-scale studies in China showed it to be well tolerated in AD patients. It is considered to be a very promising drug against AD and has been approved by the SFDA as a prescription drug in China.

A post-marketing trial conducted from December 1999 to December 2001 at 15 sites in China used a strict double-blind randomization design to evaluate the efficacy and safety of the drug [9]. Results showed that compared with baseline, patients treated with huperzine A had significant improvement in cognitive assessments (4.6 points by ADAS-Cog and 2.7 points by MMSE), behavioral assessment (1.5 points by ADAS-non-Cog), activities of daily living (2.4 points by ADL), and global impression rating (70% patients scored 1 to 3 points). There was also significant improvement compared with the placebo group. Most frequent adverse events (AE) were gastrointestinal disorders, which were mild and transient and the AE rate was low (3%). This study was qualitatively better than previous trials. However, there was no testing on the maximal tolerated dose and the treatment period was still short. Further studies are needed with a bigger sample size, longer treatment period, different doses, and patients with varied disease severities.

In 2007, the "Technical Guidance on Clinical Trials of Medicinal Products for the Treatment of Alzheimer's Disease" was drafted by AD experts in China to provide a good reference for the design, implementation and evaluation of AD trials in China. In 2010, the SFDA organized AD experts and translated the EMEA 2008 guidance ("Medicinal Products for the Treatment of Alzheimer's Disease and other Dementias"). However, at the time of writing, the local technical guidance published in 2007 is still in the process of soliciting feedback and has not been formally issued by the SFDA.

It is expected that with more attention from the SFDA, China's capacity and capability in conducting AD trials will achieve higher standards [12] and attract global pharmaceutical companies to conduct their trials here. In 2007, the clinical study of rosiglitazone (extended release tablets) as monotherapy in subjects with mild to moderate AD began recruitment in China, as the first international, multicenter Phase III clinical trial of AD in which China has participated. A search of the clinicaltrials.gov database generated 1026 AD clinical studies worldwide and only 14 AD clinical trials originated from, or included, mainland China. This small number may be due to many local trials not being registered in the database. Of the trials that are registered, five are sponsored by global pharmaceutical companies and three are sponsored by local pharmaceutical companies. Some other studies have been initiated by academic institutions in collaboration with global or local pharmaceutical companies [13]. There are only three international, multicenter AD clinical trials that have included sites in China. The current status suggests that although several global pharmaceutical companies have started to expand their AD trials into China, given the large patient pool, China has ample capacity to conduct additional global AD trials.

15.3 CLINICAL TRIAL CENTERS FOR AD IN CHINA

During the past 30 years, China has established and streamlined its own drug regulatory system. The conduct of clinical trials in China has gradually been standardized and the quality has been greatly improved through regulations and guidelines on the evaluation of efficacy and safety of investigational new drugs. In 1983, the Ministry of Health of China (MOH) accredited the first group of clinical pharmacology sites from the healthcare institutions with relatively better clinical research capabilities. Good clinical practice (GCP) guidelines were introduced into China by the MOH in 1998, and were revised in 1999 by the former State Drug Administration (SDA). In 2003, the SFDA of China was founded to replace SDA with expanded functions, and published a new version of GCP, the currently effective version. The SFDA has promoted GCP by reinforcing the quality standards in clinical trials and introducing compulsory GCP training in April 2004. The Chinese GCP is essentially in line with other international GCPs for most technical aspects, and has been modified for some local differences.

Under the Chinese GCP, clinical trials must be approved by the SFDA and the SFDA has mandated that effective from 1 Mar 2005, clinical trials can only be conducted in SFDA-accredited clinical trial institutions with specifically approved therapeutic areas. To further ensure uniform quality and GCP compliance, the clinical trial institutions must be reaccredited every three years according to a new regulation by SFDA in 2009. If problems are identified during the SFDA reaccreditation inspection, the clinical trial institution will be asked to rectify the findings and be subject to further inspection by the SFDA; otherwise the certification of the clinical trial institution will be retracted. Clinical trial institutions are large hospitals with good facilities, experienced physicians, and easily accessible patient pools. Clinical trial institutions cannot allow the same

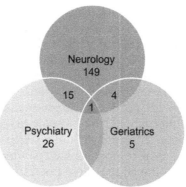

FIGURE 15.1   Numbers of clinical trial institutions able to conduct AD clinical trials (data extracted from the SFDA website in Jan 2013).

department to conduct concurrent trials using the same type of drug under different sponsors, and there is a limit to the number of different drug types that may be investigated at one time. Quality of clinical trials conducted at these centers can be ensured.

Between 2005 and January 2012, the SFDA issued 35 accreditation announcements and three reaccreditation announcements [14]. A total of 405 certificates have been issued to 378 healthcare institutions, as each certificate only covers a few therapeutic areas in one healthcare institution and some healthcare institutions applied for a second or third certificate to expand capabilities to conduct clinical trials in more therapeutic areas. Most of the clinical trial institutions are located in Beijing, Shanghai, Guangzhou, and other provincial capital cities.

Although AD and other dementias are classified under mental and behavioral disorders by international guideline (ICD-10, International Classification of Diseases, 10th Revision) and the Chinese national guideline (CCMD-3, Chinese Classification and Diagnostic Criteria of Mental Disorders, 3rd edition), in clinical practice they are treated by doctors in three specialties, namely neurologists, psychiatrists and geriatricians. The same applies in China. Clinical trial institutions that have an accredited specialty of neurology, psychiatry or geriatrics can conduct AD clinical trials in China. Through January 2012, 149 clinical trial institutions have been accredited to conduct trials in neurology, and 16 of those have concurrent accreditation in psychiatry, five have concurrent accreditation in geriatrics, and one is accredited in all three specialties. In addition, 10 clinical trial institutions are accredited to conduct clinical trials in the specialty of psychiatry alone. There are a total of 159 clinical trial institutions capable of conducting AD trials in China (Figure 15.1).

Table 15.3 shows the distribution of the clinical trial institutions capable of conducting AD clinical trials among Chinese provinces and

TABLE 15.3   The Number of Clinical Trial Institutions Capable of Conducting AD Clinical Trials in each Province or Municipality of China

Province/Municipality	Neurology	Psychiatry	Geriatrics
Anhui	1		
Beijing	20	3	
Chongqing	7		
Fujian	3		
Gansu	3		
Guangdong	14	3	
Guangxi	3		
Guizhou	1		
Hainan	3		
Hebei	6	1	
Heilongjiang	3	1	
Henan		1	
Hubei	8	2	
Hunan	11	2	1
Jiangsu	15	2	2
Jiangxi	3		
Jilin	5		1
Liaoning	3	1	
Neimenggu	2		
Shaanxi	4	3	
Shandong	8		
Shanghai	9	2	
Shanxi	3	1	
Sichuan	3	1	
Tianjin	3	1	
Xinjiang			
Yunnan	2		
Zhejiang	6	2	1
Total	149	26	5

Data extracted from the SFDA Website in January 2013.

VII. ENHANCING COUNTRIES' CAPACITY TO CONDUCT AD TRIALS

municipalities. Beijing, Jiangsu, Guangdong and Shanghai are the provinces or municipalities with strong capabilities in conducting AD clinical trials. On the city level, the top nine cities (with the number of SFDA-accredited clinical trial institutions capable of conducting AD clinical trials in brackets) are: Beijing (23), Guangzhou (12), Shanghai (11), Nanjing (11), Changsha (9), Wuhan (8), Chongqing (7), Hangzhou (7), and Xi'an (7).

15.4 CONDUCTING AD TRIALS IN CHINA

With the large patient pool, qualified clinical research institutions, and previous AD trial experience, many opportunities are available for conducting AD clinical trials in China. Yet there are many challenges, such as a poor social awareness of dementia, caregiver pressures, and a long regulatory timeline. Several factors need to be considered in order to enhance the country's capacity and capability to conduct AD trials.

15.4.1 The Patient Factor

15.4.1.1 Public Awareness of AD

In contrast to the large and increasing size of the population with dementia in China, the outpatient visit rate for dementia was very low. According to preliminary research, between 1998 and 1999, the outpatient visit rate of mild, moderate and severe dementia was 14.4%, 25.6%, and 33.6% respectively. Among dementia patients who visited outpatient departments, 46% of patients did not go to neurology or psychiatry departments. The utilization of psychometric assessment tools among general doctors was low (15%), and the rate of correct diagnosis was also low (26.9%). Only 21.3% of diagnosed patients had been given medications, and a mere 2% of patients were on acetylcholinesterase inhibitors [15].

The barriers to early diagnosis and intervention are mainly poor understanding, social stigma, and the lack of medical expertise and facilities for the elderly. The word "dementia" in Chinese (*laonian chidai*) literally means "stupid, demented elderly," so the patient and family often tend to deny the problem until the condition of the patient has worsened. There is also a common misbelief that cognitive decline is a normal part of aging, so patients do not seek early diagnosis and treatment. More recently, the Government and social groups have implemented many initiatives to educate the public about the disease and correct the misconceptions. People in cosmopolitan cities generally have a better understanding of dementia, but there are still many regions where knowledge about the disease is lacking due to the imbalanced economic and social development.

15.4.1.2 *Outpatient Medical Records and Prohibited Medicine*

In China, most outpatient medical records are still in paper form and are kept by the patients themselves and not by the hospital. As a result, patients can visit several departments of the same hospital or see different doctors in the same department concurrently, without informing the treating physician. The treating physician may not know that the patient is participating in an AD clinical trial, and may prescribe medications that are not allowed by the clinical study protocol. It is advisable that the site staff educates the patient and caregivers about the prohibited medications and asks the patient to inform the site staff immediately of any change in concurrent medications. The site staff should ask during the study visit if the patient has taken any medications which are prohibited, and ask the patient to bring their medical records so the site staff can make a photocopy to keep complete source data.

The taking of herbal remedies is another consideration that may affect the quality of AD clinical trials in China. In the Chinese culture, people have a strong belief in traditional Chinese medicines, and a number of herbal remedies have been promoted as memory enhancers or claimed to be effective in treating or preventing AD and other dementias, although there are no rigorous and large-scale clinical trials to prove the effectiveness or safety of these products. Patients and family also tend to believe in the testimonials of others. Therefore, it is crucial for the investigator to educate effectively and communicate frequently with patients in AD trials and their families.

15.4.2 The Caregiver Factor

Most of the patients with AD are cared for at home rather than in a "nursing home," community hospitals, or other institutions in China. The caregiver can be the spouse, a child of the patient, or a maid. Many caregivers for dementia patients do not receive formal caregiving-related training, and do not fully understand the course or prognosis of the illness and the associated huge financial burden. The lack of knowledge and experience needed to take care of a dementia patient may hasten the disease progression.

15.4.2.1 *Informed Consenting*

During patient recruitment for AD trials, if a patient and the family member or caregiver show great interest in "trying" the new drug since there is no approved drug on the market, it is advisable that before signing the informed consent the family member or caregiver holds a family meeting to discuss the benefit and risk of participating in the trial. It is important to reach agreement on whether the patient should participate in the trial, and discuss whether the caregiver has the time and availability to accompany the patient to the site for each visit (e.g., for completing the lengthy psychometric assessments). Patient visit compliance and follow-up is better if the family members reach a consensus, and the dropout rate will be reduced. Since the cognitive function of the patient is compromised, there is usually another informed consent form for the guardian to sign. However, the patient should still sign the informed consent form. There is a separate informed consent form for the caregiver since protocols usually require participation from the caregiver such as providing feedback on the patient's condition. Family members or caregivers who have higher educational attainment tend to understand the clinical trial better and be more cooperative.

15.4.3 The Site Factor

15.4.3.1 Site Selection and Feasibility Study

During the site feasibility phase of industry-sponsored clinical trials, in addition to assessing the experience of principal investigators (PIs) and sub-investigators, the number of outpatients, and the manpower and facility resources in the department, the sponsor companies should also pay attention to the motivation of the investigators, which is an important factor in driving the trial towards success. Generally speaking, most investigators are interested in new drugs developed by global pharmaceutical companies, which can increase the investigative site budget and provide the possibility of publishing high-impact research findings. During site selection, sponsor companies generally select sites according to previous collaborative experience and the results of a pre-study visit (PSV). Professors who are key opinion leaders (KOLs) in the field of AD will be chosen as the lead PIs, and can be consulted to recommend a few other clinical trial institutions from their extensive network to participate in the trial.

15.4.3.2 Conducting Psychometric Assessments

In China, psychometric assessments are mainly performed by the investigators themselves or trained physicians, a practice which differs from other countries where the site coordinators or research nurses may do the assessment. The advantage of this is that the investigator is more familiar with AD, and the patient will provide better cooperation due to a high level of trust in the investigator. This is helpful in accurately assessing changes in the disease state of the patient. One drawback of this feature is that the investigators usually have a busy schedule. To ensure adequate and complete assessments, before the start of the clinical trial the sponsor company should communicate the time demand for the trial to the investigator and request that the investigator plan sufficient time and resources well in advance.

In addition to the psychometric assessments performed on the patients, some trials also rely on the caregiver to give feedback and assessment on the progression/improvement of the patient's condition. Therefore, it is important to educate the caregiver on how to take care of the patient, how to comply with the required procedures in the clinical study protocol including recording of the assessment sheet, and how to communicate effectively with investigator and site staff about the patient's condition. Financial compensation for the time that caregivers spend on the trials will encourage participation.

15.4.4 Local Trials vs Global Trials

Between 2009 and 2010, one of our authors conducted a survey among 273 clinical research professionals in China to understand the differences in quality standard and their views of local trials versus global trials in the country [16]. "Local" trials are the studies conducted locally in China in order to register medicinal products which have been marketed in the USA and/or Europe, whereas "global" trials are studies conducted to get the FDA's and/or the EMEA's approval of the new medicinal product. While the majority of respondents (90%) agreed that both local and global trials should have the same quality standard, most respondents (71%) considered that in reality local trials did not meet the same standard of quality as global trials. According to the respondents, main areas where local trials are of lower quality were around study monitoring, study design, and data quality/data management. The reasons for the lower quality of local trials were thought to be low trial funding, small study grants, lack of site staff's/investigator's interest in local trials, lack of training for site staff, and fewer regulatory requirements.

In the early years, local trials of AD in China were mainly for the registration of imported drugs that were approved in other countries. Recently, more local trials have been conducted for the generic drugs produced by Chinese pharmaceutical companies. The main differences between local and global AD trials are the role of the lead PI and the trial design.

15.4.4.1 Role of Lead PI

In multicenter local trials in China, there is typically a lead investigator, whose responsibilities include trial design, identifying and recommending other investigative sites, and training of other investigators. There is no medical monitor in local trials, and the lead investigator covers some functions of the medical monitor such as answering medical queries from other investigative sites and overseeing the safety aspects of the trial. In some trials, only the institutional review board (IRB) at the lead investigator's institution needs to review the scientific and ethical aspects of the study, while in other trials all IRBs of participating institutions need to review and approve the trial. To date the SFDA has no formal guidelines for the ethical review process in multicenter trials, and a draft of "Guidelines for Ethics Committees on Drug Clinical Trial Ethical Review," issued in 2009, is still consolidating public feedback.

Having a lead investigator in a trial has several advantages. The lead investigator is usually the KOL in the field and is highly reputable. They will have a lot of experience in conducting clinical trials in China, and may help to identify any design aspect in the clinical trial protocol that may be a hurdle to implement in China. They will understand the drug evaluation and approval process in China and may give suggestions to the sponsors. They will have a good network with other investigators and can recommend other sites to participate in the trial. Therefore, the role of the lead investigator is very important in local trials. It is also recommended that global pharmaceutical companies consider involving a Chinese investigator in the planning of international multicenter trials, as the local considerations in China are usually different from the Western countries due to the culture differences.

15.4.4.2 Trial Design, Operation and Quality Control

Local trials are generally designed by the lead investigator. Most local AD trials in China have been aimed at demonstrating short-term improvement in AD. However, the treatment period is still shorter than global trials. As can be seen in Tables 15.1 and 15.2, the treatment period usually lasted only 12 or 16 weeks in trials conducted in the early years of AD. The FDA and EMEA guidelines require that the treatment period should be at least six months. In local trials, there is no follow-up period to evaluate long-term safety of the experimental drug. More recently, the Chinese technical guidance drafted in 2007 states that the double-blind treatment period should last at least six months and recommends a one-year or longer open-label extension period to evaluate the maintenance of efficacy and assess safety over the long term.

Global trials usually have a standard training program for the site staff involved in the trial, including employing a third party consulting company to conduct training on the assessment instruments and answer queries from the site staff during the trial. In contrast, local trials usually do not have such training, which may affect the reliability and accuracy of the ratings, especially if a site is not experienced in AD trials. In a multicenter local trial of memantine, [11] the placebo group from one site showed treatment effect with improvement in the Severe Impairment Battery (SIB) scores, which is contradictory to the degenerative characteristic of AD, and the SIB results from this group had a large and significant deviation from other sites. Post-hoc analyses had to be performed excluding the results from this site in order to demonstrate the efficacy of memantine.

It is expected that as opportunities increase to participate in global AD trials, training will improve, and research capabilities will be strengthened in implementing AD trials. As a result, all clinical research, including local clinical trials, will have improved design, better quality, and higher standards for the new drugs developed by Chinese pharmaceutical companies in the future.

15.5 SUMMARY

AD is a challenging therapeutic area, and the development of effective treatment requires the successful design and implementation of clinical trials. While AD trials in many developed countries are competing for sites and patients, China offers abundant opportunities for efficient and cost-effective AD trials. Patient recruitment can be accelerated in light of the large pool of treatment-naïve patients. Most clinical trial institutions are big hospitals with good infrastructure and experienced physicians, and are sought after by patients, making it easier to enroll many patients at one site. Investigators are highly motivated to participate in well-planned and monitored clinical trials of novel drugs.

However, China still needs to overcome barriers to strengthen its capacity and capabilities to conduct AD trials. The country needs to raise social awareness for dementia and encourage early diagnosis and early intervention. Clinical research professionals are required to pay more attention to the quality of clinical trials, follow evidence-based medicine principles and local and international guidelines to design trials, and ensure high standards in clinical trial implementation. The national technical guidance of AD trials is under development and its implementation is expected to improve the overall quality standard in the conduct of AD trials. Global pharmaceutical companies can strategically plan to venture into China early in the development phase of their drug, if they wish to market their drugs for AD in this important market.

With concerted efforts from the government, healthcare institutions, clinical research professionals and the clinical research industry, the country will realize its potential as an attractive destination for AD clinical trials and new drugs can be developed there for the benefit of AD patients.

Acknowledgments

The authors are indebted to Dr. Suzanne Gagnon, MD, FACP, former Chief Medical Officer and Executive Vice President of ICON Clinical Research, and Dr. Peter Schueler, MD, Senior Vice President, Medical and Safety Services at ICON Clinical Research who spent their time and effort in helping review this chapter. Without their help, this chapter would not have reached the standards set for it.

We wish to mention a special appreciation to Hilda Cheng, Project Manager, ICON Clinical Research and Shanshan Zhan, Clinical Research Associate, ICON Clinical Research for sharing their experience on the operation of AD clinical trials in China.

References

[1] National Bureau of Statistics of China. China Statistical Yearbook. [Jan 2013]. Available from: <http://www.stats.gov.cn/tjsj/ndsj/2012/indexch.htm>; 2012.

[2] Zhang ZX, Zahner GE, Roman GC, Liu J, Hong Z, Qu QM, et al. Dementia subtypes in China: prevalence in Beijing, Xian, Shanghai, and Chengdu. Arch Neurol 2005;62:447–53.

[3] World Health Organization Dementia: a public health priority. Geneva: World Health Organization—Alzheimer's Disease International; 2012.

[4] Zhang ZX, Li L. The important clinical trials changing the therapeutic methods of Alzheimer's disease in the last 10 years in China [in Chinese]. J Intern Med Concepts Pract 2009;4:261–4.

[5] Xu YF, Gao ZX, Tang HC, Weng Z, Jin HM, Ma X, et al. Tacrine in treatment of Alzheimer disease: a multicenter, double-blind study in China [in Chinese]. Chin J New Drugs Clin Rem 2000;19:7–9.

[6] Peng DT, Xu XH, Hou QY, Wang LN, Xie HG, Zhang ZX, et al. The safety and efficacy of aricept in patients with Alzheimer disease [in Chinese]. Chin J Neurol 2002;35:19–21.

[7] Wang YH, Chen QT, Zhang ZX, Shu L, Yao JL, Yu HZ, et al. The treatment by using rivastigmine for patients with Alzheimer disease: results of a multicenter, randomized, open-labeled, controlled clinical trial [in Chinese]. Chin J Neurol 2001;34:210–3.

[8] Hu HT, Zhang ZX, Yao JL, Yu HZ, Wang YH, Tang HC, et al. Clinical efficacy and safety of akatinol memantine in the treatment of mild to moderate Alzheimer's disease: a donepezil-controlled, randomized trial [in Chinese]. Chin J Intern Med 2006;45:277–80.

[9] Zhang ZX, Wang XD, Chen QT, Shu L, Wang JZ, Shan GL. Clinical efficacy and safety of huperzine A in treatment of mild to moderate Alzheimer disease, a placebo-controlled, double-blind, randomized trial [in Chinese]. Natl Med J China (Beijing, China) 2002;82:941–4.

[10] Hong X, Zhang ZX, Wang LN, Shao FY, Xiao SF, Wang YH, et al. A randomized study comparing the effect and safety of galantamine and donepezil in patients with mild to moderate Alzheimer's disease [in Chinese]. Chin J Neurol 2006;39:379–82.

[11] Chen X, Zhang ZX, Wang XD, Yao JL, Chen SD, Qian CY, et al. Multicenter research on efficacy and tolerance of memantine in Chinese patients with Alzheimer's disease [in Chinese]. Chin J Neurol 2007;40:364–8.

[12] Zhao JZ, Zhang ZX. Attach importance to clinical pharmaceutical trial of Alzheimer's disease [in Chinese]. Chin J Neurol 2007;40:361–3.

[13] ClinicalTrials.gov. <http://www.clinicaltrials.gov>; [Last accessed 31.01.12].

[14] The State Food and Drug Administration, the People's Republic of China. Drug Clinical Trial Institution Qualification Announcement. [cited Jan 2013]. Available from: <http://www.sfda.gov.cn/WS01/CL0069/>.

[15] Zhang MY. *Senile Dementia Prevention and Treatment Guide* [in Chinese]. Beijing: Peking University Medical Press; 2007.

[16] Fan J. Global and local trials in China: do they have the same quality standards? *Bull, Pharm Contract Manage Group* 2010;11:9–11.

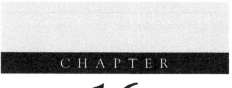

CHAPTER

16

Lessons Learned: Alzheimer's Disease Clinical Trials in Eastern Europe

Lynne Hughes

Quintiles, Reading, Berkshire, UK

16.1 INTRODUCTION: EASTERN EUROPE

Eastern Europe (EEu), as defined by the United Nations Statistics Division in 2007 [1], primarily includes the countries of Bulgaria, Czech Republic, Hungary, Poland, Romania, Russian Federation, and Slovakia as well as the Slavic republics of Belarus, Moldova and the Ukraine.

However, EEu can also be defined as the nations bordered by the Baltic and Barents seas on the north; the Adriatic, Black, and Caspian seas and the Caucasus Mountains on the south; and the Ural Mountains. Using this definition, the nations of Albania, Bosnia and Herzegovina, Croatia, Serbia and Montenegro (formerly Yugoslavia) would also be included. This definition also includes the Baltic republics of Estonia, Latvia, and Lithuania, considered by the UN as Northern Europe. The Transcaucasian countries of Armenia, Azerbaijan, and Georgia are included in this definition, though they are defined by the UN as western Asia. Finally, Turkey is often considered as a part of EEu.

Key countries:
- Belarus
- Bulgaria
- Czech Republic
- Hungary
- Moldova
- Poland
- Romania

M. Bairu & M.W. Weiner (Eds):
Global Clinical Trials for Alzheimer's Disease.
DOI: http://dx.doi.org/10.1016/B978-0-12-411464-7.00016-X
263
© 2014 Elsevier Inc. All rights reserved.

- Russia
- Slovakia
- Ukraine
- Albania
- Bosnia and Herzegovina
- Croatia
- Montenegro
- Serbia
- Slovenia

Baltic States:
- Estonia
- Latvia
- Lithuania

Eurasia:
- Armenia
- Azerbaijan
- Georgia
- Kazakhstan
- Turkey.

For the purposes of this review, we will be focusing primarily on Bulgaria, the Czech Republic, Hungary, Poland, the Baltics, Russia, Serbia, Romania, the Ukraine, and Turkey, as these countries have made the most significant contribution to global clinical trials in Alzheimer's disease (AD) to date.

There is significantly less experience in countries such as Belarus, Moldova, Albania, Bosnia and Herzegovina, and Montenegro, as well as most of the countries within Eurasia—except for Turkey. Many of these countries have not been involved in global AD trials but are involved in local trials. Even relative "newcomers" to the global AD trial arena—including Slovakia, Serbia and Slovenia—are able to make a good input to a global trial in terms of their patient contribution, and these countries will be increasingly important to trials over the coming years.

In terms of the investigators in EEu—the majority have English as a good second (or third) language and a high percentage have spent some time training, or on sabbaticals, in either the USA or in Western European countries. Thus, they are well aware of trial expectations and able to ensure their patients comply with the global requirements dictated by the trial protocols.

16.2 PREVALENCE OF AD

AD poses possibly the largest future medical challenge to developed countries and the challenge is also increasing in developing countries (Table 16.1).

TABLE 16.1 Prevalence of AD vs. Total Dementia Cases Per Country [2,3]

Country	Total Population Per Country 2008	Calculated Actual AD Cases in 2005	Prevalence Eurodem	Country	Total Population Per Country 2008	Calculated Actual AD Cases in 2005	Prevalence Eurodem
India	1,142,780,000	3,542,618	0.003	Germany	82,127,000	1,116,927	0.014
Japan	127,704,000	1,711,234	0.013	France	64,473,140	876,835	0.014
Australia	21,550,000	172,400	0.008	Italy	59,619,290	757,165	0.013
New Zealand	4,293,500	19,321	0.005	UK	61,186,000	673,046	0.011
South Africa	47,850,700	NA		Spain	46,063,500	626,464	0.014
Turkey	70,586,256	1,270,553	0.018	Netherlands	16,490,950	209,435	0.013
Russia	145,500,000	1,091,250	0.008	Belgium	10,666,866	144,003	0.014
Ukraine	46,191,022	586,626	0.013	Portugal	10,617,600	134,844	0.013
Poland	38,115,967	484,073	0.013	Sweden	9,248,805	117,460	0.013
Romania	21,528,600	273,413	0.013	Austria	8,340,924	105,930	0.013
Greece	11,215,000	142,431	0.013	Switzerland	7,689,100	97,652	0.013
Hungary	10,035,000	127,445	0.013	Denmark	5,506,000	69,926	0.013
Serbia	9,527,100	120,994	0.013	Finland	5,327,490	67,659	0.013
Czech Rep	10,446,157	107,595	0.010	Norway	4,802,050	60,986	0.013
Israel	7,373,000	100,273	0.014	Ireland	4,422,100	56,161	0.013
Bulgaria	7,640,238	86,335	0.011	Luxembourg	483,800	6,144	0.013
Slovakia	5,404,784	68,641	0.013	Iceland	319,765	4,061	0.013

(Continued)

TABLE 16.1 (Continued)

Country	Total Population Per Country 2008	Calculated Actual AD Cases in 2005	Prevalence Eurodem	Country	Total Population Per Country 2008	Calculated Actual AD Cases in 2005	Prevalence Eurodem
Lithuania	3,361,100	42,686	0.013	Brazil	188,453,000	1,507,624	0.008
Latvia	2,268,000	28,804	0.013	Mexico	106,682,500	949,474	0.009
Slovenia	2,041,050	25,921	0.013	Colombia	44,660,000	397,474	0.009
Estonia	1,340,600	17,026	0.013	Peru	28,750,770	241,506	0.008
Malta	410,600	5,215	0.013	Chile	16,850,000	149,965	0.009
Croatia	4,435,400	NA		Ecuador	13,867,761	123,423	0.009
China	1,335,740,000	5,209,386	0.004	Argentina	39,745,613	55,246	0.001
Hong Kong	9,960,000	38,844	0.004	Costa Rica	4,468,000	39,765	0.009
Egypt	75,730,000	204,471	0.003	Puerto Rico	3,991,000	30,132	0.008
Lebanon	4,099,000	30,743	0.008	Indonesia	229,005,000	503,811	0.002
Jordan	5,924,000	NA		Philippines	90,457,200	90,457	0.001
Kuwait	2,851,000	NA		Korea	72,014,000	82,816	0.001
Morocco	31,343,359	NA		Malaysia	27,757,000	31,921	0.001
Saudi Arabia	24,735,000	NA		Taiwan	23,027,672	26,482	0.001
Tunisia	10,327,000	NA		Singapore	4,839,400	5,565	0.001
UAE	4,380,000	NA		Thailand	63,038,247	NA	
USA	306,070,000	4,591,050	0.015				
Canada	33,512,000	360,000	0.011				

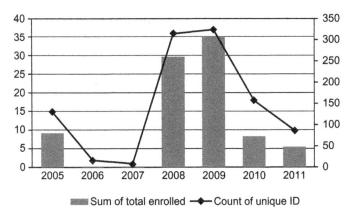

FIGURE 16.1   Eastern Europe contribution to AD studies. (Quintiles has developed an internal, proprietary database using illustrative, de-identified data from many sources. These data are referenced throughout the text.)

EEu consists of many countries with different languages, each country with different sociodemographic and socio-economic characteristics, different cultural, legal, social and healthcare system-related traditions, and different psychopathological traditions [4].

All of these factors can complicate both the conduct of studies—in terms of standardization of care, and interpretation and completion of scales—as well as interpretations of findings. Unlike the long US and Western European tradition of fairly regular, large-scale community and general population studies with uniform methods and designs, there is no such tradition yet in all countries within EEu. However, the available AD data suggest prevalence rates of dementia in EEu similar to those in Western Europe.

16.3 INCREASING ROLE OF EMERGING COUNTRIES IN THE DEVELOPMENT AND EXECUTION OF TRIALS

Data from Quintiles' proprietary database[*] shows that countries in EEu started significant participation in global AD trials from 2005 and made significant contributions in 2008 and 2009 in symptomatic trials (Figures 16.1 and 16.2). Of interest, there was also a reasonable

---

[*]Quintiles has developed an internal, proprietary database using illustrative, de-identified data from many sources. These data are referenced throughout the text.

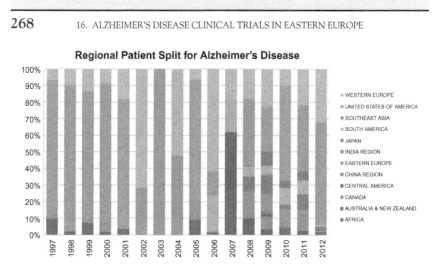

FIGURE 16.2 Regional patient split for Alzheimer's Disease. (Quintiles has developed an internal, proprietary database using illustrative, de-identified data from many sources. These data are referenced throughout the text.)

contribution made to trials which utilized potential disease-modifying drugs (DMDs)—even though these countries were unable to participate in the positron emission tomography (PET) imaging addenda due to the lack of availability of this ligand in this region.

When taken into account with the prevalence data shown in Table 16.1, it is more apparent why these regions are being considered for global trial participation, as their recruitment rates are on a par with those in Western Europe and the USA, and thus there is a robust population of accurately diagnosed subjects for trial participation. Thus, the efficiency of clinical trial conduct is enhanced due to the increased numbers of subjects at each site—minimizing the challenges of site variability.

Access to MRI facilities in all the countries is not usually a problem although there may be differences in magnet strength. If the required field strength is greater than a three tesla, then there may be challenges in a number of sites/countries. In addition, overall compliance with imaging is higher when the imaging center is on the same site as the main hospital or clinic where the subjects are being seen. When subjects have to leave the hospital premises and drive to an off-site imaging facility, there is a risk that they will not complete this procedure, especially if it is at the end of a long and tiring day for subject and caregiver alike. This is not usually the case for sites within EEu as, due to their centralized healthcare system, the hospitals usually consist of large, all-encompassing facilities whereby subjects can undertake all the necessary assessments without having to venture to off-site departments.

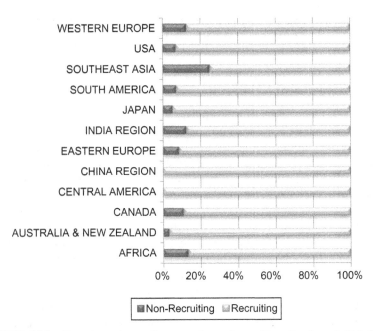

FIGURE 16.3   Recent metrics on the percentage of recruiting sites from initiated sites per region. (Quintiles has developed an internal, proprietary database using illustrative, de-identified data from many sources. These data are referenced throughout the text.)

The use of ApoE4 genotyping is becoming more commonplace in AD studies. For the most part, this is not an issue and all countries and sites in EEu are able to comply with this request for clinical trial purposes. ApoE4 genotyping is not, for the most part, routinely performed in EEu as part of a patient's work-up for AD; whereas it is being used more routinely in other areas of the world.

There are currently a number of restrictions regarding ApoE testing in certain countries: Those countries not allowing ApoE genetic testing include Turkey and Israel. Some countries, e.g., Italy, allow ApoE sampling but their ethics committees often mandate sharing of the results with the patients.

In terms of trial efficiency, a key parameter here is to attempt to limit the number of non-recruiting sites, as these cost both time and money to the sponsoring company. Figure 16.3 shows that, in general, there is quite a low percentage overall of non-recruiting sites within EEu and that this region has better metrics with respect to this parameter than sites in Western Europe and Canada, and is almost equivalent to sites in the USA. This, coupled with an overall higher recruitment rate, makes EEu a very attractive region for the conduct of trials in AD.

16.4 OPPORTUNITIES FOR EMERGING MARKETS: FOCUS ON EASTERN EUROPE

16.4.1 New Symptomatic and Disease-Modification Treatment Trials

Approximately 30% of ongoing trials are targeting symptomatic therapy and this figure is likely to increase over the next few years. Many of these trials are targeting the mild to more moderate population range (Mini-Mental State Examination (MMSE) 20–12) and are requesting a stable dose of 10 mg donepezil at baseline; many exclude memantine.

This is a very challenging patient population to recruit. As their disease progresses, many subjects are prescribed an increased dose of donepezil and/or the addition of memantine. Thus, these products are being seen more as the "standard of care" for AD subjects, in particular in Western Europe and within the USA. Therefore, a key to successful completion of such trials will be the inclusion of countries from outside these regions; EEu countries are ideally placed to support such trials.

Of note, in a number of countries in EEu, a subject might well have utilized their healthcare providers' limit for reimbursement of donepezil by the time their MMSE score decreases to below 20. At this stage, they would need to pay for additional treatment themselves and thus any trial-related request for stable background therapy could be a challenge for some subjects. Provision of the requested add-on therapy by the sponsoring company will expand the potential number of subjects available to the trial in this region.

In terms of participation in trials utilizing potential DMDs, the limiting factor here, as mentioned in previous chapters, is the availability of the mandated PET ligand. In a number of countries within EEu, there is availability of PET scanners—e.g., Russia, Poland, the Czech Republic, Turkey, etc. The MRI mandated procedures pose no challenges for the sites—except that the protocol has to permit a reasonable time period for the scheduling of such procedures. The lumbar punctures (LPs) can be performed and the principal investigators need to work closely with the study coordinator to explain the purpose of these procedures in order to aid subject compliance. Thus, sites in this region are able to contribute, more and more, to trials requesting the sophisticated biomarkers that are being required by regulatory agencies and/or pharmaceutical companies.

There are a number of very large specialist neurology sites in EEu, which have contributed significantly to recent studies sponsored by major pharmaceutical companies. These sites have a huge catchment area and thus have access to a large number of patients. As a result of the historical influence of the centralized healthcare systems, these sites

TABLE 16.2   Average Recruitment Rates in Mild to Moderate AD Trials Observed in Eastern Europe

Country	Recruitment Rate (psm)
Bulgaria	0.47
Czech Republic	0.75
Hungary	0.46
Israel	0.43
Lithuania	0.50
Poland	0.47
Romania	0.77
Russia	0.59
Serbia	0.36
Turkey	1.11
Ukraine	0.56
USA	0.58
UK	0.46

retain enormous patient populations, and the low reimbursement rates of available treatments in these countries contribute to a remarkable opportunity for patient enrolment.

These countries have participated in numerous Phase III trials in neurology which utilize rating scales as primary endpoints and have contributed significantly to a number of Phase III and Phase IIIb line extension trials in AD, as well as in earlier Phase II trials.

In terms of overall recruitment rates to trials for symptomatic therapies, Table 16.2 shows the average recruitment rates observed during recent trials. These are average rates and show that countries within EEu have recruitment rates on a par with, or exceeding those, observed in the USA or in the UK.

Mild to moderate AD patients are primarily seen and treated by neurologists in EEu. In some cases, they are treated by psychiatrists. Donezepil, rivastigmine, galantamine, and memantine are amongst the commonly prescribed treatments for this patient population. The percentage of treatment-naïve patients varies amongst the EEu countries, and the cost of available treatment could play a huge role in the availability of this sub-group.

Most (if not all) of the clinical scales are used routinely in EEu countries. The majority of countries also have good access to MRI scanners

CEE AD Patient Contribution

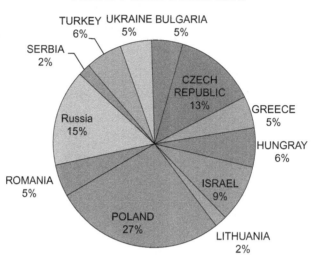

FIGURE 16.4 Central and Eastern Europe AD patient contribution. (Quintiles have developed an internal, proprietary database using illustrative, de-identified data from many sources. These data are referenced throughout the text.)

and reasonable access to PET scanners—with at least one in the majority of CEE countries.

Overall, there are no anticipated regulatory/EC issues in EEu countries; however it is important to be aware that:

- There could be ethical issues or delays in approvals if there is no rescue treatment for treatment-naïve patients in the protocol.
- Concerns may be raised about a long duration study (six months or more) which is a pure placebo trial.

16.4.2 Eastern European Countries

The most experienced EEu countries in the conduct of trials in AD are the Czech Republic, Russia and Poland (Figure 16.4), countries that have been involved in the global trials arena for more than 15 years. Quintiles was one of the first global contract research organizations (CROs) to enter this region and incorporate sites in pivotal Phase III trials in AD. These countries are now used for most global strategies for AD trials, as their recruitment rates are usually fairly high and dependable, the investigators are well versed in all the common scales, and their standard of care is similar to countries within Western Europe.

However, other countries—including Bulgaria, Romania, Serbia and the Ukraine—are regularly part of pivotal strategies for trials in AD at all stages of mild, moderate and severe. These countries are more limited for some trials utilizing DMDs, because manufacturers of the assigned PET ligands do not yet have distribution to these countries, but they are able to conduct PET imaging using Fluorodeoxyglucose (FDG) and PIB (Pittsburgh Compound B) at selected centers.

The Baltics—Estonia, Latvia and Lithuania—have played an increasingly important role in global clinical trials, although there has been less involvement in Phase III trials. These countries have well-developed healthcare systems and a centralized structure, so that a few sites have access to a very high population of patients. Therefore, utilizing just a few sites in these countries can provide access to a sizeable percentage of the country's population. Estonia, however, is changing to a decentralized system and from a state-funded system to one funded by health insurance organizations. It is likely that other countries will follow this approach.

One of the main challenges for these countries is managing the reimbursement of trial-mandated concomitant medications, especially if the trial requires a more moderate stage of AD when subjects may have utilized their healthcare-reimbursed amounts of funding for donepezil and are then being asked to provide this at their own cost. Thus, sponsor companies should be aware of this and factor it into their budget if they wish to include these countries.

In general, data from Quintiles[†] over the past 10 years shows that the countries in CEE have, on average, consistently higher recruitment rates of subjects for AD trials at the mild to severe stages when compared with sites in Western Europe and in the USA. (There are too few trials currently completed in prodromal AD [pAD] to draw any conclusions at this time.) In addition, the quality of the subjects has been good, the investigators have been experienced and have understood the aims of the trial and the need for compliance, and the patient recruitment has been extremely dependable. As such, they have already made a significant contribution to many of the completed and ongoing trials in AD.

Another key player now in the global AD clinical trials arena is Russia. There are an estimated 1.1 million people suffering from dementia in this country and it is thought to be one of the top five countries worldwide in terms of dementia prevalence. Hospice care is fairly new in Russia, starting in the early 1990s. Thus, most subjects live at home and are cared for by their family. Donepezil and memantine are the most widely used medications—but are rarely covered by healthcare insurance. Thus, if an add-on design, reimbursement of mandated concomitant medication will usually be requested by the ethics committee. The majority of sites used for clinical trials lie within the key cities in Russia—but the recruitment levels to trials are high.

[†]Quintiles has developed an internal, proprietary database using illustrative, de-identified data from many sources. These data are referenced throughout the text.

VII. ENHANCING COUNTRIES' CAPACITY TO CONDUCT AD TRIALS

For the majority of countries in EEu, LPs are not used routinely in the work-up of a subject with AD and thus compliance with this assessment can be low. Therefore, should these be required, then it is strongly recommended that efforts are made, and tools put in place, to educate the subject and their family as to the benefit of this procedure—whether directly to the subject or to AD research in general. With such a potentially large catchment of subjects, time spent in educating and supporting the sites, study coordinators, subjects and their families can be well spent in terms of compliance as well as high recruitment.

Turkey is a fairly recent arrival to the global AD trials arena, although it has been involved in many local trials in AD with pharmaceutical companies previously. It is difficult to obtain sufficiently detailed population statistics for the number of people in Turkey over the age of 74 and thus the estimated incidence of 129,715 (0.18%) is probably an underestimation. Placebo-controlled trials will be questioned, especially if required in treatment-naïve subjects. LPs are rarely used—unless there is an urgent medical requirement for such a procedure—but sites are familiar with MRI scans and PET scanning in AD trials. The scales are generally available in the appropriate languages and, again, the potential recruitment rate is higher than in Western Europe and in the USA.

16.5 CONCLUSION

The current AD clinical trials arena is extremely congested and there are a substantial number of AD trials, in planning or in progress, from many sponsors, and therefore careful site selection is essential. In general:

- There is a notable shift towards earlier stage AD trials—to the mild cognitive impairment or mild stage of AD.
- Generally, recruitment rates are significantly lower than those observed even three years ago.
- Trials are becoming more complex—with a number of additional assessments and, often, substantial requirements for biomarker assessments. This accounts for the observed reduction in recruitment rates as the sites are unable to process a high patient flow through the ever-increasing complexities of the trial procedures.

Investigators in EEu are extremely keen and motivated to expand on their clinical trials experience in AD and contribute to global, pivotal trials. These regions all have access, at varying levels, to the commonly used medications for AD and, as such, are not keen to participate in trials which other regions will not support, such as pure placebo-controlled trials. These regions have an increasingly sophisticated healthcare system, knowledgeable and experienced investigators, study support staff, and a huge opportunity for subject recruitment. They want their subjects to have the same trial opportunities as subjects in Western Europe and the USA, and will contribute significantly to global trials when given the opportunity.

In terms of "lessons learned," these can be summarized as follows:

- Understand reimbursement of background medication(s) before starting a trial in EEu to ensure that the appropriate subjects are available; allow time to plan for suitable reimbursement if required.
- State the tesla strength of the MRI, if imaging is required.
- Allow for a reasonable screening period—to permit scheduling of imaging assessments—of at least six weeks for a DMD trial.
- Provide hand-outs for the study coordinators explaining the trial rationale and critical nature of biomarker assessments: Provide support as needed for LPs.
- Discuss whether LP data can "substitute" for any specific PET ligand imaging if availability of PET ligand is limited.
- Scales have been discussed in previous chapters, but all of the most widely used scales are translated and validated into the key EEu languages and there are experienced raters available. It is critical to factor in the time for scale acquisition and plan for the option of scale training in local languages.

Finally, many sponsors are also looking at other, exploratory, end-points which require a significantly lower number of subjects in order to determine a response to treatment, e.g., changes in brain volume. However, until a sponsor undertakes such a trial—with the full support of the regulatory agencies—then it is up to the pharmaceutical company and CRO (as indicated) to work with the countries and sites to determine the best options for timely recruitment, quality subjects, confirmed diagnosis of subjects, and high quality data. This provides tremendous opportunities for the countries within EEu.

References

[1] United Nations Statistics Division. Composition of Macro Geographical (Continental) Regions, Geographical Sub-regions, and Selected Economic and Other Groupings. Retrieved September 18, 2007.
[2] Alzheimer's Disease International. The prevalence of dementia worldwide. <http://www.alz.co.uk/adi/pdf/prevalence.pdf>.
[3] Brookmeyer R, Johnson E, Ziegler-Graham K, Arrighi, HM. Forecasting The Global Burden Of Alzheimer's Disease. Johns Hopkins University, Dept. of Biostatistics Working Paper. January 2007. Available from: <http://biostats.bepress.com/jhubiostat/paper130/>.
[4] Hofman A, Rocca WA, Brayne C, Breteler MM, Clarke M, Cooper B, et al. The prevalence of dementia in Europe: a collaborative study of 1980–1990 findings. Eurodem Prevalence Research Group. Int J Epidemiol 1991;20:736–48.

CHAPTER 17

Experience in Alzheimer's Disease Clinical Trials in Turkey

Yağız Üresin[1], Hilal İlbars[2], İbrahim Hakan Gürvit[3] and Murat Emre[3]

[1]Istanbul University Faculty of Medicine Department of Medical Pharmacology, Istanbul, Turkey [2]Turkish Medicines and Medical Devices Agency, Ankara, Turkey [3]Istanbul University Faculty of Medicine, Department of Neurology, Istanbul, Turkey

17.1 INTRODUCTION

Turkey straddles the continents of Europe and Asia, borders seven countries—Greece and Bulgaria in the north-west, Syria in the south, Iraq in the south-east, and Armenia, Georgia, and Iran in the east. Due its unique geographical location, it has been seen as a bridge to Europe from Asia and the Middle East.

Soon after the foundation of the Republic of Turkey in 1923 from the Turkish remnants of the Ottoman Empire, a series of political, legal, cultural, social, and economic policy amendments were introduced that were designed to convert the new Republic of Turkey into a secular nation state. In 1945 Turkey joined the United Nations, and in 1952 it became a member of the North Atlantic Treaty Organization (NATO). In 1995, Turkey and the European Foreign Ministers decided to implement the final phase of the Ankara Agreement to establish a Customs Union with Turkey. In this framework, a Customs Union Agreement came into force on January 1, 1996. The Customs Union between Turkey and the European Union ensures free circulation of goods, capital, and services, as well as the coordination of economic and financial policies. The Customs Union also involves the elimination of all custom duties and the abolition of all quantitative restrictions.

Turkey is in the review phase for joining the European Union (EU) and has undergone many important reforms in the areas of patient

M. Bairu & M.W. Weiner (Eds):
Global Clinical Trials for Alzheimer's Disease.
DOI: http://dx.doi.org/10.1016/B978-0-12-411464-7.00017-1

277

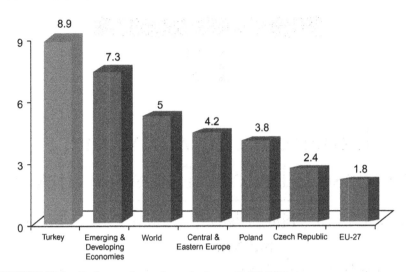

FIGURE 17.1   Real gross domestic product growth (%), 2010.

rights, criminal law, specialized biotech drug dispending acts, and others. It was formally accepted as a candidate for EU membership in December, 2004.

Turkey has a population of 75 million people (median age is 29.7 years). The country has reputable research sites with strong technical infrastructure capabilities complying with international standards.

17.1.1 The Turkish Economy

The Turkish economy has shown remarkable performance with its steady growth over the past decade. Significant improvements over such a short period have registered Turkey on the world economic scale as an exceptional emerging economy—the 16th largest economy in the world and the sixth largest economy as compared with EU countries, according to gross domestic product (GDP) figures (at purchasing power parity) in 2010 (Figure 17.1). Turkey stood out as the fastest growing economy in Europe and one of the fastest growing economies in the world. In addition, according to OECD (Organization for Economic Co-operation and Development), Turkey is expected to be the fastest growing economy among OECD members between 2011 and 2017, with an annual average growth rate of 6.7% [1].

17.1.2 The Pharmaceutical Industry

Turkey accounts for roughly 42% of the total Middle Eastern pharmaceutical market. While the overall pharmaceutical market size is among the top 30 largest in the world, per capita spending on pharmaceuticals remains low. Given the possible accession to the EU, the potential for growth is very promising compared with more established and mature markets in Western Europe.

Pharmaceutical products were produced on a small scale in Turkish laboratories between 1928 and 1950. Production increased with the establishment of local and foreign-investment plants from 1952, which is seen as the start of the "fabrication period" of the Turkish pharmaceuticals industry. Investment by foreign capital companies has been increasing since 1984, and 19 foreign capital firms have entered the Turkish pharmaceuticals market since 1990. Today, there are approximately 300 entities operating in Turkey, out of which 42 manufacturing facilities belong to multinational companies. The Turkish prescribed pharmaceutical market reached €6.54 billion and 1.42 billion units by volume in 2009. The growth rate of the market is 3.1% in terms of Euros and 3.9% by volume. The market size for original drugs in Turkey was US$4.1 billion in 2009 and US$4 billion in 2010. The production structure of the pharmaceutical industry has a high level of technology and automation. Approximately 25,000 people are employed in the sector.

Innovative drugs and new treatments which can help prevent diseases and reduce treatment costs will become important over time. Hence both developed and developing countries consider pharmaceutical research and development for discovery and production of new treatments a priority area for investment and strategic growth. The Turkish government aims to make Turkey one of the world's top 10 economies in health services by 2023 by increasing research and development (R&D) expenditures to 3% of GDP and by increasing exports to US$ 500 billion.

The Association of Research-Based Pharmaceutical Companies (AIFD), established in 2003 by international pharmaceutical companies operating in Turkey, has become a part of this objective for 2023. According to AIFD's "Turkey's Pharmaceutical Sector Vision 2023 Report" published in 2012, the average lifespan in Turkey increased by 24% in the last 30 years and has now reached 74 years. Based on a study conducted by Professor Lichtenberg of Columbia University and the National Bureau of Economic Research, innovative drugs accounted for 75% of the increase in life expectancy in the 30 countries surveyed, including Turkey. However, in order to achieve sustainable progress in health services, the country must also focus on improving its competitive position. Currently, Turkey lags behind other emerging pharmaceutical markets (now referred to as "pharmerging" countries, such as Brazil, Russia, India, and China) in global pharmaceutical investment. According to the World Economic Forum's Global Competition Index (2011–2012), Turkey ranked 59 out of 142 countries, and ranked 71 in the Innovation Capacity Index (Figure 17.2).

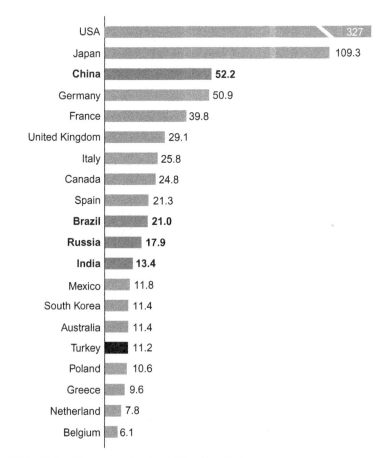

FIGURE 17.2   Pharma market size (billion $) in 2011.

While the Turkish pharmaceutical sector is ranked 16th in terms of market value, it is 36th in terms of clinical research conducted and the volume of pharmaceutical exports. Currently, pharmaceutical production in Turkey is focused around low value-added products, with high value-added products being imported. Turkey, which is currently the strongest and most dynamic economy in the region, can become a formidable player in the pharmaceutical sector. It has the necessary knowledge base, infrastructure, and geostrategic location to attract global pharmaceutical R&D and could become a global player in the pharmaceutical industry [2].

In 2010, an analysis was carried out by the Istanbul Faculty of Medicine based on clinical trial applications to the ethics committee (EC). Because of unknowns during the introduction of new regulations on clinical research, the Istanbul University Ethics Committee was the only operating EC in the country at this time, providing robust statistics

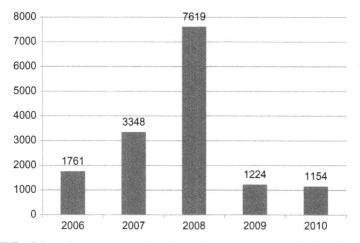

FIGURE 17.3   Industry-supported clinical trials according to Istanbul Medical Faculty EC applications by year.

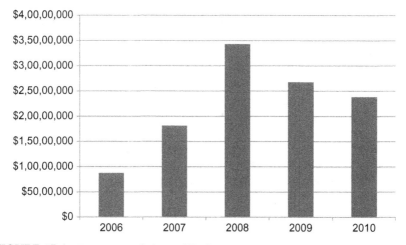

FIGURE 17.4   Ex ante intended overall budget assumption on commercial drug trials in Turkey according to Istanbul Medical Faculty EC applications by year.

on industry-sponsored studies during this period. During this period 15,106 patients were recruited to industry-supported trials in Turkey (Figure 17.3); the total budget was estimated to be US$ 111 million between 2006 and 2010 (Figure 17.4) [3].

17.2 CLINICAL TRIALS LEGISLATION, REFORM, AND AMENDMENTS

Turkey has a long tradition of clinical trial legislation, regulation, and guidelines. The country has taken major steps towards harmonizing its legislation with the EU in the field of clinical research; currently Turkish regulations are totally in line with EC Directives (EC 2001/20 and EC 2005/28).

The history of clinical trials in Turkey dates back to the beginning of the twentieth century. The beginning of the modern era of clinical trials in Turkey, however, was in 1993 with the introduction of the "Drug Research Bylaws" which regulated the conduct of clinical trials in Turkey. They were in line with the initial drafts of the International Conference on Harmonization (ICH)-GCP Guidelines. A good clinical practice (GCP) guideline document was introduced in 1995, followed by good laboratory practice (GLP) and good manufacturing practice (GMP) guidelines. The growing number of clinical trials over time, however, necessitated new and updated regulations. This was partly covered by documents such as regulations on compassionate use, observational trials, patient rights, and articles in the Turkish penal law. Thereafter, major changes in Turkey's national policies occurred, aligning with those of the EU. A new period began that required a complete revision of all legal documents and adaptation to EU rules and regulations.

The latest regulation on clinical trials in Turkey was introduced in August 2011. This regulation aimed to regulate the procedures in clinical trials—by providing scientific and ethical standards for the design, conduct, record-keeping, and reporting, and for other matters relating to clinical trials conducted on human volunteers—in order to protect volunteers' rights in accordance with the international agreements and conventions to which Turkey is a party and in accordance with EU standards. This legislation has 18 guidelines, all of which are in line with EU legislations.

The scope of this legislation spans clinical trials to be performed on humans with products or drug preparations, even if they are:

- registered or licensed, observational clinical trials, or trials on observational medical devices;
- clinical trials with any other substances or products which may be studied on humans, including medical devices, advanced therapy medicinal products, traditional herbal medicinal products, or cosmetic raw materials or products;
- bioavailability and bioequivalence studies;
- comparability studies for biosimilar products;
- trials with industrial or non-industrial advanced medicinal products;

- stem cell transplantation trials on humans, organ and tissue transplantation trials, surgical trials, and gene therapy trials; as well as trial facilities, persons or institutions that will conduct these trials.

Non-interventional clinical trials are not covered by this regulation, except observational drug studies and observational medical device studies. According to current legislation, after receiving approval from ECs, permission is needed from the Turkish Medicines and Medical Devices Agency (TMMDA) in order to conduct clinical trials in Turkey.

17.2.1 Ethics Committees

According to Turkish regulations, ECs (comprised of not less than seven and not more than 15 members, with at least one of them a non-healthcare professional and one a jurist, and the majority consisting of healthcare professionals holding a doctorate or medical degree) should be assembled in order to perform a scientific and ethical assessment of the trial protocol, the design and suitability of the trial, the inclusion and exclusion criteria, the suitability of investigators, the adequacy of the clinical trial sites, and the methods and documents used to inform the volunteers and obtain consents from the individuals, as well as any other aspects pertinent to the clinical trial, with a view to ensure that the volunteers' rights, safety and well-being are protected and that the study is conducted and monitored according to the regulations. ECs are established within universities on the proposal of the rector, within RSH Centers on the proposal of the President of RSH Center, or at training and research hospitals on the proposal of the chief physician. They must be approved by the Ministry and commence functioning as of the approval date thereof. ECs are independent in their function of reviewing and approving clinical trial applications from a scientific and ethical perspective.

Clinical trials may only be conducted at centers for health practice and research established within universities, approved centers for research and development subordinate to universities, and the Ministry's teaching and research hospitals which are suitable for and possess appropriate staff, equipment, and laboratory facilities that enable ensuring the safety of research subjects and proper conduct and monitoring of a clinical trial; appropriate emergency care is necessary. Clinical trials that have been granted scientific and ethical approval by the EC require the permission of the Ministry and may not be commenced without the permission of TMMDA.

As well as the GCP, GLP, and GMP guidelines already mentioned, Turkey has additional guidelines for clinical trials including ones for:

- the application format and documentation to be submitted to ECs and the Ministry of Health (MoH);

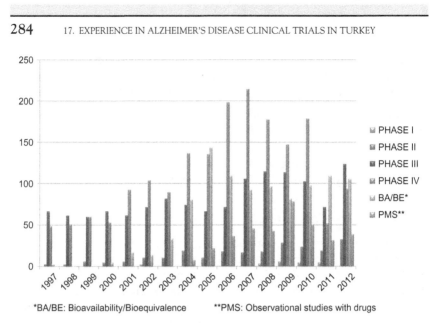

*BA/BE: Bioavailability/Bioequivalence   **PMS: Observational studies with drugs

FIGURE 17.5   The distribution of clinical drug trials conducted in accordance with legislation in Turkey between January 1, 1997 and December 31, 2012.

- advanced treatments;
- the collection, verification, and presentation of adverse reaction reports occurring during clinical trials;
- pediatric trials;
- investigational medicinal products (IMP);
- insurance of volunteers;
- inspections;
- data monitoring committees;
- observational studies conducted with drugs;
- compassionate use programs; and
- standard operating procedures (SOPs) for ECs.

In order to standardize EC SOPs and applications, TMMDA is working intensively. The clinical trials department of TMMDA reviews clinical trials; in this department there is a phase evaluation unit, a bioequivalence/bioavailability evaluation unit, and a post marketing surveillance evaluation unit. The distribution of clinical drug trials conducted in accordance with legislation in Turkey between January 1, 1997 and December 31, 2012 is shown in Figure 17.5. These include studies in oncology, anesthesiology, the central nervous system, the cardiovascular system, endocrinology, and infectious diseases, in rank order.

17.3 CLINICAL TRIALS FOR ALZHEIMER'S DISEASE AND DEMENTIA IN TURKEY

A number of large, randomized clinical trials as well as experimental studies on Alzheimer's disease (AD) and other dementia have been conducted in several centers in Turkey. A representative list of such trials conducted in Turkey from 1997 until today is provided below.

17.3.1 Phase II/III Randomized Clinical Trials

EXPRESS: A RANDOMIZED PLACEBO-CONTROLLED TRIAL OF RIVASTIGMINE IN PATIENTS WITH PARKINSON'S DISEASE DEMENTIA

This was a large, randomized international study in 68 sites involving 560 patients with mild to moderate dementia associated with Parkinson's disease. The cholinesterase inhibitor rivastigmine was compared with placebo over a six month treatment period. The co-primary endpoints were the Alzheimer's Disease Assessment Scale-cognitive portion (ADAS-Cog) and Alzheimer's Disease Cooperative Study-Clinical Global Impression of Change (ADAS-CGIC). The Department of Neurology in the Istanbul Faculty of Medicine at Istanbul University was the international coordinating center in this study. After completion of the study, Turkish centers underwent a successful site inspection by the Food and Drug Administration. The successful completion of this study with a positive outcome led to the registration of rivastigmine as the first medication for the treatment of dementia associated with Parkinson's disease [4].

MEMANTINE FOR PATIENTS WITH PARKINSON'S DISEASE DEMENTIA OR DEMENTIA WITH LEWY BODIES: A RANDOMIZED, DOUBLE-BLIND, PLACEBO-CONTROLLED TRIAL

This was a randomized, controlled, multicenter international trial in which patients with Parkinson's disease dementia or dementia with Lewy bodies with mild to moderate severity were recruited. Patients were randomized to receive either memantine or placebo for six months. A number of efficacy parameters were assessed. The Department of Neurology at Istanbul Faculty of Medicine at Istanbul University was the international coordinating center. A total of 199 patients were recruited in 30 specialist centers in eight countries. This study was successfully completed and demonstrated that memantine may have mild benefits in patients with Lewy body-related dementias [5].

IDENTITY II: EFFECT OF LY450139, A Υ-SECRETASE INHIBITOR, ON THE PROGRESSION OF AD AS COMPARED WITH PLACEBO

AD is thought to be caused by an excess of beta amyloid that forms amyloid plaques. Inhibiting the enzyme gamma-secretase lowers the production of beta amyloid. Semagacestat (LY450139), a functional gamma-secretase inhibitor shown to lower beta amyloid in blood and spinal fluid in humans, was tested in a randomized, double-blind, placebo-controlled Phase III safety and efficacy trial. A number of Turkish sites were also part of this large multicenter study. This was an add-on study in which the use of approved AD drugs was permitted. Men and women 55 years and older, with mild to moderate AD were eligible. This study was terminated prematurely, due to worsening of the active group in an interim analysis of IDENTITY I data [6].

CONCERT: A PHASE III MULTICENTER, RANDOMIZED, PLACEBO-CONTROLLED, DOUBLE-BLIND, 12-MONTH SAFETY AND EFFICACY STUDY EVALUATING DIMEBON IN PATIENTS ON DONEPEZIL WITH MILD TO MODERATE AD

Dimebon, a putatively mitochondrial stabilizer, was shown to be effective in a European study in mild to moderate AD patients. A number of Phase III studies were started in order to further prove its efficacy. The CONCERT study was one of these large-scale multinational studies in which a number of Turkish sites also took part. The purpose of this study was to assess the safety and efficacy of Dimebon in patients with mild to moderate AD who were on donepezil. This study was prematurely terminated due to the lack of efficacy shown in a similarly designed previous study (CONNECTION) [6].

SCARLET ROAD: A MULTICENTER, RANDOMIZED, DOUBLE-BLIND, PLACEBO-CONTROLLED, PARALLEL-GROUP TWO-YEAR STUDY TO EVALUATE THE EFFECT OF SUBCUTANEOUS RO4909832 ON COGNITION AND FUNCTION IN PRODROMAL AD

This ongoing interventional, safety/efficacy study with a passive immunization agent is evaluating the effect of gantenerumab (RO4909832) on cognition and functioning as well as its safety and pharmacokinetics in patients with prodromal AD. Patients are randomized to receive subcutaneous injections of either gantenerumab or placebo. The anticipated time on study treatment is 104 weeks. The inclusion criteria for this study includes patients aged 50–85 with prodromal AD who are not receiving memantine or cholinesterase inhibitors. A patient with prodromal AD is defined as a cognitively impaired, but not demented, person with an abnormal cerbrospinal fluid (CSF) Aβ42 level.

Primary outcome measures of this study include the effect on the change in the Clinical Dementia Rating scale Sum of Boxes (CDR-SOB), a global measure of cognition and functional ability. A number of Turkish sites are involved in this study, but recruitment has turned out to be slow due to difficulties persuading patients to enroll. The major reason for patients to decline is the requirement of a lumbar puncture; the stringent inclusion/exclusion criteria gave rise to a very high number of randomization drop-outs—in some countries the drop-out rate exceeded 90% of all screened patients. The performances of the Turkish sites were above average, and at the time of writing the two initial sites had reached their recruitment quotas [6].

17.3.2 Open-label Clinical Trials

CARE: A 24-WEEK, MULTICENTER, OPEN-LABEL EVALUATION OF COMPLIANCE AND TOLERABILITY OF THE ONCE-DAILY 10 CM² RIVASTIGMINE PATCH FORMULATION IN PATIENTS WITH PROBABLE AD

This multicenter, multinational study aimed to evaluate compliance, tolerability, safety, efficacy, and caregiver burden of rivastigmine patch $10\,cm^2$ treatment in patients with AD (Mini-Mental State Examination (MMSE) 10–26), initiating therapy for the first time with a cholinesterase inhibitor, and in patients who were unresponsive to previous cholinesterase inhibitor treatment in a community setting. Primary outcome measures were the proportion of patients who reached the target rivastigmine patch size of $10\,cm^2$ and stayed on it for at least eight weeks.

EDSE: AN OBSERVATIONAL STUDY IN A NATURALISTIC SETTING ON THE EFFICACY OF MEMANTINE ON BEHAVIORAL SYMPTOMS OF AD

This study was performed to assess the efficacy of memantine on the behavioral symptoms of AD in a naturalistic setting. This was a 12-week, open-label, multicenter, observational national study. The inclusion criteria included a diagnosis of probable AD, and a relatively high score in a behavioral rating scale. A total of 556 patients received a once daily dose of 20 mg memantine, reached after 5 mg-weekly increase. Altogether 67 centers, mainly Neurology and Psychiatry departments of universities and public hospitals across the country, participated. This study was successfully completed and proved the feasibility of a large-scale dementia trial on a national scale.

17.4 CONCLUSIONS

Turkey has fully implemented legislation and guidelines on clinical trials, compatible with those of the EU. The approval process for clinical trials involves firstly approval from an EC followed by approval from the TMMDA.

A number of large, multicenter, international, randomized, controlled clinical trials for AD and other dementias have been conducted in several centers in Turkey. These studies have been successfully completed; Turkish sites proved their potential to recruit large numbers of patients and to produce high quality data, as endorsed by inspection from foreign agencies. They are fully equipped and experienced in running large-scale international clinical trials, meeting high demands in logistics and coordination.

Currently, the field is adapting to changing definitions in AD. Targeting early pre-dementia stages, i.e., conducting clinical trials in patients with prodromal AD, even in at-risk subjects at the preclinical stage, is in progress. Turkish sites must also adapt themselves to this "brave new AD world" and develop innovative ways to recruit patients for these new types of studies. They must also have easy access to biomarkers, which are indispensible for the diagnosis of these early phases of AD. More experience with early stage AD clinical trials will ensure that such new expertise is acquired.

References

[1] Asenaoktar M, Asenaoktar S. Lessons learned in Turkey. In: Bairu M, editor. Global clinical trials playbook. Elsevier; 2012. p. 117–25.
[2] PricewaterhouseCoopers. Turkey's Pharmaceutical Sector Vision 2023 Report. Cited 2012. Available from: <www.aifd.org.tr> .
[3] Kockaya G, Demir M, Uresin AY. Economic effect of clinical trials for Turkey. Value in Health 2012;15:a277–575. (Poster at PMD44 ISPOR 15th Annual European Congress, Berlin, Germany, Nov 5, 2012.)
[4] Emre M, Aarsland D, Albanase A, et al. Rivastigmine for dementia associated with Parkinson's disease. N Engl J Med 2004;351:2509–18.
[5] Emre M, Tsolaki M, Bonuccelli U, et al. Memantine for patients with Parkinson's disease dementia or dementia with Lewy bodies: a randomised, double-blind, placebo-controlled trial. Lancet Neurol 2010;9(10):969–77.
[6] Data available from: www.clinicaltrials.gov.

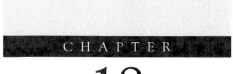

CHAPTER

18

Strengthening/Building Alzheimer's Disease Global Clinical Trial Site Capabilities and Capacity in and for Emerging Markets. Lessons Learned from Japan

Yoko Fujimoto[1] and Takeshi Iwatsubo[2]

[1]Pfizer Japan Inc, Japan [2]Tokyo University, Japan

18.1 THE HISTORY OF CLINICAL TRIALS FOR THE TREATMENT OF ALZHEIMER'S DISEASE IN JAPAN

18.1.1 The Genesis for Developing Donepezil

Donepezil, the most widely used cholinesterase inhibitor for treating symptoms of Alzheimer's disease (AD), was originated and developed by Eisai, a Japanese pharmaceutical company, and Japan was the first country to initiate the clinical development. Japan Phase I development was initiated in 1989, followed by US development starting in 1991. Following a general rule required by the Japanese regulatory authority in those days, Japan independently conducted Phase II dose-finding studies and Phase III confirmatory studies, as well as a study to evaluate the safety of long-term treatment and proved efficacy and safety in Japanese patients. All clinical trials of the four approved drugs for AD conducted in Japan are listed in Table 18.1.

For clinical development of donepezil, most of the major university hospitals and academic medical centers, which specialized in dementia treatment, participated in these clinical trials and most of the experts

M. Bairu & M.W. Weiner (Eds):
Global Clinical Trials for Alzheimer's Disease.
DOI: http://dx.doi.org/10.1016/B978-0-12-411464-7.00018-3

289

TABLE 18.1 All Clinical Trials of Four Approved Drugs for Alzheimer's Disease Conducted in Japan

Investigational Drug	Phase	Study Number	Brief Description	PK/PD	Objectives Efficacy	Safety
Donepezil Aricept®	I	001	Single-dose oral administration PK study in healthy male subjects	X	–	X
		002	Meal study	X	–	X
		003	Repeated-dose study	X	–	X
		005	Repeated-dose study	X	–	X
		004	PK study in elderly subjects	X	–	X
		006	BE study and PK study of enantiomer	X	–	X
	II	111	Dose finding study in mild to moderate AD	–	X	X
		112	Dose finding study in mild to moderate AD	–	X	X
		131-A	Dose finding study in mild to moderate AD	–	X	X
		131-B	Long-term study in mild to moderate AD	–	X	X
		132	Long-term study study in mild to moderate AD	–	X	X
		133	Dose finding study in mild to moderate AD	–	X	X
		134	Dose finding study in mild to moderate AD	–	X	X
	III	161	Mild to moderate AD	–	X	X
		231	Dose finding study in severe AD	–	X	X
		232	Continuous administration study in severe AD	–	X	X

Drug	Phase	Study No.	Description			
Rivastigmine Exelon Patch®	I	1101	PK study in healthy subjects	X	–	X
	II	1201	Dose finding study in mild to moderate AD	–	X	X
	II/III	1301	Dose finding study in mild to moderate AD	–	X	X
		1301E1	Continuous administration study in mild to moderate AD	–	X	X
Galantamine Hydrobromide Reminyl®	I	GAL-BEL-26	Single-dose oral administration PK study in Japanese and non-Japanese	X	–	X
		GAL-JPN-1	Repeated-dose study in healthy male subjects	X	–	X
	III	GAL-JPN-2	PK study in elderly subjects	X	–	X
		GAL-JPN-3	Mild to moderate AD	–	X	X
		GAL-JPN-5	Mild to moderate AD	–	X	X
		GAL-JPN-4	Mild to moderate AD	–	X	X
		GAL-JPN-6	Effect of meal on PK	X	–	X
		JNS023-JPN-01	BE study of Reminyl® tablets vs Reminyl® OD tablets	X	–	X
Memantine MEMARY®	I	IE1301	BE study of 5 mg vs 10 mg	X	–	X
		IE1602	BE study of 10 mg vs 20 mg	X	–	X
		IE1801	PK study in healthy subjects Single-dose oral administration	X	–	X
		IE2201	PK study in AD	X	X	X
		IE1601	PK study in subjects with renal dysfunction	X	–	X
		IE1302	PK study in elderly Japanese and elderly Caucasian	X	–	X

(Continued)

TABLE 18.1 (Continued)

Investigational Drug	Phase	Study Number	Brief Description	Objectives PK/PD	Objectives Efficacy	Safety
	II	IE2901	Exploratory study in severe AD	–	X	X
		IE2101-DB	Dose finding study in severe AD	–	X	X
	III	IE3501	Confirmatory study in severe AD	–	X	X
		MA3301	Dose-finding study in mild to moderate AD (Confirmatory study)	–	X	X
		IE2101-OL	Continuous administration study in AD who have completed participation in IE2101-DB	–	X	X
		MA3302	Continuous administration study in AD who have completed participation in MA3301	–	X	X
		I E2301	Continuous administration study in AD who have completed participation in IE2901, IE2101-OL and IE2201	–	–	X
		IE3604	Drug adherence study of 20mg	–	–	X

AD: Alzheimer's disease BE: Bioequivalence PD: Pharmacodynamics PK: Pharmacokinetics.

for AD treatment were involved all over Japan. Thus, clinical development of donepezil became the underpinning for future clinical trials for AD in Japan. However, it is unfortunate for the future development of AD drugs that the clinical development is not fully aligned with the USA and EU countries. For example, the Japanese version of Alzheimer's Disease Assessment Scale-cognitive component (ADAS J-Cog) was developed for evaluating cognitive function in the clinical trials; however, ADAS J-Cog was not intended to be comparable with the US version of ADAS-Cog and the comparability was not validated. In addition, interview-based measurement by the Clinician's Global Impression of Change, which was used as a co-primary endpoint together with ADAS J-Cog, was also not intended to achieve comparability with the USA and EU countries. This makes subsequent clinical development for AD drugs in Japan more difficult.

18.1.2 Difficulties with the Clinical Development of Rivastigmine, Galantamine, and Memantine

Japan's development and approval of three widely prescribed drugs—rivastigmine, galantamine and memantine—was considerably slower than in other developed countries: All three drugs were approved in 2011. Development of rivastigmine oral was dropped in Japan and the patch was approved in 2011. Galantamine and memantine were also approved in 2011, about 10 years behind US approval. Three key reasons why Japan was so behind in terms of the development and approval were: (1) delayed initiation of clinical development, (2) high regulatory requirements; and (3) failure of clinical trials. All three factors are closely related to each other.

If we talk about the delayed initiation of clinical development, Japanese Phase I study for memantine was initiated in 2000, after the efficacy was confirmed in global Phase III studies. Japanese Phase I study for galantamine was initiated in 2003 after the initial approval in Sweden. As for rivastigmine, development of the patch formulation was launched in 1993 after global Phase III was initiated.

The Japanese regulatory authority, the Ministry of Health, Labor and Welfare (MHLW), and the Pharmaceuticals Medical Devices Agency (PMDA) generally request pharmaceutical companies to show dose–response efficacy and safety of investigational drugs in the Japanese population as well as pharmacokinetic data, although other countries did not request their own country's data and approved these drugs with data mainly generated in the USA and EU.

In 1998, the International Conference on Harmonization E5 (ICH E5) guideline was issued and a bridging development strategy was introduced [1], which encouraged the use of foreign data in the clinical data package for Japanese filing [2]. Thereafter, drug applications based on bridging studies began to increase. The "bridging strategy" consists of conducting "mirror studies" in Japan to obtain clinical data on efficacy, safety, and dosage regimen to allow extrapolation of foreign clinical data to the Japan data package. It must be noted that PMDA accepts "bridging strategy" only on the condition that Japanese studies show a similar dose–response result to global studies, and that the bridge between studies in two different regions are established.

All three AD programs pursued a bridging strategy and conducted Japanese Phase II bridging studies, however none of these studies was successful, for example: a positive ADAS-J Cog result and a negative result of the Clinician's Interview-Based Impression of Change plus caregiver input-Japan (CIBIC plus-J) for rivastigmine; a positive result of Severe Impairment Battery (SIB) and a negative result of AD Cooperative Study-Activities of Daily Living inventory-Japan (ADCS-ADL-J) for memantine; and an inconsistent result in dose–response for galantamine. Following PMDA's request, Phase III studies were repeated for galantamine and memantine. Efficacy data for both programs repeated negative with CIBIC plus-J, however eventually all three drugs were approved in 2011 because of high medical needs and alignment with other countries. It was a tough experience for Japanese regulatory authorities. The situation behind the approval was that drug lag in AD treatment had become a significant social concern in Japan. Understanding of the difficulties of bringing out AD drugs was widespread due to the fact that these trials failed although the efficacy and safety had already been proved in other countries. While developing these three drugs, Japanese experts and medical staff involved in the clinical studies realized that the true challenge of AD clinical trials is not overcoming operational hurdles themselves but confirming the efficacy result of the drug. The difficulties experienced in developing these drugs helped Japan a lot in establishing a foundation for developing AD disease-modifying drugs.

One controversial outcome of this experience is that a Japan-specific path for AD clinical trials was built up and strengthened, which causes additional challenges for the future. In order to develop these programs, a global standard of questionnaire such as CIBIC-plus was introduced, however it is not aligned with global questionnaires but with a Japanese modified version. The Japanese version of CIBIC-plus used for these programs consists of three measurements—Disability Assessment for Dementia (DAD), Behave-AD, and Mental Function Impairment Scale (MENFIS)—and is different from the widely used ADCS-CIBIC.

18.1.3 The New Era of Global Clinical Trials of Disease-Modifying Drugs for AD

In the past decade, multiple programs for potential disease modifying drugs were initiated globally by multiple pharmaceutical companies and

Japan was part of this movement. Japan has a "super-aging society" and is still the second largest market in the pharmaceutical business. Global pharmaceutical companies intended to develop AD drugs simultaneously in Japan using US standard procedures, including questionnaires.

In a nod to the situation, MHLW issued the "Basic Principles on Global Clinical Trials" guidance in 2008, which outlines the basic concepts for planning and implementing multiregional trials in Japan to promote participation from the early stages of drug development [1]. The global strategy increases the opportunities for simultaneous drug submissions and approvals worldwide. Since its publication, the number of multiregional studies in Japan has greatly increased, including those for anti-AD drugs [2]. Multiple-dose studies to evaluate safety and pharmacokinetics in Japanese are required by PMDA for joining multinational large studies in order to confirm there is no significant intrinsic ethnic difference. Therefore, small Japanese studies were generally conducted in parallel with global early-phase studies for potential AD disease-modifying drugs, including two advanced programs of anti-AD monoclonal antibodies, bapineuzumab and solanezumab, both of which failed to show positive results from Phase III studies in 2012. Clinical trials for AD disease-modifying drugs conducted in Japan are shown in Table 18.2.

As for bapineuzumab, a Japanese standalone Phase I study was conducted and more than 300 Japanese patients were enrolled in two multinational studies. The number of Japanese patients was about 15% of the total patients enrolled in two Phase III multinational studies, which is generally the minimum requirement to assess Japanese patients' efficacy and safety required by PMDA.

If we take ACC-001, a vaccine to produce antibodies to amyloid protein, as an example of the ongoing global development program for AD, Japan is heavily involved from the early stage of development. Two multiple ascending dose studies had been conducted in parallel with global early Phase II studies. The development plan was built to fully meet PMDA's requirements of timely participation in global Phase III studies. Eventually, dosing experience of ACC-001 in Japan is second only to the USA; retrospectively, however, the strategy plan is a subject to be carefully evaluated from the international perspective of efficiency in clinical development.

It is also the time when the Japanese Alzheimer's Disease Neuroimaging Initiative (J-ADNI) started the activities, aiming at conducting a longitudinal work-up of standardized neuroimaging, biomarker and clinico-psychological surveys, when a series of large global Phase III programs of AD disease-modifying drugs started in Japan. The research protocol was designed to maximize compatibility with that of US-ADNI, including structural magnetic resonance imaging analysis for the evaluation of brain atrophy, fluorodeoxyglucose and amyloid

TABLE 18.2 List of all Clinical Trials of Potential Disease-Modifying Drugs for Alzheimer's Disease Conducted in Japan

Investigational Drug	Phase	Study Number	Region	Brief Description	PK/PD	Objectives Efficacy	Safety	Source
Avagacestat BMS-708163 (withdrawn)	I	CN156-012	Japan	Placebo-controlled, ascending multiple-dose study to evaluate the safety, tolerability, PK, and PD of BMS-708163 in healthy male Japanese subjects and a comparison to healthy elderly Japanese subjects	X	–	X	JapicCTI-090845 NCT00828646
Semagacestat LY450139 (withdrawn)	III	11271, H6L-MC-LFBC	Global	Effects of LY450139, on the progression of AD as compared with placebo	–	X	X	NCT00762411
		7666, H6L-MC-LFAN	Global	Effect of LY450139 on the long term progression of AD	–	X	X	NCT00594568
		5930, H6L-MC-LFBF	Global	Open-label extension for AD who complete one of two Semagacestat double-blind studies (H6L-MC-LFAN or H6LMC-LFBC)	–	X	X	NCT01035138
Bapineuzumab AAB-001 (withdrawn)	I	3133K1-102	Japan	Study evaluating single ascending doses of AAB-001 vaccine SAD Japanese AD	X	–	X	NCT00397891
	III	3133K1-3000, B2521001	Global	Efficacy and safety trial of Bapineuzumab in mild to moderate AD who are apolipoprotein Eε4 non-carriers	–	X	X	NCT00667810
		3133K1-3002, B2521003	Global	Long-term safety and tolerability trial of Bapineuzumab (AAB-001, ELN115727) in AD who are apolipoprotein E e4 noncarriers and participated in study 3133k1-3000	–	–	X	NCT00996918

Drug	Phase	Study code	Region	Description			NCT/Registry
		3133K1-3001, B2521002	Global	Efficacy and safety trial of Bapineuzumab in mild to moderate AD who are apolipoprotein E ε4 carriers	–	X	NCT00676143
		3133K1-3003, B2521004	Global	Long-term safety and tolerability trial of Bapineuzumab (AAB-001, ELN115727) in AD who are apolipoprotein E ε4 carriers and participated in study 3133k1-3001.	–	–	NCT00998764
Solanezumab LY2062430	II	12025, H8A-JE-LZAK	Japan	Multiple-dose safety in mild-to-moderate AD	X	–	JapicCTI-080636 NCT00749216
	III	6747, H8A-MC-LZAM	Global	Effect of LY2062430 on the progression of AD	–	X	NCT00905372
		11934, H8A-MC-LZAN	Global	Effect of LY2062430 on the progression of AD	–	X	NCT00904683
		11935, H8A-MC-LZAO		Open-label extension study in AD who have completed participation in either Solanezumab clinical trial H8A-MC-LZAM (NCT00905372) or H8A-MC-LZAN (NCT00905683).	–	X	NCT01127633
Gantenerumab RO4909832	I	JP22431	Japan	A multi-center, multiple-ascending dose, randomized, doubleblind, placebo-controlled, parallel-group study to investigate the safety, tolerability and PK of Gantenerumab following subcutaneous injection in Japanese AD	X	–	JapicCTI-121849 NCT01656525

(Continued)

TABLE 18.2 (Continued)

Investigational Drug	Phase	Study Number	Region	Brief Description	Objectives PK/PD	Objectives Efficacy	Objectives Safety	Source
Ponezumab PF-04360365 (withdrawn)	I	A9951005	Japan	Single intravenous dose study of PF-04360365 in Japanese mild to moderate AD	X	–	X	JapicCTI-080533 NCT00607308
		A9951016	Japan	Multiple intravenous dose study of PF-04360365 in Japanese mild to moderate AD	X	–	X	NCT01125631
Vanutide cridificar ACC-001	II	3134K1-2202, B2571006	Japan	Multicenter, randomized, third-party unblinded, adjuvant and placebo controlled, multiple ascending dose, safety, tolerability, and immunogenicity trial of ACC-001 with QS-21 adjuvant in Japanese mild to moderate AD	–	X	X	JapicCTI-101213 NCT00752232
		3134K1-2206, B2571009	Japan	Multicenter, randomized, third-party unblinded, adjuvantcontrolled, multiple ascending dose, safety, tolerability, and immunogenicity trial of ACC-001 with QS-21 adjuvant in Japanese mild to moderate AD	–	X	X	JapicCTI-101214 NCT00959192
		3134K1-2207, B2571001	Japan	Long term extension study evaluating safety, tolerability and immunogenicity of ACC-001 in Japanese mild to moderate AD	–	X	X	JapicCTI-111413 NCT01238991

AD: Alzheimer's disease BE: Bioequivalence PD: Pharmacodynamics PK: Pharmacokinetics.

positron emission tomography, cerebrospinal fluid sampling, and ApoE genotyping, together with a set of clinical and psychometric tests that were prepared to achieve the highest compatibility to those used in the United States [4]. J-ADNI significantly contributed to the development of infrastructure in Japan for global clinical trials for AD.

18.2 HOW TO STRENGTHEN QUALITY AND EFFICIENCY OF CLINICAL TRIALS FOR ANTI-AD DRUGS

18.2.1 Consideration of Ethnic Difference

Ethnic difference is generally a critical factor in terms of global drug development and AD is an area where more attention should be paid. Ethnic factors are generally classified as either intrinsic or extrinsic. Japan is one of the most sensitive countries for ethnic difference in drug development, mainly because of the racial uniformity of the country as well as the long history of drug development in the country. PMDA and pharmaceutical companies, which have developed global programs of anti-AD drugs, intensively discussed the ethnic differences and there are vague but some common opinions about the intrinsic or extrinsic ethnic difference surrounding AD drug development.

Intrinsic ethnic factors are those that help to define and identify a sub-population and may influence the ability to extrapolate clinical data between regions. Examples of intrinsic factors include genetic polymorphism, height, weight, organ dysfunction, as well as pathological background of the target disease. It is widely understood that there is no significant intrinsic ethnic difference in AD itself, since no difference is observed in the pathology of the AD brain, and data on biomarkers and demographics from US-ADNI and J-ADNI data also support the consistent pathophysiology of AD. Active and passive immunotherapy targeting amyloid beta peptides seems less likely to be affected by ethnic differences because it is directly linked to the nature of immunological response. Meanwhile, small chemical entities such as secretase inhibitors are more likely to be affected by intrinsic factors related to absorption, distribution, metabolism, and excretion.

Extrinsic ethnic factors are those associated with the environment and culture in which patients reside. Examples of extrinsic factors include the social and cultural aspects of a region such as medical practice, diet, socio-economic status, etc. Drug development of AD is likely to be highly affected by extrinsic factors, since clinical symptoms of AD are heavily affected by multiple extrinsic factors, for example family structure, housing accommodation, caregiver, and cultural and social stimulation.

Most of them are not directly related to ethnic difference but personal variation; however, there are some common characteristics of each item based on ethnicity and Japan is not an exception.

Japanese people have a common tendency not to talk a lot about personal matters to people they are not familiar with, and it becomes a hurdle for physicians or medical staff to assess cognitive dysfunction, behavior, or ADLs of AD patients. In addition, the public nursing care insurance system called "Kaigo-Hoken" was implemented in Japan in 2000. Elderly people with dementia are a population who need intensive support by caregivers who are employed by the municipal government; therefore care for patients by family members has been minimized recently in some families, which makes it more difficult for physicians, nurses, and neuropsychologists to evaluate the condition of AD patients.

In addition to such AD-specific factors, standard treatment in a country is a typical extrinsic ethnic factor to be considered. In Japan, donepezil had been the only anti-AD drug prescribed for a long period, although other countries prescribed memantine and other cholinesterase inhibitors as well. Chinese medicine is widely used in China and some Asian countries, although the influence is limited in Japan. In addition to the variety of drugs, difference in standard drug dosage is an important factor to be considered. In Japan, relatively lower dosages are prescribed compared with other countries [5]. The reason is not only due to the difference in pharmacokinetics or pharmacodynamics, but also to the cultural preference of Japanese people for insufficient efficacy rather than minor side effects [6].

18.2.2 Study Preparation

One of the difficulties of AD drug development is that two primary efficacy endpoints, cognitive function and global evaluation, need to be achieved and both of the efficacy endpoints were, to a greater or lesser extent, evaluated mainly by interview with patients and caregivers using questionnaires. The challenge to evaluate AD symptoms with a questionnaire is significantly increased when we conduct multinational studies, mainly because of cultural and linguistic differences.

Linguistic validation is critical to develop questionnaires to deal with multiple languages in clinical trials and it is far from a general translation process. Translation by linguistic expertise for both English and Japanese is just the first step in developing country- and/or language-specific questionnaires comparable with the original English version. For example, to select words for word recall tests, we need to select a word comparable to an English word in terms of word frequency and impact as well as the meaning itself. In addition to linguistic validation, psychometric validation is critical to appropriately evaluate AD clinical symptoms in multinational trials. It is a very time-consuming process and dedicated work by experts who fully understand neuropsychology in both English and Japanese is essential. It is not a task for a vendor to handle multiple languages with little support from experts in each country for limited time periods.

Implementation of the questionnaire is another critical process. Training for raters of neuropsychological tests is generally provided by pharmaceutical companies or the contract organization. Trainers should be native speakers who are very familiar with the questionnaire so that they can ensure that raters understand the method correctly. The other issue is that training is generally given for each program and a rater will sometimes be given multiple directions by multiple companies; this can cause much confusion in their rating of clinical trials for AD and may negatively affect the quality of their rating. A consistent method should be developed and for this purpose the role of an academic society is critical.

18.2.3 Study Operation

Considering the difficulty of AD clinical trials, understanding of the country-specific situation is an important first step to reduce the operational burden on clinical trials for AD while maintaining the quality of the study. Japan has several unique points and it is important to understand the situation, maximize the benefits, and minimize the negative aspects.

Japan has a universal health-insurance system that covers all of its citizens, and patients have a right of free access. AD patients visit doctors at outpatient practices at large hospitals such as university or general hospitals as well as clinics. Thus, AD patients are generally dispersed throughout the hospitals and clinics and it is difficult to select a clinical site to enroll a great number of AD patients. The trial sites which enroll high numbers of AD patients within a short period are not always the sites of high AD expertise. Considering the balance between speed and quality, selecting trial sites for AD is difficult.

The characteristics of the nursing system in Japan are unique, as described in the section on ethnic difference earlier. There is also a system to allow patients with dementia to stay in hospital or in a nursing home for few days or weeks to reduce the burden on the caregiver and patients enrolled in clinical trials. These supporting systems narrow down the eligible population for AD clinical trials.

Psychiatrists and neurologists are key players in the treatment of AD patients in Japan, similar to other major countries in Asia, and the weight is moving from psychiatrists to neurologists. The collection of cerebrospinal fluid in clinical trials for AD is becoming more important, since the focus is more on finding a disease modifier than symptomatic treatment. Psychiatrists generally do not use lumbar punctures for collecting cerebrospinal fluids. At the moment there is a tendency for an elderly person who has dementia symptoms to be treated by a psychiatrist as they have more expertise to deal with the behavioral and psychological symptoms of dementia. The current situation where experts from both departments see AD patients independently is not efficient and a system to enable their collaboration should be developed at both hospital and academic organization level.

The positive aspect of clinical trials for AD in Japan is that magnetic resonance imaging (MRI) is very common all over the country and there is no difficulty in using MRI for screening or following up the changes during trials. Amyloid imaging is also becoming common, although none of the probes have been approved yet and most of them do not meet good manufacturing practice (GMP) criteria required for use in clinical trials; an initiative to build the infrastructure has recently started.

Due to its long history of drug development, Japan has a lot of experience for clinical trials. At the same time, the uniqueness of Japan sometimes presents a challenge. In particular, clinical trials managed by foreign companies or English-speaking organizations create problems for the investigators and staff at the trial sites, since they are only familiar with trials domestically handled in Japanese. A little language support may sometimes help the situation. Thus, it is important to be aware of local customs from the outset, otherwise there will be problems throughout.

18.2.4 Consideration of Regulatory Requirements

As already mentioned, PMDA has their specific opinion regarding Japanese data in clinical data packages for filing, especially with regards to Japan's participation in multinational studies. Intrinsic ethnic similarities generally need to be evaluated prior to joining multinational studies and if the initiation of Japan Phase I studies are delayed, Japan may lose the chance to participate in multinational studies. Sample sizes of Japanese patients required in multinational studies is another important discussion point with PMDA. Based on the guidance, the number of Japanese patients which can show similar tendency of the efficacy and safety to the whole study data is generally required in a multinational study. Thus, pre-discussion with PMDA is important when proceeding with AD drug development in Japan and the timing of the discussion is also critical.

18.3 FUTURE PERSPECTIVE

The difficulty of conducting clinical trials for AD is significantly increased by targeting disease-modifying drugs, and is becoming more difficult by initiating early intervention for prodromal AD [7], mild cognitive impairment (MCI) due to AD, or even preclinical AD [8]. In Japan, additional attention needs to be paid to global development and multinational studies, which is the current global standard of drug development for AD.

To deal with the recent situation facing such drastic changes of drug development for AD, efficiency is becoming more important. A wide range of collaboration should be strongly promoted, including global collaboration, East Asian collaboration, industrial collaboration among pharmaceutical and imaging companies, academic collaboration including neurology, psychiatry, geriatrics and radiology, and, more importantly, collaboration among academia, industries and regulatory bodies. Unfortunately, barriers among each group seem relatively high in Japan compared with the USA and major EU countries.

In order to promote collaboration, strong leadership by academic society is important, because academic societies are in the position to access and manage the collaborations across each player. J-ADNI is an epoch-making initiative in this perspective and follow-up action is significantly important. The value depends on the subsequent implementation of the initiative in the area of research and drug development for AD.

18.4 CONCLUSION

The challenges of developing clinical trials for AD in Japan have been highlighted in this chapter. Such knowledge and realization come from Japan's long history of clinical trials for AD. The authors hope these experiences are taken advantage of for the future success of clinical development of AD, especially in emerging markets which are newly participating in the global clinical development for AD.

References

[1] Harmonized Tripartite Guideline. Ethnic factors in the acceptability of foreign clinical data. International Conference on Harmonization. ICH-E5 (R1). Available from: http://www.ich.org/fileadmin/Public_Web_Site/ICH_Products/Guidelines/Efficacy/E5_R1/Step4/E5_R1__Guideline.pdf.
[2] Uyama Y, Shibata T, Nagai N, Hanaoka H, Toyoshima S, Mori K. Successful bridging strategy based on ICH E5 guideline for drugs approved in Japan. Clin Pharmacol 2005;78:102–13.

[3] Ministry of Health, Labour and Welfare of Japan. Basic principles on global clinical trials. Available from: http://www.pmda.go.jp/english/service/pdf/notifications/0928010-e.pdf.

[4] Iwatsubo T. Japanese: Alzheimer's disease neuroimaging initiative: present status and future. Alzheimers Dement 2010;6:297–9.

[5] Malinowski HJ, Westelinck A, Sato J. Same drug, different dosing: differences in dosing for drugs approved in the United States, Europe, and Japan. J Clin Pharmacol 2008;48:900–8.

[6] Nakashima K, Narukawa M, Takeuchi M. Approaches to Japanese dose evaluation in global drug development: factors that generate different dosages between Japan and the United States. Clin Pharmacol Ther 2011;90:836–43.

[7] Dubois B, Feldman HH, Jacova C, Cummings JL, Dekosky ST, Barnerger-Gateau P. Revising the definition of Alzheimer's disease: a new lexicon. Lancet Neurol 2010;9:1118–27.

[8] Jack Jr CR, Albert MS, Knopman DS, McKhann GM, Sperling RA, Carrillo MC. Introduction to the recommendations from the National Institute on aging-Alzheimer's association workgroups on diagnostic guidelines for Alzheimer's disease. Alzheimers Dement 2011;7:257–62.

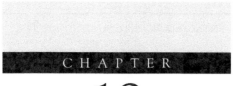

CHAPTER
19

Strengthening/Building Alzheimer's Disease Global Clinical Trial Site Capabilities and Capacity in and for Developing/Emerging Markets. Lessons Learned from Korea†

Seong Yoon Kim

Asan Medical Center, Seoul, Korea

19.1 DEMENTIA IN KOREA

19.1.1 Prevalence of Dementia in Korea

In Korea, the percentage of elderly people in the population is rapidly increasing (Figure 19.1) due to improved medical services, and partly due to a decreasing childbirth rate [1]. The average age of marriage is being postponed and the number of children per newly-wed couples is very low due to the burdens of higher education and housing. Social issues related to the elderly population are also increasing: less job opportunities, the social burdens of elderly care, soaring medical expenditures, social isolation, and psychiatric issues such as depression and suicide.

The prevalence of dementia in Korea is estimated to be 6.3–13.0% of the elderly population, and dementia due to Alzheimer's disease (AD)

---

†All references to 'Korea' in this chapter are to 'South Korea'.

M. Bairu & M.W. Weiner (Eds):
Global Clinical Trials for Alzheimer's Disease.
DOI: http://dx.doi.org/10.1016/B978-0-12-411464-7.00019-5

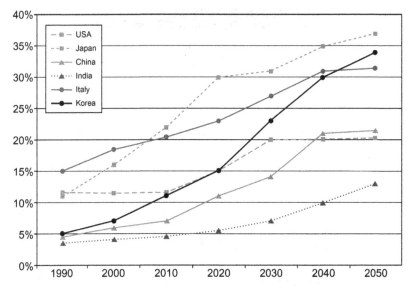

FIGURE 19.1 Anticipated percentages of elderly people in the populations of several countries. Compared with other countries, the percentage of elderly in the Korean population has steeply increased in the last 20 years and this is expected to speed up.

comprises 45–75%, while vascular dementia comprises 12–37% (Table 19.1) [2–7]. According to a recent national survey conducted in 2012, the prevalence of dementia among the elderly population is 9.1%, and the estimated number of dementia patients is expected to be over 740,000 [8]. Considering the life expectancy of Koreans at birth (79.3 years in total: 76.1 for men, 82.7 for women), the prevalence of dementia patients will exceed 13% of the elderly population by 2050 (Figure 19.2).

Dementia is considered one of the major medical and social challenges for the Korean government, and is thus given a top priority in health policymaking as in other countries. The government has established nationwide dementia counseling centers, based on the Welfare Law for the Elderly in the 1990s. The Ministry of Health and Welfare announced a Comprehensive Dementia Policy in 2008, followed by the legislation of the Dementia Management Law in 2012.

19.1.2 Characteristics of Korean Dementia Patients

The wide range in levels of education in the Korean elderly population, which is probably due to the unstable educational system between 1940 and 1970, is an important issue in evaluating elderly people (in their

TABLE 19.1 Dementia Prevalence Studies in Korea

Authors	Region	Age	Sample	Screening	Diagnosis	Prevalence by Sex			Prevalence by Type		
						Male	Female	Total	AD	VaD	Other
Jhoo et al. [2]	Seongnam	>65	1,118	–[a]	DSM-IV	2.6	8.8	6.3	75.7	18.9	5.4
Kim et al. [3]	Busan	>65	1,230	MMSE-K	DSM-III-R	2.7	10	8	–	–	–
Suh et al. [4]	Yeoncheon	>65	1,217	PAS-K	DSM-III-R	6.3	7.1	6.8	61.7	35.3	3
Lee et al. [5]	Seoul	>65	953	MMSE-KC	DSM-IV	4.5	10.4	8.2	65.4	24.7	9.9
Woo et al. [6]	Yeoncheon	>65	1,674	MMSE-K	DSM-III-R	8.8	9.9	9.5	47.4	26.3	22.7
Park et al. [7]	Youngil	>65	766	MMSE-K	DSM-III-R	7.2	14.5	10.8	60	12	38

MMSE-K: Korean version of mini-mental state examination PAS-K: Korean version of psychogeriatric assessment scale MMSE-KC: Korean version of mini-mental state examination included in CERAD-K packet

AD: Dementia of Alzheimer's disease type

VaD: Vascular Dementia

[a]: Single phase design: No screening tests were carried out, and the subjects were evaluated with CERAD-K.

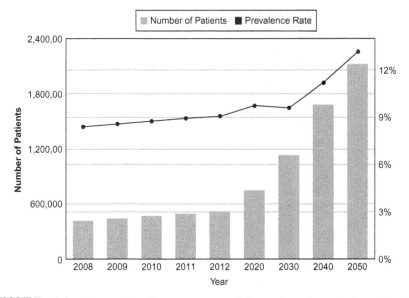

FIGURE 19.2   The anticipated steep increase of dementia patients: In line with the increasing elderly population in Korea, the number of dementia patients is expected to soar.

70s or over). (This may be particularly true for women, as they had less social and educational privileges compared with men.)

The prevalence of mild cognitive impairment (MCI) is about 2.5–3 times higher than AD prevalence, i.e., around 24–26% (20–22% for men, 25–30% for women) of the elderly population. Since the definition of MCI is largely dependent on cognitive assessment, the educational level exerts greater influence on the prevalence of MCI.

Due to the diagnostic heterogeneity of vascular cognitive impairments, the prevalence of vascular dementia varies widely according to the surveys, and this is also true of Korean studies. Alhough the number of people with obesity and other vascular risk factors is increasing, the greater possibilities of prevention and treatment options for vascular cognitive impairments make this category of dementia an important target for health policymaking. Vascular risk factors, such as hypertension, diabetes, dyslipidemia, lack of exercise, and obesity, are of great social concern, though the smoking rate is decreasing in Korea.

The relationship between Apolipoprotein E (ApoE) genotype and the epidemiology of sporadic AD is well known. In a Korean study for centenarians and the general population [9], the distribution of ApoE genotypes was as shown in Table 19.2.

TABLE 19.2   Distribution of ApoE Genotypes in Centenarian and Control Groups

Genotype	Centenarians (n = 103) Number (frequency)		Controls (n = 6,435) Number (frequency)	
E2/2	0	(.0%)	27	(.4%)
E2/3	11	(10.7%)	690	(10.7%)
E3/3	78	(75.7%)	4,585	(71.3%)
E4/2	2	(1.9%)	78	(1.2%)
E4/3	12	(11.7%)	1,005	(15.6%)
E4/4	0	(.0%)	50	(.8%)
p value	0.702			

19.2 THE NATIONAL MEDICAL SYSTEM AND INSURANCE SYSTEM IN KOREA

19.2.1 Korean Medical Service System

After the Korean War, Korean society experienced radical reconstruction of the economy, education, and social infrastructures. The medical service system was also included in this overall social reform.

The resultant medical insurance system in Korea is composed of three main services; the National Health Insurance Service, the Medical Aid Program, and the Long-term Care Insurance Program. The National Health Insurance Service is the compulsory public insurance system, which covers the whole population. It was revised several times throughout the 1970s and 1980s, and all Koreans except the lower-income group are enrolled in this program. The coverage of medical expenditures by this program is generally 50–60%, but some high-cost illnesses such as cancer, or chronic diseases like mental disorders, are covered up to 90–95%. The Medical Aid Program is a form of public assistance for those from low income households. The insurance coverage is almost 100%. The Long-term Care Insurance Program was established in 2008, and covers the financial burden of caring for senior citizens with geriatric illnesses. Part of the dementia care expenditures is covered by this program on a severity basis.

The number of the healthcare facilities in South Korea are shown in Table 19.3 [10,11].

TABLE 19.3   Healthcare Facilities in South Korea in 2011

Hospitals and Treatment Centers	
Tertiary hospitals	44
General hospitals	275
Hospitals	2,363
Clinics	27,837
Dental Care	
Dental hospitals	199
Dental clinics	15,058
Oriental Medicine	
Oriental health hospitals	184
Oriental health clinics	12,401
Public Health Services	
Public health hospitals	17
Public health centers	240
Health sub-centers	1,294
Primary healthcare posts	1,917
Midwifery clinics	40
Pharmacy	
Pharmacist offices	21,079
Total	82,948

19.3 RECENT ADVANCES IN CLINICAL TRIALS IN KOREA

19.3.1 Increased Network among Korean Dementia Researchers

Before 2000, most of the studies on dementia had been conducted in individual medical centers or institutions. With the outbursts of web-based technology, however, collaborative studies among several medical institutions became very active. The launch of several public-funded dementia cohort projects also greatly enhanced the chance and possibility of multisite collaborative studies and drug trials. The use of electronic data capture systems and application of common evaluation protocol for dementia subjects also heightened the collaborative productivity. Some of the representative projects are the Clinical Research Centers for Dementia (CRCD)[12,13], the Korean Longitudinal Study on Health and Aging (KLoSHA) [2], and the Gwangju Dementia and Mild Cognitive Impairment Study (GDEMCIS) [14]. Current ongoing national projects, such as the Korean Alzheimer Dementia Neuroimaging Initiative (K-ADNI) or the Korean Longitudinal Study on Cognitive Ageing and Dementia (KLoSCAD), will also serve as a research network and database from which various clinical research projects and drug trials can be conducted.

19.3.2 National Supports: KFDA and Other Organizations and National Projects

The Korean Food and Drug Administration (KFDA) was founded in 1998 to support food and drug safety evaluation and approval of new drugs. Another public organization for drug development is the KoNECT (Korean National Enterprise for Clinical Trials), which was set up in 2007 by the Korean Ministry of Health Welfare and Family to foster clinical trials and to enhance the national drug development capability. The Korea Drug Development Fund (KDDF) was launched in 2011 to expedite the drug development process and support training for human resources with a budget of US$1 billion.

Furthermore, to enhance biotechnology and the health industry the government designated 10 "research-driven hospitals" in 2013, so that these medical institutes can invest more resources into basic and clinical research.

19.3.3 Clinical Trials in Korea

Though the medical service system in daily practice has been steadily stabilized for the last 50 years, the infrastructure for basic and clinical research was relatively underdeveloped until 20 years ago. According to KoNECT reports [15], the number of clinical trials approved by KFDA has been steeply increasing in the last 10 years. Major areas of medicine with steep increases are allergy-rheumatology, central nervous system (CNS), cardiovascular (CV), endocrine, gastroenterology, and oncology (Figure 19.3).

The earlier phases of drug trials are growing in the areas of CNS and oncology as shown in Figure 19.4.

19.3.3.1 Clinical Trials for Dementia and Alzheimer's Disease

CNS disorders like strokes or epilepsy, and psychiatric disorders such as depression, schizophrenia, and anxiety disorders are the most active

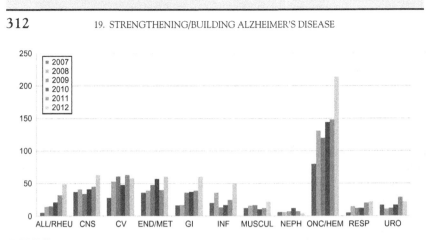

FIGURE 19.3　Trends in the number of clinical trials in major areas of medicine in Korea from 2007 to 2012. (The number of clinical trials submitted to KFDA has increased four-fold since 2003.)

area of research and clinical trials. Dementia accounts for about 10–15% of all CNS trials, but most of them are for AD [16] (Figure 19.5).

The market size of dementia drugs in Korea was US$ 400 million in 2012. This is estimated to expand up to four times by 2020, i.e., to more than US$ 1,700 million [17] (Figure 19.6). Currently, approved drugs for AD and some vascular dementias in Korea include three acetylcholine esterase inhibitors (donepezil, rivastigmine, galantamine), and memantine.

New development of anti-dementia drugs is still in its infancy in Korea. The number of investigational new drugs hitherto submitted to the KFDA is less than 20, some of which are listed in Table 19.4.

19.4 EVALUATION OF THE SUBJECTS IN DRUG TRIALS FOR DEMENTIAS

19.4.1 Subject Evaluation Process

The diagnostic process generally applied for thorough dementia evaluation involves: medical history for cognitive dysfunction and functional impairment; physical and neurological examination; evaluation for accompanying psychiatric and behavioral symptoms; laboratory tests; neuroimaging such as magnetic resonance imaging (MRI) or fludeoxyglucose positron emission tomography (FDG-PET) and ApoE genotyping.

Most of the general hospitals or tertiary referral hospitals use a predefined series of MRI protocol for evaluating dementia. A series of T1, T2, fluid attenuated inverse recovery (FLAIR), gradient echo (GRE), and diffusion weighted image (DWI) tests are routinely performed, and some institutes add volumetric acquisition for research purposes. Most of the

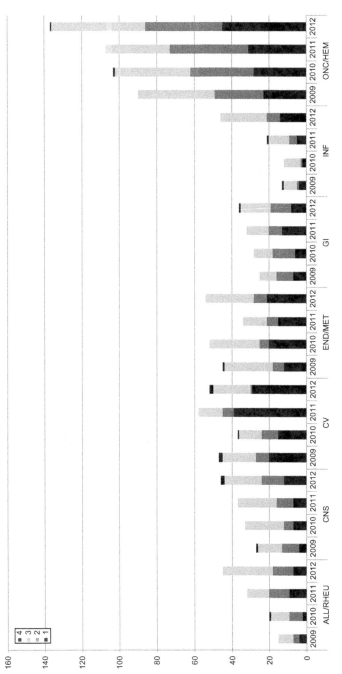
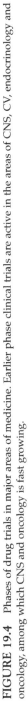

FIGURE 19.4 Phases of drug trials in major areas of medicine. Earlier phase clinical trials are active in the areas of CNS, CV, endocrinology and oncology, among which CNS and oncology is fast growing.

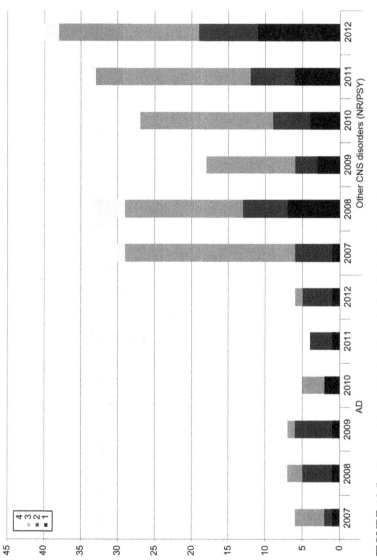

FIGURE 19.5 Phases of drug trials for AD and other CNS disorders. Of the 40+ clinical trials for dementia submitted to the KFDA since 2007, all except three were for AD. Three exceptions were one study on alcoholic dementia, one for vascular dementia, and one on diffuse Lewy body dementia.

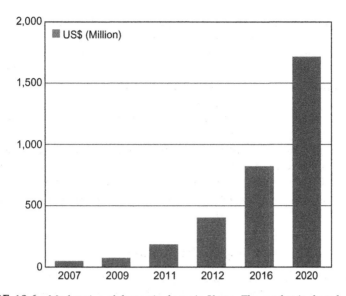

FIGURE 19.6   Market size of dementia drugs in Korea. The market is shared with oriental medicine, OTC medications, functional food, and oral supplements, which are also rapidly increasing.

TABLE 19.4   Current Status of Dementia Drug Development in Korea as of 2012

Pharmaceutical Company	Research Laboratory	Ingredient	Development Stage
Kwangdong Pharma	Elcom Science	Natural product	Phase II
SK Chemical		Natural product	Phase III
Whanin Pharmaceutical	Scigenic	Natural product	Phase III
Hanwha Dream Pharma	Newmed	Natural product	Phase II
Daewoong Pharma	Medifron	Synthetic chemical (DWP09031)	Approved
	Neurotech	Synthetic chemical (AAD-2004)	Phase I
	Bioland	Natural product(BL153)	Phase II
	Medipost	Stem cell (Neurostem AD)	Patent acquired

tertiary referral hospitals are equipped with 3.0T scanners and picture archiving and communication systems (PACS).

Some centers use amyloid PET for research purposes. The application of PET imaging to detect the amyloid deposition using Pittsburgh Compound B (PIB) or flutemetamol was approved by the KFDA in 2011, but, as of the time of writing, only for research purposes.

The measurement of amyloid beta or tau in the cerebrospinal fluid (CSF) is not routinely carried out in clinical practice. This is the same for ApoE genotyping, although it is included in initial diagnostic procedures in some Korean dementia clinics. The autopsy rate of unconfirmed deaths in Korea is very low, so neuropathological confirmation of various neurodegenerative disorders is a field most Korean dementia researchers think needs to be established.

19.4.2 Neuropsychological Evaluation

Usually a neuropsychologist is assigned to perform neuropsychological tests in most of the general hospitals. For research purposes, sometimes a certified study coordinator (usually a registered research nurse) can also evaluate study subjects.

Various standardized versions of cognitive tests are employed as screening tools. The Mini-Mental State Examination (MMSE), MoCA (Montreal Cognitive Assessment) [18,19], and Hasegawa Scale [20] are some of these. There exist at least four versions of the Korean MMSE, according to different correction methods for education, sex, and age [21–24]. Differences between these tests are summarized in Table 19.5.

For detailed neuropsychological evaluation, Seoul Neuropsychological Screening Battery (SNSB) [25] and its dementia version SNSB-D [26], or the Korean version of Consortium to Establish a Registry for Alzheimer's Disease Assessment Packet (CERAD) [23,27] are frequently used. While these test batteries are used for clinical use, the Korean version of Alzheimer's Disease Assessment Scale—Cognitive domain (ADAS-Cog-K) [28] is used in the majority of drug trials for AD (Table 19.6).

Some dementia screening tools rate the cognitive decline and functional impairment together; some examples include the Korean versions of Informant Questionnaire on the Cognitive Decline in the Elderly (IQCODE) [29]; AD8 [30]; Short form Samsung Dementia Questionnaire (S-SDQ) [31]; and Korean Dementia Screening Questionnaire (KDSQ) [32].

19.4.3 Evaluation of Functional Impairment

There are several functional (activities of daily living [ADL]) assessment tools used to evaluate functional impairment: the Korean versions of instrumental ADL (K-IADL) [33], Bayer ADL (B-ADL) [34], Disability

TABLE 19.5 Comparison of Different Versions of the Korean MMSE Tests

	MMSE-K (1989)	K-MMSE (1987)	MMSE-KC (2002)	MMSE-DS (2010)
Features	Partially modified for illiterate subjects	Translated true to the original MMSE. Age and years of education-adjusted norms are provided	Age and years of education-adjusted norms are provided	Age and years of education-adjusted norms are provided
Orientation (10 points)	Time orientation (5 points)	Time orientation (5 points)	Time orientation (5 points)	Time orientation (5 points)
	Spatial orientation (5 points); the home address and the present location are questioned together	Spatial orientation (5 points); "What kind of a place is this?" The home address is not questioned	Spatial orientation (5 points); same as MMSE-K	Spatial orientation (5 points); geographic position, floor, name of the place
Memory registration (3 points)	Tree, car, hat	Airplane, pencil, pine tree	Tree, car, hat	Tree, car, hat
Memory recall (3 points)	Tree, car, hat	Airplane, pencil, pine tree	Tree, car, hat	Tree, car, hat
Attention and calculation (5 points)	100–7 (5 times), if unable to perform, the respondent is asked to say "samcheon lee kang san" backward	Only 100–7 is questioned, "saying a word backward" is left out due to the varying level of difficulty	No calculation question, the respondent is asked to say "samcheon lee kang san"[a] backward	Only 100–7 is questioned
Language (8 points)	Pencil, clock "Receive with the right hand/ fold in half/ put on your lap". Say "ganjang kongjang kongjang jang"[b] Reasoning/ writing tasks are offered	Clock, ballpoint pen "Flip the paper over/ fold in half/ give it to me." Say "Bak muni bulyeo ilkyun"[c]. Writing of a simple sentence is asked	Key, stamp Same as MMSE-K	Pencil, clock Same as MMSE-K

(Continued)

TABLE 19.5   (Continued)

	MMSE-K (1989)	K-MMSE (1987)	MMSE-KC (2002)	MMSE-DS (2010)
Visual construction (1 point)	Interlocking Pentagon copy	Interlocking Pentagon copy	Interlocking Pentagon copy	Interlocking Pentagon copy

[a]"sam cheon lee kang san" is a Korean idiom meaning beautiful county. The five syllables are equivalent to five items of 100–7.
[b]"ganjang kongjang kongjang jang" is a kind of Korean tongue twister. It is the equivalent of "No ifs, ands, or buts". Although not very difficult to pronounce, this phrase has been used to test vocalization ability.
[c]"Bak muni bulyeo ilkyun" is a Korean idiom meaning "seeing is believing." It substitutes "No ifs, ands, or buts."

Assessment for Dementia scale (DAD-K) [35], the Seoul-activities of daily living (SADL) [36], and the Seoul-instrumental activities of daily living (S-IADL) [37], etc.

19.4.4 Evaluation of Behavioral and Psychological Symptoms

Delusion, hallucination, depression, anxiety, wandering, aggression, aberrant eating or sexual behaviors are frequently encountered during the course of dementia. These behavioral and emotional symptoms are not only frequent, but also a major source of caregiver burden and main reasons for the early institutionalization of patients. Usual clinical and research assessment tools for these symptoms include: Korean versions of Neuropsychiatric Inventory (K-NPI) [38], geriatric depression scale (GDS-K) [39], BEHAVE-AD Korean version [40], and Behavior Rating Scale for Dementia (BRSD) in CERAD Packet [41].

19.5 LESSONS LEARNED FROM PREVIOUS AND ONGOING AD TRIALS IN KOREA

19.5.1 Changing Public View on Clinical Trials

The general public's view on clinical research in Korea was not positive a few decades ago. This notion might be related to the deep-rooted Confucian tradition, which cherishes the body parts endowed from parents; this also explains the very low autopsy rate in Korea. But this view has been changing in recent years. Thanks to education and public awareness promoted by public or private organizations, the younger generation tends to acknowledge the importance of medical research and clinical trials in expanding medical knowledge and treatment options.

TABLE 19.6 Subtests in the Seoul Neuropsychological Screening Battery (SNSB)

Cognitive Domain	Neuropsychological Tests
Attention	Digit span: forward/backward
	Letter cancellation
Language and related functions	Spontaneous speech/comprehension/repetition
	K-BNT
	Reading/writing
	Finger naming/right–left orientation/calculation/ body part identification
	Praxis test: Buccofacial, Ideomotor
Visuospatial functions	K-MMSE: Drawing
	RCFT: Copy
Memory	K-MMSE: Registration/recall
	SVLT
	RCFT: Immediate and delayed recalls/recognition
Frontal/executive functions	Contrasting program/Go–No go test
	Fist-Edge-Palm/Alternating hand movement
	Alternating square and triangle/Luria loop
	COWAT
	—Semantic (animal, supermarket)
	—Phonemic (3 Korean alphabets: "Kiuk," "Eeung," "Siot")
	Korean-Color Word Stroop Test (K-CWST)
Other Index	K-MMSE
	Geriatric Depression Scale
	B-ADL
	CDR

SNSB: Seoul Neuropsychological Screening Battery; K-BNT: Korean version of the Boston Naming Test; K-MMSE: Korean version of the Mini-Mental Status Examination; RCFT: Rey Complex Figure Test; SVLT: Seoul Verbal Learning Test; COWAT: Controlled Oral Word Association Test; K-CWST; Korean-Color Word Stroop Test; B-ADL: Barthel Activities of Daily Living; CDR: Clinical Dementia Rating.

19.5.2 Legislation Regarding Medical Research and Clinical Trials

Together with the recent boom in biotechnology and health technology in Korea, the laws and regulations regarding research ethics have been much strengthened and revised. The Bioethics and Biosafety Law effective from 2012, together with the Personal Information Protection Act enforced in 2011, works as a safeguard for human research subject protection. This change of clinical research environment will work as both an advantage and a disadvantage at the same time. The positive aspects are: protected research environment and ensured data quality; better human research protection, especially for vulnerable subjects like dementia patients; and a better environment for earlier phase trials and monitoring. The negative aspects may be: a tougher and longer review process by the institutional review board (IRB), KFDA, and other regulatory bodies; increased budget and longer study periods per clinical trials; and a transient shortage of human resources and facilities that meet the high standards of qualification.

19.5.3 The Importance of Cognitive Tests and ADL Evaluation

The main issue in anti-dementia drug development and evaluation is the reliability and validity of cognitive and behavioral assessments. Contrary to Western countries, the wide range of educational levels in the elderly population in Korea has raised some issues in the interpretation of cognitive test results. Recently, there has been some international effort to validate and harmonize dementia evaluation instruments such as ADAS-Cog, DAD, MMSE, NPI, clinical dementia rating (CDR), etc [42]. Regional and global collaboration of this kind will enhance the feasibility of multisite clinical trials for dementia subjects, and greatly expedite drug development and the approval process.

The rapid industrialization of Korea and the resultant urban–rural lifestyle discrepancy make standardized ADL assessment very difficult. This may be critical in deciding the conversion point from MCI to AD, which relies solely on the decline of functional impairment in a current diagnostic system. Development of reliable biomarkers and applications to clinical practice will make the diagnostic process less dependent on the current operational diagnosis of AD.

19.5.4 Experiences for Research Network

As information technology (IT) has been a national strategic industry in Korea for a long time, the utilization of high-tech IT in the medical research field seems natural and much recommended. The mandatory medical insurance system covering the whole population, together with electronic medical record systems in most hospitals, will be a solid base on which various dementia research collaborations can be established. The above-mentioned CRCD, K-ADNI, and KLoSCAD are some of those examples of dementia research collaborations.

Collaboration between industry and academia has not been very active until now. Many of the bio-venture companies are now eagerly seeking to field-test their diagnostic and therapeutic products. Several "research-driven hospitals," recently designated by the government to enhance such academia–industry collaborations, will work as a test-bed for such developments.

19.6 CONCLUSION

The rapid increase of the elderly population in Korean society raises several social and medical issues. The establishment of a public medical system since the 1960s has enabled us to provide people with high quality medical care, but the relatively underdeveloped infrastructure for clinical research and drug trials remains to be set up.

Clinical research on AD in Korea has been improved both in quality and quantity, but summarizing some of the lessons learned from past experiences will give us some insight and help in designing future trials: 1) cognitive tests and function measurements need careful interpretation due to the unstable educational system between 1940 and 1970, and the rapid industrialization of modern Korean society; 2) in a governmental drive to encourage clinical research, several national collaborative research networks will work as a solid base for future clinical trials; 3) recent revision of clinical research-related regulations, and a change in the general public's view on drug trials, can be an advantage and a disadvantage for drug trials at the same time.

References

[1] United Nations. World Population Prospects: The 2010 Revision. Department of Economic and Social Affairs, New York, 2011. [Cited April 2013]. Available at: <http://esa.un.org/wpp/index.htm>.
[2] Jhoo JH, Kim KW, Huh Y, Lee SB, Park JH, Lee JJ, et al. Prevalence of dementia and its subtypes in an elderly urban Korean population: results from the Korean Longitudinal Study on Health And Aging (KLoSHA). Dement Geriatr Cogn Disord 2008;26:270–6.
[3] Kim J, Jeong I, Chun J-H, Lee S. The prevalence of dementia in a metropolitan city of South Korea. Int J Geriatr Psychiatry 2003;18:617–22.
[4] Suh G-H, Kim JK, Cho MJ. Community study of dementia in the older Korean rural population. Aust N Z J Psychiatry 2003;37:606–12.

[5] Lee DY, Lee JH, Ju Y-S, Lee KU, Kim KW, Jhoo JH, et al. The prevalence of dementia in older people in an urban population of Korea: the Seoul study. J Am Geriatr Soc 2002;50:1233–9.

[6] Woo JI, Lee JH, Yoo KY, Kim CY, Kim YI, Shin YS. Prevalence estimation of dementia in a rural area of Korea. J Am Geriatr Soc 1998;46:983–7.

[7] Park J, Ko HJ, Park YN, Jung CH. Dementia among the elderly in a rural Korean community. Br J Psychiatry J Ment Sci 1994;164:796–801.

[8] Cho M, Kim K, Kim M, Kim M. Nationwide study on the prevalence of dementia in Korean Elders, Ministry of Health, Welfare and Family, Seoul, 2009.

[9] Choi Y-H, Kim J-H, Kim DK, Kim J-W, Kim D-K, Lee MS, et al. Distributions of ACE and APOE polymorphisms and their relations with dementia status in Korean centenarians. J Gerontol A Biol Sci Med Sci 2003;58:M227–31.

[10] Kim DS. Introduction: health of the health care system in Korea. Soc Work Public Heal 2010;25:127–41.

[11] Kim JD, Kang YK. National Health Insurance Statistical Yearbook 2011. National Health Insurance Service, Seoul, 2011.

[12] Park HK, Na DL, Han S-H, Kim J-Y, Cheong H-K, Kim SY, et al. Clinical characteristics of a nationwide hospital-based registry of mild-to-moderate Alzheimer's disease patients in Korea: A CREDOS (Clinical Research Center for Dementia of South Korea) study. J Korean Med Sci 2011;26:1219–26.

[13] An H, Chung C-S, Lee J, Kim DK, Lee J-H, Kim SY, et al. The prevalence and severity of neuropsychiatric symptoms in Alzheimer's disease and subcortical vascular dementia: the CREDOS study. J Korean Geriatric Psychiatry 2011;15:70–5.

[14] Lee KS, Cheong H-K, Kim EA, Kim KR, Oh BH, Hong CH. Nutritional risk and cognitive impairment in the elderly. Arch Gerontol Geriatr 2009;48:95–9.

[15] Korea National Enterprise for Clinical Trials. Available at: <http://www.konect.or.kr/eng/>.

[16] Home–ClinicalTrials.gov. Available at: <http://www.clinicaltrials.gov/ct2/home>.

[17] Health Chosun website. [Cited April 2013] Available at: <http://health.chosun.com/>.

[18] Lee JY, Dong WL, Cho S-J, Na DL, Jeon HJ, Kim S-K, et al. Brief screening for mild cognitive impairment in elderly outpatient clinic: validation of the Korean version of the montreal cognitive assessment. J Geriatr Psychiatry Neurol 2008;21:104–10.

[19] Kang Y. Reliability validity, and normative study of the korean-montreal cognitive assessment (K-MoCA) as an instrument for screening of vascular cognitive impairment (VCI). Kor J Clin Psychology 2009;28:549–62.

[20] Kim KW, Lee DY, Jhoo JH, Youn JC, Suh YJ, Jun YH, et al. Diagnostic accuracy of mini-mental status examination and revised hasegawa dementia scale for Alzheimer's disease. Dement Geriatr Cogn Disord 2005;19:324–30.

[21] Kwon Y, Park J. Korean version of mini-mental state examination (MMSE-K) Part I: development of the test for the Elderly. J Korean Neuropsychiatr Assoc 1989;28:125–35.

[22] Kang Y, Na DL, Hahn S. A validity study on the Korean mini-mental state examination (K-MMSE) in dementia patients. J Korean Neurol Assoc 1997;15:300–8.

[23] Lee JH, Lee KU, Lee DY, Kim KW, Jhoo JH, Kim JH, et al. Development of the Korean version of the Consortium to Establish a Registry for Alzheimer's disease Assessment Packet (CERAD-K): clinical and neuropsychological assessment batteries. J Gerontol B Psychol Sci Soc Sci 2002;57:P47–53.

[24] Kim TH, Jhoo JH, Park JH, Kim JL, Ryu SH, Moon SW, et al. Korean version of mini-mental status examination for dementia screening and its short form. Psychiatry Investig 2010;7:102–8.

[25] Kang Y, Na DL. Seoul neuropsychological screening battery (SNSB). Human Brain Research and Consulting Co., Seoul, 2003.

[26] Ahn H, Chin J, Park A, Lee BH, Suh MK, Seo SW, et al. Seoul Neuropsychological Screening Battery-dementia version (SNSB-D): a useful tool for assessing and monitoring cognitive impairments in dementia patients. J Korean Med Sci 2010;25:1071–6.

[27] Lee DY, Lee KU, Lee JH, Kim KW, Jhoo JH, Kim SY, et al. A normative study of the CERAD neuropsychological assessment battery in the Korean elderly. J Int Neuropsychol Soc Jins 2004;10:72–81.

[28] Youn JC, Lee DY, Kim KW, Lee JH, Jhoo JH, Lee KU, et al. Development of the Korean version of Alzheimer's disease Assessment Scale (ADAS-K). Int J Geriatr Psychiatry 2002;17:797–803.

[29] Lee DW, Lee JY, Ryu SG, Cho SJ, Hong CH, Lee JH, et al. Validity of the Korean version of informant Questionnaire on the cognitive decline in the elderly (IQCODE). J Korean Geriatr Soc 2005;9:196–202.

[30] Ryu HJ, Kim H-J, Han S-H. Validity and reliability of the Korean version of the AD8 informant interview (K-AD8) in dementia. Alzheimer Dis Assoc Disord 2009;23:371–6.

[31] Choi SH, Na DL, Oh KM, Park BJ. A short form of the samsung dementia questionnaire (S-SDQ): development and cross-validation. J Korean Neurol Assoc 1999;17:253–8.

[32] Yang DW, Cho B, Chey J, Kim S, Kim B. The development and validation of Korean Dementia Screening Questionnaire (KDSQ). J Korean Neurol Assoc 2002;20:135–41.

[33] Kang SJ, Choi SH, Lee BH, Kwon JC, Na DL, Han SH, et al. The reliability and validity of the Korean instrumental activities of daily living (K-IADL). J Korean Neurol Assoc 2002;20:8–14.

[34] Choi SH, Na DL, Lee BH, Kang SJ, Ha C-K, Han S-H, et al. Validation of the Korean version of the Bayer activities of daily living scale. Hum Psychopharmacol 2003;18:469–75.

[35] Suh GH. Development of the Korean Version of Disability Assessment for Dementia Scale (DAD-K) to assess function in Dementia. J Korean Geriatr Soc 2003;7:278–87.

[36] Ku HM, Kim JH, Lee HS, Ko HJ, Kwon EJ, Jo S, et al. A study on the reliability and validity of seoul-activities of daily living (S-ADL). J Korean Geriatr Soc 2004;8:206–14.

[37] Ku H, Kim J, Kwon E, Kim S, Lee H, Ko H, et al. A study on the reliability and validity of Seoul-Instrumental Activities of Daily Living (S-IADL). J Korean Neuropsychiatr Assoc 2004;43:189–99.

[38] Choi SH, Na DL, Kwon HM, Yoon SJ, Jeong JH, Ha CK. The Korean version of the neuropsychiatric inventory: a scoring tool for neuropsychiatric disturbance in dementia patients. J Korean Med Sci 2000;15:609–15.

[39] Bae JN, Cho MJ. Development of the Korean version of the Geriatric Depression Scale and its short form among elderly psychiatric patients. J Psychosom Res 2004;57:297–305.

[40] Suh GH, Park JH. The behavior pathology in Alzheimer's disease rating scale, Korean Version (BEHAVE-AD-K): factor structure among Alzheimer's disease inpatients. J Korean Geriatr Psychiatry 2001;5:86–95.

[41] Youn JC, Lee DY, Lee JH, Kim KW, Jhoo JH, Choo IH, et al. Development of a Korean version of the behavior rating scale for dementia (BRSD-K). Int J Geriatr Psychiatry 2008;23:677–84.

[42] Qi S. Alzheimer's Disease Instrument Validation Study, Poster Number 16402. Alzheimer's Association International Conference; 2011.

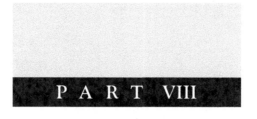

PART VIII

PHARMACOGENETICS AND PHARMACOGENOMICS CONSIDERATIONS

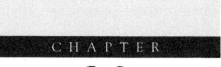

CHAPTER 20

Pharmacogenomics in Developing Countries: Challenges and Opportunities

Sidney A. Spector

Department of Neurology, VA Medical Center, Phoenix, Arizona, USA, and Global Biopharma, Scottsdale, Arizona, USA

20.1 INTRODUCTION

In June 2003, the European Agency for the Evaluation of Medicinal Products (EMEA) implemented guidelines developed by an expert panel of scientists for the benefit of stakeholders, including government regulatory bodies, the pharmaceutical industry, academia, and healthcare professionals and patients, to offer regulatory clarity to the popular definitions of *pharmacogenetics* and *pharmacogenomics*, as well as other terms used in the handling of samples and data from pharmacogenetic testing [1]. Contemporaneously, similar efforts were underway at the Food and Drug Administration (FDA) in the United States [2]. It had been recognized by all concerned that the burgeoning science of pharmacogenetics and pharmacogenomics could offer considerable insight into the genetic influences underlying inter-individual differences in response to drug therapies, and offer pathways toward identifying more genetically homogeneous sample populations for participation in clinical trials to improve the chances of demonstrating effectiveness and safety of drugs through clinical development programs.

It was acknowledged by the regulatory agencies that the design of future drug development programs might likely reflect the discoveries in this new field of study. Then, in 2005, the FDA and EMEA jointly issued their "Guidance for Industry: Pharmacogenetic Data Submissions" [3], and subsequently published "General Principles: Processing Joint FDA

M. Bairu & M.W. Weiner (Eds):
Global Clinical Trials for Alzheimer's Disease.
DOI: http://dx.doi.org/10.1016/B978-0-12-411464-7.00020-1

EMEA Voluntary Genomic Data Submissions" in April 2007 to outline the process by which sponsors might have joint FDA/EMEA briefings to discuss voluntary submission of pharmacogenetic and pharmacogenomic data as part of their clinical development programs [4]. The overarching goal of these guidelines was to provide precise definitions and guidance for the use of pharmacogenetic and pharmacogenomics research in drug development programs in harmony across regulatory regions throughout the world that would lead to the development of safer and more effective medicines.

20.2 DEFINITIONS AND HISTORICAL PERSPECTIVE

The scientific disciplines of pharmacogenetics and pharmacogenomics address the role of heredity in determining the genetic contributions to disease and drug responses in humans. In the context of developing and characterizing genomic biomarkers based on specific DNA and/or RNA variations that would predict drug efficacy and/or safety, the regulatory agencies defined *pharmacogenetics* as the study of "variations in DNA sequences as related to drug response." DNA variations include single nucleotide polymorphisms (SNPs), variability of short sequence repeats, haplotypes, DNA modifications, deletions or insertions of one or more single nucleotides, copy number variation, and cytogenic rearrangements such as translocations, duplications, deletions or inversions. Pharmacogenetics was considered a subset of *pharmacogenomics*, which was defined as "the study of variation of DNA and RNA characteristics as related to drug response," which also include, for example, RNA variations related to sequences, gene expression levels, processing (e.g., splicing and editing) and microRNA levels [1,5].

More commonly, *pharmacogenetics* is the study of the impact of single genes on an individual's response to a drug, and *pharmacogenomics* is the study of the complex interaction between genetic and environmental factors responsible for the variability of more common diseases across populations, and how these populations, ethnic and racial groups, and individuals respond to medicines [6–8]. Pharmacogenomics got its impetus from the sequencing of the human genome, and the development of technologies to study relatively large samples of genetic material in a more efficient, cost-effective manner. This has led to the identification of numerous metabolic enzyme variants, as well as polymorphisms of genes encoding drug transporters and drug targets that contribute to individualized drug responses [9]. Most recently, polymorphisms that control gene expression in portions of DNA previously thought to have negligible function have been described, and are now thought to act as switches that modulate other genes and which ultimately influence phenotypic traits and susceptibility to disease [10]. Further, the new technologies that have facilitated the study of relatively large populations for genetic variants related to common, complex human diseases are now being incorporated into the design of clinical drug trials to optimize the potential for maximizing drug effects and minimizing drug toxicities in more homogeneous populations through the process of clinical drug development.

The notion that there might be "chemical individuality in man" was proposed over 100 years ago [11]. A half century later, the observation that the abnormally prolonged muscle relaxation in individual family members after exposure to the muscle relaxant succinycholine [12], and the individual responses to the anti-malarial drug primaquine due to inherited variants of glucose-6-phosphate dehydrogenase [13], supported the concept that inheritance might be responsible for variability in response to these drugs [14]. Indeed, the same defect in glucose-6-phosphate dehydrogenase was found to be responsible for hemolytic anemia due to fava bean ingestion in Mediterranean communities, and over 100 variants of this enzyme have been described, putting over 400 million people at risk of various drug and environmentally induced causes of hemolysis [8].

Pharmacogenetics was coined in 1959 to describe the role of heredity in determining the way by which various doses of drugs provide the range of effectiveness and toxicity observed in clinical practice [15]. The science of pharmacogenetics relies on objective pharmacokinetic (absorption, metabolism, excretion) and pharmacodynamic measures of drug exposure, clinical efficacy, and toxicity to help explain unique clinical phenotypes. By the 1980s over 100 examples of heterogeneity of drug responses and toxicities in clinical practice were found to be associated with individual monogenic Mendelian hereditary traits, based on the discoveries of genetic examples of polymorphisms of drug metabolizing enzymes, including, but not limited to, N-acetyltransferase, pseudocholinesterase, and the cytochrome P450 enzymes [16,17].

In the 1990s ongoing efforts by geneticists to identify underlying hereditary traits that lead to both rare and common disorders were concurrent with the exponential growth of pharmacogenetic research. The search for genetic variants through linkage disequilibrium (LD) analysis of families was relatively successful in identifying the genetic underpinnings of rare single-gene disorders [18]. For Alzheimer's disease (AD), mutations linked to chromosomes 14, 1 and 21 were identified through LD analysis and sequence comparisons implicating the presenilin-1 (PSEN1 [19]), presenilin-2 (PSEN2 [20]) and amyloid precursor protein (APP [21]) genes, respectively. However, LD studies are not effective in identifying genetic variants that are less penetrant, or contributions of multiple genes responsible for more complex common diseases such as cancer, diabetes and obesity, cardiovascular disease, psychiatric disorders and AD [22].

Complementary association studies which compare a control group with affected individuals with a particular disease for the frequency of specific genetic variants have provided additional value in identifying modest gene effects that cannot be uncovered with LD studies, leading, for example, to the identification of ApoE4 allele as a genetic risk factor in individuals with the sporadic form of AD [23–25]. The identification of a gene that increases the risk for the disease phenotype becomes a potential pharmacogenic target for drug development, especially if the gene product can be biologically tied to the pathogenesis of the disease. Potential therapeutic strategies have been proposed to prevent formation of the ApoE4 allelic protein, or modify its structural properties to render it non-toxic, though such approaches have yet to be translated into a viable clinical treatment [26].

Ongoing attempts to identify hereditary markers responsible for, or contributing to, both rare and common diseases and individual drug response phenotype received further impetus from the sequencing of the human genome in 2001 [27,28]. As a result, genomic studies have demonstrated that although humans are nearly identical in their DNA repertoire, subtle changes in coding sequences, accounting for less than 0.1% of the 3 billion DNA bases, are responsible for the variety of heritable differences in an individual's susceptibility to disease and response to drugs [29,30]. The most frequent type of genomic variability, SNPs, accounts for over 90% of genetic variability so far observed [6,31]. The genetic mechanisms of variation which may contribute to an individual's response to a drug vary, and may include changes in the primary sequence of the coding, in the regulatory regions, and splice regions of the gene. In addition, other genetic variations, for example, those affecting mRNA splicing [32], duplications or deletions of genomic segments of 1 kb or larger, called copy number variation [33], and genetic variation in downstream pathways from the drug target reflect this genetic diversity [34].

Most recently, the Encyclopedia of DNA Elements Project (ENCODE) has begun to decipher regions of the genome that contain "junk" DNA, previously thought to be non-functional, which are now thought to control which genes are expressed throughout various stages of life [10]. Coupled with the potential role of environmental agents (ecogenetics) such as food components (e.g., grapefruit juice), pollutants, industrial chemicals, pesticides and other chemicals, the overall response of an individual to a particular drug is even more complex than previously thought. *Pharmacogenomics* has now become the scientific discipline that studies the complex interactions between genetic and environmental influences that cause disease and an individual's response to drugs.

20.3 PHARMACOGENOMICS AND BIOINFORMATICS

There are now over 1,380 biological databases accessible on the world wide web illustrating the prodigious growth in the fields of molecular biology and genetics during the past 20 years [35]. The mapping of the human genome and the development of high throughput technologies [36–38] for the screening of large samples with large numbers of polymorphisms in a cost-effective and time-efficient manner certainly has been the primary impetus for the exponential increase of such specific databases and genomic research [39]. One of the first post-genomic databases, the Pharmacogenomics Knowledge Base (*PharmGKB*), begun in 2000 at Stanford University, California, USA with support from the National Institutes of Health, has become a vital centralized and global resource that curates and disseminates current knowledge in pharmacogenomics about the complex relationships between genes, variants, drugs, diseases and pathways [40,41]. *PharmGKB* continues to serve as a data repository for complementary data supplied by investigators worldwide. This facilitates the development of collaborative consortia along common research interests to combine diverse data sets that provide ample statistical power to detect complex genetic associations that might explain inter-individual variability to drug response.

Another global collaboration led to the development of the International HapMap Project in 2003, designed to produce a haplotype map of the human genome that would provide a database that describes common patterns of variation with population frequencies of 5% or more that potentially influence susceptibility to the common, complex diseases and inter-individual response to medicine [42,43]. Within this database are genome-wide maps which include identities, positions and frequencies of polymorphisms for six populations across North America (Canada, United States), Europe (United Kingdom), Africa (Nigeria) and the Far East (China, Japan), based on ancestral geography, in an effort to maximize the chance of identifying most of the common variation and some of the less common variation among these different populations. Over 3.5 million SNPs had been genotyped through this project [44]. Comparison between specific populations has led to the discovery of ethnically variant SNPs that differentiate these studied populations and have shed light on the evolution of genetic diversity from the original migration out of Africa [45,46]. This collaboration has also facilitated the study of vast numbers of SNPs across the genome that has provided substantial insight into common genetic variants associated with disease and drug phenotype response [47–49]. By 2008, more than 250 genetic loci in which common genetic variation occurs were found to be associated with a variety of diseases, including diabetes, obesity, cardiovascular and inflammatory disorders, and AD [50–55].

The fact that studies implementing *HapMap* genomic data could not explain fully the heritability of common disease led researchers to establish the *1000 Genomes* Project, an international effort (China, Germany, United Kingdom, and United States) launched in 2008 to provide the most comprehensive map of human genetic variation, looking for rare SNPs that are present at 1% or greater frequency and which may not have been identified in the *HapMap* Project [56]. Initially mandated to sequence the genomes of 1000 individuals from five ancestries (West African, European, American, and East and South Asian), this project is now collecting genomic data comprising 2,500 samples from 27 populations around the world. The ability to collect these data depended on the development of high throughput sequencing platforms, one of the initial goals of the *1000 Genomes* Project that has allowed researchers to pinpoint novel and rare variants [38,39].

Comparison between the *HapMap* and pilot *1000 Genomes* data sets found considerable overlap between the two resources, though not all variants cataloged in *HapMap* are noted in the *1000 Genomes* pilot database, suggesting that the current differences between the information derived from the two data sets might affect decisions about which resource to use for SNP validations and candidate gene research [44]. In addition, other databases such as the *Human Genome Diversity Panel*, which represents 1,064 individuals from 51 populations from Europe, the Middle East, South/Central Asia, East Asia, Oceania and the Americas, and the *Perlegen* database, which catalogs 71 Americans of European, African and Asian descent, are available for research investigation [57,58]. Though these genomic databases provide information regarding genetic variability across the ethnic and racial groups designated to be studied in these projects, most of the non-Asian and non-white populations throughout the world are under-represented in these genomic databases. The collection of genomic data in underdeveloped nations has been limited to some degree by the scarcity of expensive and highly technical high throughput sequencing equipment and technical expertise [59].

Prior to sequencing the genome, geneticists traditionally implemented linkage disequilibrium and candidate gene studies to localize genes responsible for heritable traits and disease [47]. These approaches have been most successful in identifying single Mendelian genes with high penetrance responsible for a few specific diseases such as, for example, Huntington's disease [60], cystic fibrosis [61], and cardiovascular diseases [62], though there has been some limited success in identifying polygenic traits in some more common disorders. Indeed, such studies led to the identification of the PSEN-1, PSEN-2 and APP genes responsible for a small proportion of early-onset AD [19–21]. However, these approaches are limited in their ability to identify polygenic influences which cumulatively, along with environmental factors, are responsible for much of the variability of common and complex diseases. Identification of genes of modest penetrance requires analysis of vastly larger numbers of genetic samples to achieve statistically significant power [63], which was not feasible before the mapping of the genome.

By leveraging genomic information from, for example, the *HapMap* and the *1000 Genomes* projects during the past half decade, genome-wide association (GWA) studies have increased our knowledge of the genetic basis for many common, complex diseases [48,50–53]. GWA studies are a powerful alternative to LD and candidate gene studies. These studies are not hypothesis driven, but rely on systematic search of SNPs across pre-specified regions of the genome to identify genetic associations with phenotypic traits of common diseases [47,48,64]. Next-generation and third-generation sequencing technologies have made such analyses less expensive and faster to complete. Genetic variation of specific SNPs within the population can theoretically be pinpointed with high sensitivity and accuracy. As costs of such analyses have diminished, much larger sample sizes can now be studied to attain adequate statistical power. Thus, the early concerns about the validity, sensitivity and reliability of GWA studies has waned with improved technology and study design, and this genomic investigative approach now facilitates greater understanding of the complexity of the genetics of human diseases caused by multiple variants with modest effects [64–66]. GWA studies are now curated by the National Human Genome Research Institute (NHGRI) and the Centers for Disease Control and Prevention (CDC) [67,68].

While significant insight has been gleaned from GWA studies of the more frequently cataloged populations of mostly European descent (for up to 75% of the GWA studies published by 2011), it is not clear to what extent these findings may be extrapolated to other ethnic and racial groups. For example, even within a population of Americans, frequency of genetic risk for particular traits varies between those of European descent and those of other ancestral populations, reinforcing the concern for study of more homogeneous populations due to this stratification issue [6,69,70]. More national and regional efforts in developing and developed countries, as in Far Eastern Asia (Singapore Genome Variation Project; Japanese Millennium Genome Project, Beijing Institute of Genomics), India (Indian Genome Variation Database Consortium, IGVdb Consortium), Iran (Human Genome Diversity Project of Iran, HGDPI), Mexico (Mexican National Institute of Genomic Medicine, INMEGEN), Brazil (Brazilian National Pharmacogenetic/Pharmacogenomic Network: REFAREN), and sub-Saharan Africa (Malaria Genomic Epidemiology Network—MalariaGEN) are being undertaken to gather genomic information from more homogeneous samples about ancestral lines, heritable traits, and genetic diseases [71–77].

Collaborations between developed and developing regions within Asia (e.g., The Human Genome Organization, HUGO, Pan-Asian SNP

Consortium), and between Mexico and other Latin American countries, are ongoing [74,78]. As a result, over the past few years there has been an exponential rise of GWA studies and meta-analyses of GWA studies performed in many non-European populations such as those from Gambia, China, South Korea, Taiwan, Japan, Singapore, and the Pacific Island of Kosrae [56,69]. The greatest challenge will be to study sub-Saharan African populations, which are considered the most ancestral and demonstrate the most genetic diversity requiring more sophisticated genotyping tools and statistical methods to uncover rare causal variants [79].

20.4 GENETICS OF AD

The genetic mutations that lead to a portion of rare early-onset familial AD (FAD) account overall for less than 1% of the cases of this common neurodegenerative disorder [80,81]. Nevertheless, identification of these mutations has provided support for the amyloid hypothesis invoked to explain the pathogenesis of AD [82]. PSEN1 and PSEN2 are trans-membrane proteins that form the catalytic core of the gamma secretase complex responsible for cleavage of APP in the production of beta amyloid protein [83,84]. Their mutations, of which over 200 have been cataloged, lead to increased ratios of toxic forms of $Abeta_{42}$ relative to $Abeta_{40}$, confirming the role of these presenilins in normal cleavage of APP. The gene responsible for normal production of APP is located on chromosome 21q [20,85]. APP is a trans-membrane protein thought to be involved in signal transduction in neurons [86]. Patients with FAD with an APP mutation accumulate excess $ABeta_{42}$ compared with other amyloid protein species. Over expression of APP in individuals with Down's syndrome due to an extra chromosome 21 in which the APP gene is found is thought to cause premature Alzheimer's dementia in these individuals [87–89].

In contrast, late-onset Alzheimer's disease (LOAD) develops sporadically later in life [90–92] and is considered a typical example of a common disorder with complex heritability. Indeed, LOAD was the first such disease in which a susceptibility gene was identified through an association with a DNA variant [23–25]. The apolipoprotein E (ApoE) gene is found on chromosome 19q13.2, and is associated with both LOAD and FAD [23]. The gene product is the major apolipoprotein of the chylomicron of the brain and includes three isoforms (ApoE2, ApoE3, ApoE4) that are determined by two coding SNPs [80]. The presence of one or two alleles of ApoE4 invokes a two to three times greater risk of developing LOAD (in European populations) and lowers the age of onset [24,25]. The frequency of ApoE4 carriers varies across ethnic groups [93], but the qualitative effect of the presence of the ApoE4 allele is the same. The mechanism by which the ApoE4 allele increases risk of LOAD is not known, though ApoE4-mediated toxicity causing amyloid aggregation and/or tau hyperphosphorylation has been proposed [94]. In contrast, the presence of the ApoE2 allele appears to exert a protective effect by a yet unidentified mechanism [95]. The discovery of the ApoE susceptibility gene and its association with increased risk of AD provided initial support for the common disease-common variant hypothesis on which subsequent candidate gene association and GWA studies have been based [91].

Candidate gene association studies in LOAD patients have led to the identity of additional susceptibility genes. SORL1 (neuronal sortilin-related receptor), located on chromosome 11q23.2-q24.2, is a member of the vacuolar protein sorting receptor family, which plays a role in trafficking and processing of APP [96]. Initially found in the autopsied brains of LOAD patients, it is thought that under-expression of SORL1 affects APP processing which leads to overproduction of AB42. Variants in this gene have been shown to be associated with risk of LOAD in several ethnic groups including Caucasians, Asians, Caribbean's, Hispanics, African Americans and Israeli-Arabs [97], Han Chinese [97,98], and Caucasians with Down's syndrome [99], though their effect size is small and there is substantial allelic heterogeneity across these ethnic groups. Others have not identified a true association between the SORL1 gene and LOAD in Caucasian American or Japanese cohorts, possibly because the cohorts studied were too small in some cases to reveal an effect, or the penetrance of the SORL1 gene is so modest in certain ethnic groups that it is not always detected [100,101]. A recent meta-analysis of association studies investigating the relationship between SORL1 and risk for LOAD supports the association in Caucasian and Asian populations [102].

A review of literature to date has identified publication of 21 GWA studies (see Table 20.1) looking for systematic genetic variation in either case-control studies or assessments in families with LOAD [103–123]. Most of these studies are curated on the publicly accessed Alzheimer Research Forum website [124], and most have been reviewed elsewhere [125–128]. Newly identified genes have been linked mechanistically to Abeta amyloid production (ATXN1, BIN1, GAB2, TNKI, PCDH11X, PICALM, GALP), aggregation (ApoE, CLU), clearance (ApoE, BIN1, CLU, CR1, PICALM), tau phosphorylation (GAB2, GALP), synaptic transmission (PCDH11X, PICALM), inflammation and immune function (ApoE, CD33, CLU, CR1, ABCA7, EPHA1, TREM2), cell membrane processes (PICALM, BIN1, CD33, CD2AP, MS4A family) and lipid biology (ApoE, CLU, ABCA7)). A mis-sense mutation in the gene encoding the triggering receptor expressed on myeloid cells 2 (TREM2), thought to play a role in inflammation, has recently been found to confer a significant risk of AD [122].

Not all of the genes identified in these GWA studies have yet to be pathogenically linked with LOAD (e.g., EXOC3L2, MTHFD1L). Based

TABLE 20.1 Genome-wide Association Studies in Alzhiemer's Disease[1]

GWAS	Design	Population	Replicated Genes[2]	Biological Mechanism(s) in AD	Nominated Genes[3]
Grupe et al. [103]	Case-control	USA, UK	TNK1	Phospholipid signal transduction; abeta production	ACAN, BCR, CTSS, EBF3, FAM63A**, GALP, GWA_14q32.13, GWA_7p15.2, LMNA, MYH13, PCK1, PGBD1, TRAK2, UBD
			LOC651924	(unknown)	
Coon et al. [104]	Case-control	USA, Netherlands	GAB2	Abeta production; tau phosphorylation	
Reiman et al. [105]	Case-control	USA/Netherlands	GAB2	Abeta production; tau phosphorylation	
Li et al. [106]	Case-control	Canada/USA			GOLM1, GWA_15q21.2, GWA9p24.3
Abraham et al. [107]	Case-control	UK			LRAT
Betram et al. [108]	Family-based	USA	ATXN1	Abeta production	
			CD33	Inflammation	
			GWA 14q31	(unknown)	
Poduslo et al. [109]	Family-based / Case-control	USA			TRPC4AP
Harold et al. [110]	Case-control	USA/Europe	CLU	Abeta aggregation and clearance; immune function; lipid metabolism	
			PICALM	Abeta production and clearance; synaptic transmission	

Study	Design	Population	Gene	Function	Additional genes
Lambert et al. [111]	Case-control	Europe	CLU	Abeta aggregation and clearance; immune function; lipid metabolism	
			CR1	Abeta clearance; inflammation (complement receptor)	
			PICALM	Abeta production and clearance; synaptic transmission	
Potkin et al. [112]	Case-control	USA (ADNI)			ARSB, CAND1, EFNA5, MAG12, PRUNE2
Heinzen et al. [113]	Case-control	USA			CHRNA7
Beecham et al. [114]	Case-control	USA			FAM113B
Carrasquillo et al. [115]	Case-control	USA	PCDH11X	Abeta production; synaptic transmission	
Seshadri et al. [116]	Case-control	Europe/USA	BIN1	Abeta production and clearance	
			CLU	Abeta aggregation and clearance; immune function; lipid metabolism	
			EXOC3L2	(unknown)	
			PICALM	Abeta production and clearance; synaptic transmission	
Naj et al. [117]	Case-control	USA/Europe	MTHFD1L	Mitochondrial function	
Hu et al. [118]	Case-control	USA	BIN1	Abeta production and clearance	
			CR1	Abeta aggregation and clearance; inflammation	

(Continued)

TABLE 20.1 (Continued)

GWAS	Design	Population	Replicated Genes[2]	Biological Mechanism(s) in AD	Nominated Genes[3]
Hollingsworth et al. [119]	Case-control	Europe/USA	CD33	Regulates functions within cells of immune system	EPHA1
			CD2AP MS4A6A/4E	Receptor-mediated endocytosis members of cell surface proteins expressed in lymphoid tissue	
			ABCA7	trans-membrane transport	
Wijsman et al. [120]	Family-based/ Case-control	USA	CLU	Abeta aggregation and clearance; immune function; lipid metabolism	CUGBP2
			BIN1	Abeta production and clearance	
Sherva et al. [121]	Family-based	Israel			AGPAT1
Jonsson et al. [122]	Case-control	Iceland/Norway/ Netherlands/USA	TREM2	Expressed in microglia (anti-inflammatory function)	
Guerreiro et al. [123]	Case-control	UK/USA/ Portugal/Canada	TREM2	Expressed in microglia (anti-inflammatory function)	

[1]All GWA studies (excluding Ref. [109]) have confirmed the APOE gene as a susceptibility gene for LOAD.
[2]Association studies and meta-analyses support "replicated genes" as having significant association with LOAD.
[3]Nominated gene candidates require further documentation of significant association with LOAD.

on confirmatory replication and meta-analytic data, coupled with mechanistically plausible biology, BIN1, CLU, CR1, CD33, EXOC3L2, GAB2, TNK1, CD2AP, EPHA-1, LOC651924, MTHFD1L and PICALM are now thought to confer added risk for LOAD, whereas other genes (ATXN1, PCDH11X, GALP) are still considered as provisional susceptibility genes until further replication studies are completed [125–127]. Recent complementary studies involving exome sequencing have provided evidence bridging unreplicated candidate susceptibility genes discovered in GWA studies with gene expression of mRNA in autopsied brain tissue (e.g., IREB1, CREB2, MS4A4A, ABCA7) [125,126,128,129]. Further, a gene which codes for a trans-membrane glycoprotein that controls cytosolic calcium concentrations and amyloid levels in the brain (CALHM1) is highly associated with elevated CSF $Abeta_{42}$ and $Abeta_{40}$ in normal individuals at risk to develop LOAD [130,131]. Nevertheless, even for these specific genes hypothesized to enhance risk of LOAD, their effect sizes are relatively small (up to 1.5-fold increased risk in carriers), when compared with that found for ApoE4 (approximately four-fold increase) [23,132]. These potentially causal variants still do not fully explain the extent of heritability of LOAD, thought to be between 60 and 80% [133–136].

The association of a region of high linkage disequilibrium that spans ApoE, TOMM40, a translocase of the outer mitochondrial membrane and ApoC1 with LOAD supports the notion that this highly conserved region of this gene may provide an example of potential effects of multiple variant alleles expressed in tandem or sequentially [137]. In fact, the length of the polymorphic variant residing on the TOMM40 mitochondrial translocase gene appears to correlate with the age of onset of LOAD based on phylogenic analysis in Caucasian populations, as had been previously shown for the ApoE4 allele [24,136,137], though this has recently been questioned [138]. Mitochondrial dysfunction is receiving renewed consideration as an early putative mechanism in LOAD due to early accumulation of abnormal amyloid filaments in trans-membrane pores, leading to mitochondrial dysfunction and neurotoxic effects [135,139,140]. It is in this manner that it is thought that the TOMM40 gene may exert its effect. The presence and/or relevance of TOMM40 gene variation has yet to be studied in non-Caucasian populations.

20.5 PHARMACOGENOMICS AND THE FUTURE FOR PERSONALIZED MEDICINE IN DEVELOPING COUNTRIES

Clinical observations and pharmacogenetic research into the individuality of response to medicine over the past 50 years, reinforced and extended through genomic studies during the past decade in which detailed genetic variation has defined individuals and populations that are predisposed to a particular disease or respond differentially to a specific drug, are paving the way for *personalized medicine* based on these individual susceptibilities. Ideally, this concept encompasses the notion that an individual's genetic composition and particular environmental exposures would dictate a personally customized approach to disease prevention and treatment, eventually replacing the "one drug fits all" approach to medical care that has been the mainstay of clinical practice for the past 100 years with "the right drug for the right person at the right dose and at the right time" [141,142]. Concrete examples prove the success of translation of basic genetic research into clinical decisions to prevent or treat disease, such as determination of BRCA mutations that identify women destined to develop breast cancer, testing for thiopurine methyltransferase (TMPT) genotypes which guide dosing of thiopurines for treatment of leukemia and inflammatory bowel disease, and identification of breast cancer patients who over-express HER2 allele, which invokes a poorer prognosis but is predictive of better clinical response to trastuzumab [143–145].

As noted above, the EMEA and FDA have taken a proactive approach to encourage pharmacogenetic and pharmacogenomic testing by sponsors within the design of clinical drug development programs. In fact, the drug labels of over 110 currently marketed medications listed in the FDA's "Table of Pharmacogenomic Biomarkers" (about 10% of FDA-approved drugs) now include information regarding drug exposure and clinical response variability, risk of adverse events, genotype-specific dosing and polymorphic drug target and disposition genes [146,147].

However, there are formidable hurdles yet to be overcome in establishing personalized medicine as a viable alternative paradigm of medical care [7,141,147–149]. The scientific and technological advances in basic pharmacogenomic research have far outpaced clinical, social and economic areas of study that determine the ultimate utility of such knowledge in the medical care of individuals and populations. The regulatory and ethical issues of an individual voluntarily providing a vast array of genetic information that may potentially be used contemporaneously and in the future by researchers, healthcare professionals, insurance companies and governments remains to be fully vetted [150]. Design of clinical drug trials and data analyses will have to account for the multigenic origins of common diseases and environmental influences which might potentially obscure the genetic variable being studied. To facilitate this process, the National Institute of Health's (NIH) Pharmacogenetics Research Network (PGRN) was implemented as a collaborative effort of scientists with a wide range of research interests, to identify the genetic sources of individuality of drug response, exploiting diverse research strategies to facilitate collection of valid and meaningful clinical data, the results of which are curated in the *PharmGKB* database [40,151].

Validation of genetic testing procedures, laboratory quality control standards, and reliability and interpretation of results remain ongoing issues. Direct to consumer sale of genetic testing kits is an example of "premature translation" where the derived genetic information may not have immediate clinical value, and may have untoward social, economic and psychological ramifications [152]. In the United States, the FDA does not formally oversee the regulation of genetic test kits, though the NIH has recently created a voluntary genetic-testing registry for voluntary submission of genetic test information by providers, which includes the test's purpose, methodology, validity, evidence of the test's usefulness, and laboratory contacts and credentials [153]. The Center for Disease Control and Prevention has established the Genomic Applications in Practice and Prevention Network (GAPPNet) to promote the systematic review of genomic research findings and dissemination of meaningful translational information to the medical community, including clinical validity and utility of genomic testing [154]. Without valid evidence of clinical value, payers will not reimburse for genetic testing nor will governments provide such testing as part of national health plans. As the field of translational genomic medicine continues to permeate the clinical, legal, ethical, social, and economic sectors, it will be crucial that healthcare professionals have ample exposure to educational opportunities in these fields of knowledge, and that healthcare training programs incorporate this new information into curricula that provide a solid base for the practice of personalized medicine in the future.

In underdeveloped and developing countries, additional fiscal, regulatory, ethical, legal, social, technological, and scientific challenges to the translation of pharmacogenomic information into personalized medicine exist. While some emerging economies are allocating more funds for pharmacogenomic research, the underdeveloped countries are still at risk of being excluded from the new genomic scientific and technological revolution [155]. At first glance, inadequate basic services such as running water, electricity, and healthcare infrastructure in some countries would make personalized medicine in poor communities and nations seem too far out of reach. Indeed, some argue that health-related funding in these underdeveloped countries should be geared toward basic health needs and services such as hygiene, poverty, prevention of communicable diseases, malnutrition, and infant mortality, as well as the building of a sound healthcare infrastructure [156].

Unfortunately, the prevalence of chronic, non-communicable diseases in the developing world, including diabetes, obesity, cardiovascular disease, hypertension, and AD have increased significantly over the past 20 years, necessitating the same approaches to biomedical research for treatment and prevention of disease that are now taking place in the developed world [157–159]. In fact, because underdeveloped countries may not have adequate regulatory and scientific infrastructure in place to conduct independent genomic studies, "south to north" collaborations that involve collection of genetic specimens from research participants of underdeveloped countries (to be processed and analyzed by scientists from developed countries) have been designed to overcome this hurdle. Biobanks which collect and store large amounts of genetic and phenotypic information about individuals and populations now exist in many of the developed countries of the world [160,161]. Ethical concerns about informed consent, confidentiality and protection of genetic information, return of results to study participants, current and future data sharing, benefit from immediate translational outcomes, and benefit from development of new technologies and future cures based on participation in such research are under active debate [162–165] (see Chapter 21).

Nevertheless, there are concrete examples of how pharmacogenomic research might translate into clinical treatment of the most common diseases of the poorest and most vulnerable populations in the near term. Malaria, the most lethal parasitic disease which kills close to one million people annually, is currently treated worldwide with artemisinin combination therapy (ACT). Identification of individuals with a genetic predisposition to adverse effects from amodiaquine (one of the combination drugs in ACT), due to polymorphisms of one or more of the metabolizing CYP450 enzymes, holds promise for screening to direct those patients or local populations to other treatments [167]. Similarly, SNP variants associated with transport or metabolism of highly active anti-retroviral therapy (HAART), used in the treatment of AIDS, may be matched with phenotypic drug responses within homogeneous groups to predict drug efficacy and safety [168]. Isoniazid, in combination with other drugs for treatment of tuberculosis, another common disease with global impact, causes liver toxicity and peripheral neuropathy in those who acetylate this drug slowly. This phenotypic trait is directly related to the n-acetyltransferase (NAT2) allelic genotype. Genotying of individuals prior to use of isoniazid provides a personalized approach to treatment that avoids the development of serious side effects [169].

Ultimately, the inclusion of underdeveloped and developing nations in this pharmacogenomics revolution will require national political will and institutional leadership, with significant capital investment into infrastructure required for this biomedical pursuit. The Paris Declaration of Aid Effectiveness of 2005 signed by more than 100 donor and developing country governments, regional development banks, and international aid agencies recognized the need for more effective aid delivery and management than had been accomplished in the past [170,171]. With this Declaration comes the charge for the study of genetic variation in all underdeveloped communities to achieve more effective treatment and prevention of disease. Each developing country has its own set of challenges, and it is recognized that a variety of synergistic partnerships between government, the pharmaceutical industry, and non-government philanthropic organizations will continue to be required to effectively deliver aid and healthcare in underdeveloped countries. Focused investments in the regulatory, legal, and ethical underpinnings of pharmacogenomic research in these countries, coupled with the development of laboratory capacity and a specialized workforce to collect and study genomic data in large populations, will be required for developing countries to fulfill the hope of pharmacogenomics to improve the health and welfare of individuals through individualized prevention and treatment of disease.

References

[1] The European Agency for the evaluation of medicinal products: Position paper on terminology in pharmacogenetics. Available from: <http://www.emea.eu.int>; 2002.
[2] Lesko LJ, Salerno RA, Spear BB, Anderson DC, Anderson T, Brazell C, et al. Pharmacogenetics and pharmacogenomics in drug development and regulatory decision making: report of the first FDA-PWG-PhRMA-DruSafe workshop. J Clin PHarmacol 2003;43(4):342–58.
[3] US Department Health and Human Services Food and Drug Administration. Guidance for industry: pharmacogenomics data submissions. Available from: <http://www.fda.gov/cber/gdlns/phardtasub.htm>; 2005.
[4] General principles: processing joint FDA EMEA voluntary genomic data submissions (VGDSs) within the framework of the confidentiality arrangement. Available from: <http://www.ema.europa.eu/docs/en_GB/document_library/Other/2009/12/WC500017982.pdf>; 2006.
[5] US Department Health and Human Services Food and Drug Administration. Guidance for industry: E15 definitions for genomic biomarkers, pharmacogenomics, pharmacogenetics, genomic data and sample coding categories. Available from: <http://www.fda.gov/cber/guidance/index.htm>; 2008.
[6] Altman RB, Flockhart ID, Goldstein DB. Principles of pharacogenetics and pharmacogenomics. London: Cambridge Press; 2012.
[7] Wang L, McLeod HL, Weinshilboum RM. Genomics and drug response. NEJM 2011;364(12):1144–53.
[8] Meyer UA. Pharmacogenetics–five decades of therapeutic lessons from genetic diversity. Nat Rev Genet 2004;5:669–76.
[9] Goldstein DB, Tate SK, Sisodiya SM. Pharmacogenetics goes genomic. Nat Rev Genet 2003;4:937–47.
[10] The ENCODE Project Consortium Identification and analysis of functional elements in 1% of the human genome by the ENCODE pilot project. Nature 2007;44(7146):799–815.
[11] Garrod E. The incidence of alkaptonuria: a study in chemical individuality. Lancet 1902;2:1616–20.
[12] Kalow W, Staron N. On distribution and inheritance of atypical forms of human serum cholinesterase, as indicated by dibucaine numbers. Can J Med Sci 1957;35:1305–20.
[13] Clayman CB, Arnold J, Hockwald RS, Yount EH, Edgcomb JH, Alving AS. Toxicity of primaquine in Caucasians. JAMA 1952;149:1563–8.

[14] Mutulsky AG. Drug reactions, enzymes and biochemical genetics. JAMA 1957;165:835–7.

[15] Vogel F. Moderne Probleme der Jumangenetik. *Ergebn Inn Med Kinderheilkd* 1959;12:52–125.

[16] Evans WE, McCleod HL. Pharmacogenomics–drug disposition, drug targets and side effects. NEJM 2003;348:538–49.

[17] Ingelman-Sundberg M. Pharmacogenetics of cytochrome P450 and its applications in drug therapy: the past, present and future. Trends Pharmacol Sci 2004;25(4):193–200.

[18] Hamosh A, Scott AF, Amberger J, Bocchini CA, McKusick VA. Online Mendelian inheritance in man (OMIM), a knowledgebase of human genes and genetic disorders. Human Mutat 2000;15:57–61.

[19] Sherrington R, Rogaev EI, Liang Y, Rogaeva EA, Levesque G, Ikeda M, et al. Cloning of a gene bearing mis-sense mutations in early-onset familial Alzheimer's disease. Nature 1995;375:754–60.

[20] Levy-Lahad E, Wijsman EM, Nemens E, Anderson L, Goddard KA, Weber JL, et al. A familial Alzheimer's disease locus on chromosome 1. Science 1995;269:970–3.

[21] Goate M, Chartier-Harlin M, Mullan Brown J, Crawford F, Fidani L, et al. Segregation of a mis-sense mutation in the amyloid precursor protein gene with familial Alzheimer's disease. Nature 1991;349:704–6.

[22] Risch N, Merikangas K. The future of genetic studies of complex human diseases. Science 1996;273:1516–7.

[23] Strittmatter WJ, Saunders AM, Schmechel D, Pericak-Vance M, Enghild J, Salvesen GS, et al. Apolipoprotein E: high-avidity binding to beta-amyloid and increased frequency of type 4 allele in late-onset familial Alzheimer disease. PNAS USA 1993;90:1977–81.

[24] Pericak-Vance MA, Yamaoka LH, Hung W-Y, Alberts MJ, Walker AP, Bartlett RJ, et al. Linkage studies in familial Alzheimer's disease: evidence for chromosome 19 linkage. Am J Hum Genet 1991;48:1034–50.

[25] Corder EH, Saunders AM, Strittmatter WJ, Schmechel DE, Gaskell PC, Small GW, et al. Gene dose of apoliprotein E type 4 allele and the risk of Alzheimer's disease in late-onset families. Science 1993;261:921–3.

[26] Mahley RH, Weisgraber KH, Huang Y. Apolipoprotein E4: a causative factor and therapeutic target in neuropathology, including Alzheimer's disease. PNAS USA 2006;103(15):5644–51.

[27] Lander ES, Linton LM, Birren B, Nusbaum C, Zody MC, Baldwin J, et al. Initial sequencing and analysis of the human genome. Nature 2001;409:860–921. Erratum. 2001. *Nature*, 411, 565.

[28] Venter JC, Adams MD, Myers EW, Li PW, Mural RJ, Sutton GG, et al. The sequence of the human genome. Science 2001;291:1304–51. Erratum, *Science*, 2001, 292, 1838.

[29] Kruglyak L, Nickerson DA. Variation is the spice of life. Nat Rev Genet 2001;27:234–6.

[30] Reich DE, Gabriel SB, Altshuler D. Quality and completeness of SNP databases. Nat Rev Genet 2003;33:457–8.

[31] Altshuler D, Daly MJ, Lander ES. Genetic mapping in human disease. Science 2008;322:881–8.

[32] Otterness DM, Szumlanski CL, Wood TC, Weinshilboum RM. Human thiopurine methyltransferase pharmacogenetics. Kindred with terminal exon splice junction mutation that results in the loss of activity. J Clin Invest 1998;101(5):1036–44.

[33] Redon R, Ishikawa S, Fitch KR, Feuk L, Perry GH, Andrews TD, et al. Global variation in copy number in the human genome. Nature 2006;444(7118):444–54.

[34] Lievre A, Bachet JB, LeCorre D, Boige V, Landi B, Emile JF, et al. KRAS mutation status is predictive of response to cetuximab therapy in colorectal cancer. Cancer Res 2006;66(8):3992–5.

[35] Galperiin MY, Fernandez-Suarez XM. The 2012 Nucleic acids research database issue and the online molecular biology database collection. Nucleic Acids Res 2012;40(D1):D1–D8.

[36] Margulies M, Egholm M, Altman WE, Attiya S, Bader JS, Bemben LA, et al. Genome sequencing in micro-fabricated high-density picolitre reactors. Nature 2005;437:376–80.

[37] Brenner S, Johnson M, Bridgham J, Golda G, Lloyd DH, Johnson D, et al. Gene expression analysis by massively parallel signature sequencing (MPSS) on microbead arrays. Nat Biotechnol 2000;18:630–4. Erratum, Nat Biotechnol 2000, 18, 1021.

[38] Olsen M. Enrichment of super-sized resequestering targets from the human genome. Nat Methods 2007;4:891–2.

[39] King CR, Marsh S. Genotyping technologies Altman RB, Flockhart ID, Goldstein DB, editors. Principles of pharacogenetics and pharmacogenomics. London: Cambridge Press; 2012. p. 12–20.

[40] Hewett M, Oliver DE, Rubin DL, Easton KL, Stuart JM, Altman RB, et al. PharmGKB: the pharmacogenetics knowledge base. Nucl Acids Res 2002;3(1):163–5.

[41] Thorn CF, Klein TE, Altman RB. Pharmacogenomics and bioinformatics: PharmGKB. Pharmacogenomics 2010;11(4):501–5.

[42] International HapMap Consortium The International HapMap Project. Nature 2003;426:789–94.

[43] International HapMap Consortium A second generation human haplotype map of over 3.1 million SNPs. Nature 2007;449:851–61.

[44] Buchanan CC, Torstenson ES, Bush WS, Ritchie MD. A comparison of cataloged variation between International Hapmap Consortium and 1000 genomes project data. J Am Med Inform Assoc 2012;19:289–94.

[45] Park J, Hwang S, Lee YS, Kim SC, Lee D. SNP@Ethnos: a database of ethnically variant single nucleotide polymorphisms. Nucleic Acids Res 2007;35:D711–5.

[46] Relethford H. Genetic evidence and the modern human origins debate. Heredity 2008;100:555–63.

[47] Hirschhorn JN, Daly MJ. Genome-wide association studies for common diseases and complex traits. Nat Rev Genet 2005;6:95–108.

[48] McCarthy MI, Abecasi GR, Cardon LR, Goldstein DB, Little J, Ioannidis JPA, et al. Genome-wide association studies for complex traits: consensus, uncertainty and challenges. Nat Rev Genet 2008;9:356–69.

[49] Hardy J, Singleton A. Genomewide association studies and human disease. NEJM 2009;360:1759–68.

[50] Altshuler D, Daly MJ, Lander ES. Genetic mapping in human disease. Science 2008;322:881–8.

[51] Mohlke KL, Boehnke M, Abecasis GR. Metabolic and cardiovascular traits: an abundance of recently identified common genetic variants. Hum Mol Genet 2008;17:R102–8.

[52] Lettre G, Rioux JD. Autoimmune diseases: insights from genome-wide association studies. Hum Mol Genet 2008;17:R116–21.

[53] O'Donnell CJ, Nabel EG. Genomics of cardiovascular disease. NEJM 2011;365:2098–109.

[54] Hindorff LA, Sethupathy P, Junkins HA, Ramos EM, Mehta JP, Collins FS, et al. Potential etiologic and functional implications of genome-wide association loci for human diseases and traits. PNAS USA 2009;106(23):9362–7.

[55] Hindorff LA, Junkins HA, Mehta, JP, Manolio TA. A catalog of published genome-wide association studies. Available from: <http://www.genome.gov/gwastudies>.

[56] 1000 Genomes Project consortium A map of human genome variation from population scale sequencing. Nature 2010;467:1061–73.

VIII. PHARMACOGENETICS AND PHARMACOGENOMICS CONSIDERATIONS

[57] Cann HM, de Toma C, Cazes L, Legrand MF, Morel V, Piouffre L, et al. A human genome diversity cell line panel. Science 2002;296:261–2.

[58] Hinds DA, Stuve LL, Nilsen GB, Halperin E, Eskin E, Ballinger DG, et al. Whole-genome patterns of common DNA variation in three human populations. Science 2005;307:1072–9.

[59] Patterson K. 1000 Genomes: a world of variation. Circ Res 2011;108:534–6.

[60] The Huntington's Disease Collaborative Research Group A novel gene containing a trinucleotide repeat that is expanded and unstable on Huntington's disease chromosomes. Cell 1993;72:971–83.

[61] Beaudet A, Bowdock A, Buchwald M, Cavalli-Sforza L, Farrall M, King M-C, et al. Linkage of cystic fibrosis to two tightly linked DNA markers: joint report from a collaborative study. Am J Hum Genet 1986;39:681–93.

[62] Nabel EG. Cardiovascular disease. NEJM 2003;349:60–72. (Erratum, *NEJM*, 2003, 349, 620).

[63] Altmuller J, Palmer LJ, Fischer G, Scherb H, Wjst M. Genomewide scans of complex human diseases: true linkage is hard to find. Am J Hum Genet 2001;69:936–50.

[64] Evans DM, Cardon LR. Guidelines for genotyping in genome-wide linkage studies: single-nucleotide-polymorphism maps versus microsatellite maps. Am J Hum Genet 2004;75:687–92.

[65] Reich DE, Cargill M, Bolk S, Ireland J, Sabeti PC, Richter DJ, et al. Linkage disequilibrium in the human genome. Nature 2001;411:199–204.

[66] Seng KC, Seng CK. The success of the genome-wide association approach: a brief story of a long struggle. Eur J Hum Genet 2008;16:554–64.

[67] National Human Genome Research Institute (NHGRI) GWAS catalog. Available at <http://www.genome.gov/26525384>.

[68] Yu W, Gwinn M, Clyne M, Yesupriya A, Khoury MJ. A navigator for human genome epidemiology. Nat Rev Genet 2008;40:124–5.

[69] Rosenberg NA, Huang L, Jewett EM, Szpiech ZA, Jancovic I, Bhehnke M. Genome-wide association studies in diverse populations. Nat Rev Genet 2010;11(5):356–66.

[70] Pritchard JK, Rosenberg NA. Use of unlinked genetic markers to detect population stratification in association studies. Am J Hum Genet 1999;65:220–8.

[71] Teo YY, Sim X, Ong RTH, Tan AKS, Chen J, Tantoso E, et al. Singapore genome variation project: a haplotype map of three Southeast Asian populations. Genome Res 2009;19:2154–62.

[72] Haga H, Yamada R, Ohnishi Y, Nakamura Y, Tanaka T. Gene-based SNP discovery as part of the Japanese Millennium Genome Project: identification of 190562 genetic variations in the human genome. J Hum Genet 2002;47:605–10.

[73] The Malaria Genomic Epidemiology Network A global network for investigating the genomic epidemiology of malaria. Nature 2008;456:732–7.

[74] Seguin B, Hardy BJ, Singer PA, Daar AS. Genomics, public health and developing countries: the case of the mexican institute of genomic medicine (INMEGEN). Nat Rev Genet 2008;9:S5–S9.

[75] Hardy BJ, Singer PA, Mukerji M, Brahmachari SK, Daar A. From diversity to delivery: the case of the Indian Genome Variation initiative. Nat Rev Genet 2008;9:S9–S14.

[76] Hardy BJ, Seguin B, Goodsaid F, Jimenez-Sanchez G, Singer PA, Daar AS. The next steps for genomic medicine: challenges and opportunities in the developing world. Nat Rev Genet 2008;9:S23–7.

[77] Licinio J. Pharmacogenomics in admixed populations: the Brazilian pharmacogenetics/pharmacogenomics network–REFARGEN. Pharmacogenomics J 2004;4:347–8.

[78] Normile. D. Genetic diversity. Consortium hopes to map human history in Asia. Science 2004;306:1667.

[79] Teo YY, Small KS, Kwiatkowski DP. Methodological challenges of genome-wide association analysis in Africa. Nat Rev Genet 2010;11(2):149–60.

[80] Bekris LM, Yu CE, Bird TD, Tsuang DW. Genetics of Alzheimer's disease. J Ger Psych Neurol 2010;23(4):213–27.

[81] Raux G, Guyant-Marechal L, Martin C, Bou J, Penet C, Brice A, et al. Molecular diagnosis of autosomal dominant early onset alzheimer's disease: an update. J Med Genet 2005;42:793–5.

[82] Hardy J, Selkoe DJ. The amyloid hypothesis of Alzheimer's disease: progress and problems on the road to therapeutics. Science 2002;297:353–6.

[83] De Strooper B, Saftig P, Craessaerts K, Vanderstichele H, Guhde G, Annaert W, et al. Deficiency of presenilins-1 inhibits the normal cleavage of amyloid precursor protein. Nature 1998;391(6665):387–90.

[84] Wolfe MS, De Los Angeles J, Miller DD, Xia W, Selkoe DJ. Are presenilins intramembrane-cleavage proteases? Implications for molecular mechanism of Alzheimer's disease. Biochemistry 1999;38(25):11223–11230.

[85] AD and FTD Mutation Database. Available at <http://www.molgen.ua.ac.be/admutations>.

[86] Kang J, Lemaire HG, Unterbeck A, Salbaum JM, Masters CL, Grzeschik KH, et al. The precursor of Alzheimer's disease amyloid A4 protein resembles a cell-surface receptor. Nature 1987;325(6106):733–6.

[87] Iwatsubo T, Odaka A, Suzuki N, Mizusawa H, Nukina N, Ihara Y. Visualization of A beta 43(43) and A beta 40 in senile plaques with end-specific A beta monoclonals: evidence that an initially deposited species is A beta 42(43). Neuron 1994;13(1):45–53.

[88] Giaccone G, Tagliavini F, Linoli G, Bouras C, Frigerio L, Frangione B, et al. Down's patients: extracellular preamyloid deposits precede neuritic degeneration and senile plaques. Neurosci Lett 1989;97(1–2):232–8.

[89] Lemere CA, Blusztajn JK, Yanaguchi H, Wisniewski T, Saido TC, Selkoe DJ. Sequence of deposition of heterogeneous amyloid beta-peptides and APOE in Down's syndrome: implications for initial events in plaque formation. Neurobiol Dis 1996;3(1):16–32.

[90] Bird TD. Genetic aspects of Alzheimer's disease. Genet Med 2008;10:231–9.

[91] Avramopoulos D. Genetics of Alzheimer's disease: recent advances. Genom Med 2009;1:34.

[92] Betram L, Tanzi RE. Alzheimer's disease: one disorder, too many genes? Hum Mol Genet 2004;13(1):R135–41.

[93] Tang MX, Maestre G, Tsai WY, Liu XH, Feng L, Chung WY, et al. Relative risk of Alzheimer's disease and age-at-onset distributions, based on APOE genotypes among elderly African Americans, Caucasians, and Hispanics in New York City. Am J Hum Genet 1996;58(3):574–84.

[94] Huang Y. Molecular and cellular mechanisms of apolipoprotein E4 neurotoxicity and potential therapeutic strategies. Curr Opin Drug Discov Devel 2006;9(5):627–41.

[95] Corder EH, Saunders AM, Risch NJ, Strittmatter WH, Schmechel DE, Gaskell Jr PC, et al. Protective effect of apolipoprotein E type 2 allele for late-onset alzheimer disease. Nat Genet 1994;7:180–4.

[96] Rogaeva K, Meng Y, Lee JH, Gu Y, Kawarai T, Zou F, et al. The neuronal sortilin-related receptor SORL1 is genetically associated with Alzheimer's disease. Nat Genet 2007;39(2):168–77.

[97] Tan EK, Lee J, Chen CP, Teo YY, Zhao Y, Lee WL. SORL 1 haplotypes modulate risk of Alzheimer's disease in Chinese. Neurobiol Aging 2009;30(7):1045–51.

[98] Ning M, Yang Y, Zhang Z, Chen Z, Zhao T, Zhang D, et al. Amyloid-B-related genes SORL1 and ACE are genetically associated with risk for late-onset alzheimer's disease in the Chinese population. Alz Dis and Assoc Disorders 2010;24:390–6.

[99] Lee JH, Chulikavit M, Pang D, Zigman WB, Silverman W, Schupf N. Association between genetics variants in sortilin-related receptor 1 (SORL1) and Alzheimer's disease in adults with Down's syndrome. Neurosci Lett 2007;425:105–9.

VIII. PHARMACOGENETICS AND PHARMACOGENOMICS CONSIDERATIONS

[100] Minster RL, DeKosky ST, Kamboh MI. No association of SORL1 SNPs with Alzheimer's disease. Neurosci Lett 2008;440(2):190–2.
[101] Shibata N, Ohnuma T, Baba H, Higashi S, Hishioka K, Arai H. Genetic association between SORL1 polymorphisms and Alzheimer's disease in a Japanese population. Dement Geriatr Cogn Disord 2008;26:161–4.
[102] Reitz C, Cheng R, Rogaeva E, Lee JH, Tokuhiro S, Zou F, Genetic and Environmental Risk in Alzheimer's Disease 1 Consortium Meta-analysis of the association between variants of SORL1 and Alzheimer disease. Arch Neurol 2011;68(1):99–106.
[103] Grupe A, Abraham R, Li Y, Rowland C, Hollingworth P, Morgan A, et al. Evidence for novel susceptibility genes for late-onset alzheimer's disease from a genome-wide association study of putative functional variants. Hum Mol Genet 2007;16:865–73.
[104] Coon KD, Myers AJ, Craig DW, Webster DW, Pearson JA, Lince DH, et al. A high-density whole-genome association study reveals that APOE is the major susceptibility gene for sporadic late-onset alzheimer's disease. J Clin Psychiatr 2007;68:13–618.
[105] Reiman EM, Webster JA, Myers AJ, Hardy J, Dunckley T, Zismann VL, et al. GAB2 alleles modify Alzheimer's risk in APOE epsilon$_4$ carriers. Neuron 2007;54:713–20.
[106] Li H, Weten S, Li L, St. Jean PL, Upmanyu R, Surh L, et al. Candidate single-nucleotide polymorphisms from a genome-wide association study of Alzheimer's disease. Arch Neurol 2008;65(1):45–53.
[107] Abraham R, Sims R, Carrol L, Hollingworth P, O'Donovan MC, Williams J, et al. An association study of common variation at the *MAPT* locus with late-onset alzheimer's disease. Am J Med Genet Part B 2009;150B:1152–5.
[108] Bertram L, Lange C, Mullin K, Parkinson M, Hsiao M, Hogan MF, et al. Genome-wide association analysis reveals putative Alzheimer's disease susceptibility loci in addition to APOE. Am J Hum Genet 2008;83:623–32.
[109] Poduslo SE, Huang R, Spiro III A. A genome screen of successful aging without cognitive decline identifies lrpIb by haplotype analysis. Am J Med Genet B 2010;153B:114–9.
[110] Harold D, Abraham R, Hollingsworth P, Sims R, Gerrish A, Hamshere ML, et al. Genome-wide association study identifies variants at CLU and PICALM associated with Alzheimer's disease. Nat Genet 2009;41:1088–93.
[111] Lambert JC, Heath S, Even G, Campion D, Sleegers K, Hiltunen M, et al. Genome-wide association study identifies variants at CLU and CRI associated with Alzheimer's disease. Nat Rev Genet 2009;41:1094–9.
[112] Potkin SG, Guffanti G, Lakatos A, Turner JA, Kruggel F, Fallon JH, Alzheimer's Disease Neuroimaging Initiative Hippocampal atrophy as a quantitative trait in a genome-wide association study identifying novel susceptibility genes for Alzheimer's disease. PloS One 2009;4:e6501.
[113] Heinzen EL, Need AC, Hayden KM, Chiba-Falek O, Roses AD, Strittmatter WJ, et al. Genome-wide scan of copy number variation in late-onset alzheimer's disease. J Alzheimer's Dis 2009;19(1):66–77.
[114] Beecham GW, Martin ER, Li YJ, Slifer MA, Gilbert JR, Haines JL, et al. Genome-wide association study implicates a chromosome 12 risk locus for late-onset alzheimer's disease. Am J Human Genet 2009;84:35–43.
[115] Carrasquillo MM, Zou F, Pankratz VS, Wilcox SL, Ma L, Walker LP, et al. Genetic variation in PEDH11X is associated with susceptibility to late-onset alzheimer's disease. Nat Genet 2009;41:192–8.
[116] Seshadri S, Fitzpatrick AL, Ikram MA, DeStefano AL, Gudnason V, Boada M, CHARGE Consortium, GERAD1 Consortium, and EADI1 Consortium Genome-wide analysis of genetic loci associated with Alzheimer's disease. JAMA 2010;303:1832–40.
[117] Naj AC, Jun G, Beecham GW, Wang LS, Vardarajn BN, Buros J, et al. Common variants at MS4A4/MS4A6E, CD2AP, CD33AHD EPHA1 are associated with late-onset alzheimer's disease. Nat Rev Genet 2011;43:436–41.

[118] Hu X, Pickering E, Liu YC, Hall S, Fournier H, Katz E, The Alzheimer's Disease Neuroimaging Initiative Meta-analysis for genome-wide association study identifies multiple variants at the BIN1 locus associated with later-onset alzheimer's disease. PLoS ONE 2011;6(2):e16616. doi:10.1371/journal.pone.0016616.

[119] Hollingsworth P, Harold D, Sims R, Garrish A, Lambert JC, Carrasquillo MM, et al. Common variants at ABCA7, MS4A67/MS4A4E, EPHA1, CD33AND CD2AP are associated with Alzheimer's disease. Nat Rev Genet 2011;43:429–35.

[120] Wijsman EM, Pankratz ND, Choi Y, Wijsman EM, Pankratz ND, Choi Y, The NIA-LOAD/NCRAD Family Study Group Genome-wide association of familial late-onset alzheimer's disease replicates BIN1 and CLU and nominates CUGBP2 in interaction with APOE. PLoS Genet 2011;7(2):e1001308.

[121] Sherva R, Baldwin CT, Inzelberg R, Vardarajan B, Cupples LA, Lunetta K, et al. Identification of novel candidate genes for Alzheimer's disease by autozygosity mapping using genome-wide SNP data. J Alzheimer's Dis 2011;23(2):349–59.

[122] Jonsson T, Stefansson H, Steinberg S, Jonsdottir I, Jonsson PV, Snaedal J, et al. Variant of TREM2 associated with the risk of Alzheimer's disease. NEJM 2013;368:107–16.

[123] Guerreiro R, Wojtas A, Bras J, Carrasquillo M, Rogaeva E, Majournie E, et al. TREM2 variants in Alzheimer's disease. NEJM 2013;368:117–27.

[124] Alzheimer Research Forum. [Cited September 2012] Available from: <http://www.alzgene.org/largescale.asp>.

[125] Bertram L, Lill CM, Tanzi RE. The genetics of Alzheimer's disease: back to the future. Neuron 2010;68:270–81.

[126] Belbin O, Carrasquillo MM, Crump M, Culley OJ, Hunter TA, Ma L, et al. Investigation of 15 of the top candidate geners for late-onset alzhiemer's disease. Hum Genet 2011;129:273–82.

[127] Morgan K. The three new pathways leading to Alzheimer's disease. Neuropath Appl Neurobiol 2011;37:353–7.

[128] Allen M, Zou F, Chai HS, Younkin CS, Crook J, Pankratz VS, et al. Novel late-onset alzheimer disease loci variants associate with gene expression. Neurology 2012;79:221–8.

[129] Sleegers K, Lambert J-C, Bertram L, Cruts M, Amouyel P, van Broeckhoven C. The pursuit of susceptibility genes for Alzheimer's disease: progress and prospects. Cell 2009;26:84–93.

[130] Coon KD, Siegel AM, Yee SJ, Stephan DA, Kirsch WM. Preliminary demonstration of an allelic association of the IREB2 gene with Alzheimer's disease. J Alz Dis 2006;9:225–33.

[131] Li Y, Shaw CA, Sheffer I, Sule N, Powell SZ, Dawson B, et al. Integrated copy number and gene expression analysis detects CREB1 association with Alzheimer's disease. Transl Psychiatry 2012;2:e192. doi:10.1038/tp.2012.119.

[132] Dreses-Werringloer U, Lambert JC, Vingtdeux V, Zhao H, Vais H, Siebert A, et al. A polymorphism in CALHM1 influences Ca^{2+} homeostasis, AB levels, and Alzheimer's disease risk. Cell 2008;133:1149–61.

[133] Koppel J, Champagne F, Vingtdeux V, Dreses-Werringloer U, Ewers M, Rujescu D, et al. CALHM1 P86L polymorphism modulates CSF AB levels in cognitively healthy individuals at risk for Alzheimer's disease. J Mol Med 2011;17:974–9.

[134] Reitz C, Barral S, Mayeux R. Genome-wide association studies in Alzheimer's disease. Eur Neurol J 2012;4(1):49–58.

[135] Gatz M, Reynolds CA, Fratiglioni L, Johansson B, Mortimer JA, Berg S, et al. Role of genes and environments for explaining Alzheimer's disease. Arch Gen Psychiatry 2006;63:168–74.

[136] Martin ER, Lai EH, Gilbert JR, Rogala AR, Afshari AJ, Riley J, et al. SNPing away at complex diseases: analysis of single-nucleotide polymorphisms around APOE in Alzheimer's disease. Am J Hum Genet 2000;67:383–94.

VIII. PHARMACOGENETICS AND PHARMACOGENOMICS CONSIDERATIONS

[137] Roses AD, Lutz MW, Amrine-Madsen H, Saunders AM, Crrenshaw DG, Sundseth SS, et al. A TOMM40 variable-length polymorphism predicts the age of late-onset alzheimer's disease. Pharmacogenomics J 2010;10:375–84.

[138] Jun G, Vardarajan BN, Buros J, Yu CE, Hawk MV, Dombroski BA, et al. Comprehensive search for Alzheimer's disease susceptibility loci in the APOE region. Arch Neurol 2012;69:1–10.

[139] Ferencz B, Karlsson S, Kalpouzos G. Promising genetic markers of preclinical Alzheimer's disease: the influence of APOE and TOMM40 on brain integrity. Int J Alz Dis 2012 doi:10.1155/2012/421452.

[140] Ankarcrona M, Mangialasche F, Winblad B. Rethinking Alzheimer's disease therapy: are mitochondria the key? J Alz Dis 2010;20:S579–90.

[141] Khoury MJ. Interview: Dr. Muin J. Khoury discusses the future of public health genomics and why it matters for personalized medicine and global health. Cur Pharmacogenom Per Med 2009;7:158–83.

[142] Mancinelli L, Cronin M, Sadee W. Pharmacogenomics: the promise of personalized medicine. AAPS PharmSci 2002;2:4.

[143] Antoniou A, Pharoah PD, Narod S, Risch HA, Eyfjord JE, Hopper JL, et al. Average risks of breast and ovarian cancer associated with BRCA1 and BRCA2 mutations detected in case series unselected for family history: a combined analysis of 22 studies. Am J Hum Genet 2003;72(5):1117–30.

[144] Seidman EG. Clinical use and practical application of TPMT enzyme and 6-mercaptopurine metabolite monitoring in IBD. Rev Gastroenterol Disord 2003;3:30–8.

[145] Vogel CL, Cobleigh MA, Tripathy D, Gutheil JC, Harris LN, Fehrenbacher L, et al. Efficacy and safety of trastuzumab as a single agent in first-line treatment of HER2-overexpressing metastatic breast cancer. J Clin Onc 2002;20(3):719–26.

[146] US Department Health and Human Services Food and Drug Administration. Table of Pharmacogenomic Biomarkers in Drug Labels. [Cited September 2012] Available from: <http://www.fda.gov/Drugs/ScienceResearch/ResearchAreas/Pharmacogenetics/ucm083378.htm>.

[147] Hamburg MA, Collins FS. The path to personalized medicine. NEJM 2010;363(4):301–4.

[148] Hudson KL. Genomics, healthcare, and society. NEJM 2011;365:1033–41.

[149] Sadee W, Dai Z. Pharmacogenetics/genomics and personalized medicine. Hum Mol Genet 2005;14:R207–14.

[150] Burke W, Psaty BM. Personalized medicine in the era of genomics. JAMA 2007;298(14):1682–4.

[151] Giacomini KM, Brett CM, Altman RB, Benowitz NL, Dolan ME, Flockhart DA, et al. The pharmacogenetics research network: from SNP discovery to clinical drug response. Nature 2007;81(3):328–45.

[152] Hunter DJ, Khoury MJ, Drazen JM. Letting the genome out of the bottle–will we get our wish. NEJM 2008;358(2):105–7.

[153] US Department Health and Human Services National Center for Biotechnology Information [cited 2012 Sept]. Available from:<http://www.ncbi.nlm.nih.gov/gtr>.

[154] Khoury MJ, Reyes M, Gwinn M, Feero WG. A genetic test registry: bringing credible and actionable data together. Pub Health Genom 2010;13:360–1.

[155] Seguin B, Hardy BJ, Singer PA, Daar AS. Genomic medicine and developing countries: creating a room of their own. Nature Rev Genetics 2008;9:487–93.

[156] Holm S. Pharmacogenetics and global (in)justice Cohen JC, Illingworth P, Schuklenk IJ, editors. The power of pills: social, ethical and legal issues in drug development, marketing and pricing. Ann Arbor, Michigan: Pluto Press; 2006. p. 98–109.

[157] Hossain P, Kawar B, El Nahas M. Obesity and diabetes in the developing world–a growing challenge. NEJM 2007;356:213–5.

[158] Daar AS, Singer PA, Persad DL, Pramming SK, Matthews DR, Beaglehole R, et al. Grand challenges in chronic non-communicable diseases. Nature 2007;450:494–6.

[159] Kalaria RN, Maesre GE, Arizaga R, Friedland RP, Galasko D, Hall K, et al. Alzheimer's disease and vascular dementia in developing countries: prevalence, management and risk factors. Lancet Neurol 2008;7(9):812–26.

[160] Cambon-Thomsen A. The social and ethical issues of post-genomic human biobanks. Nature Rev Genet 2004;5:866–73.

[161] Asslaber M, Zatloukal K. Biobanks: transnational, European and global networks. Brief Funct Genom 2007;6(3):193–201.

[162] Pace CA, Emanuel EJ. The ethics of research in developing countries: assessing voluntariness. Lancet 2005;365:11–12.

[163] Nyika A. Ethical and practical challenges surrounding genetic and genomic research in developing countries. Acta Trop 2009;1125:S21–31.

[164] Glickman SW, McHutchison JG, Peterson ED, Cairns CB, Harrington RA, Califf RM, et al. Ethical and scientific implications of the globalization of clinical research. NEJM 2009;360(8):816–23.

[165] de Vries J, Bull SJ, Doumbo O, et al. Ethical issues in human genomics research in developing countries. BMC Medical Ethics, 12, 5. Available from: <http://www.biomedicalcentral.com/1472-6939/12/5>; 2011.

[166] Matimba A, Oluka MN, Ebeshi BU, Sayi J, Bolaji OO, Guantai AN, et al. Establishment of a biobank and pharmacogenetics database of African nations. Eur J Hum Genet 2008;16:780–3.

[167] Kerb R, Fux R, Morike K, Kremsner PG, Gil JP, Gleiter CH, et al. Pharmacogenetics of antimalarial drugs: effect on metabolism and transport. Lancet Infec Dis 2009;9(12):760–74.

[168] Mannello F. MMP polymorphism and HIV antiretroviral drugs. Pharmacogen J 2009;9:3550–7.

[169] Kinzig-Schippers M, Tomalik-Scharte D, Jetter A, Scheidel B, Jakob V, Rodame M, et al. Should we use N-acetyltransferase type 2 genotyping to personalize isoniazid doses? Antimicrob Agents Chemother 2005;49(5):1733–8. 2005.

[170] Borda-Rodriguez A, Huzair F. Revisiting the Paris declaration: pharmacogenomics and personalized medicine as accelerators for development aid and effectiveness. Cur Pharm and Pers Med 2011;9:240–2.

[171] OECD. Paris Declaration and Accra Agenda for Action. Available from: <www.oecd.org/development/aideffectiveness/parisdeclarationandaccraagendaforaction.htm>.

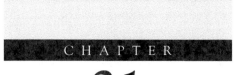

21

Application of Pharmacogenomics in Global Alzheimer's Disease Clinical Trials and Ethical Implications

Sidney A. Spector

Department of Neurology, VA Medical Center, Phoenix, Arizona, USA,
and Global Biopharma, Scottsdale, Arizona, USA

21.1 INTRODUCTION

Pharmacogenomics has the potential to play a vital role in clinical drug development by providing the methods and tools to: 1) better identify the genetic underpinnings of inter-individual phenotypic drug responses (i.e., efficacy and toxicity) based on the pharmacokinetic and pharmacodynamic effects resulting from genetic variation of drug metabolizing enzymes, transporters and targets; 2) enrich clinical trials with study subjects more likely to respond favorably to the experimental drug based on identification of disease-associated genetic polymorphisms; and 3) provide insight based on such genetic variation that might explain why a promising drug in early phase development does not show efficacy in later phase study or is withdrawn after coming to market due to untoward serious adverse effects that might be explained by an individual's or ethnic population's underlying genetic characteristics. Indeed, applied pharmacogenomics during various phases of drug development and after marketing has now demonstrated the utility of genomic medicine in the identification of individuals and ethnic or racial groups more likely to suffer from a variety of common diseases,

M. Bairu & M.W. Weiner (Eds):
Global Clinical Trials for Alzheimer's Disease.
DOI: http://dx.doi.org/10.1016/B978-0-12-411464-7.00021-3

and who are destined to respond more favorably and safely to medicines based on underlying genetic factors. To date, the abundance of pharmacogenomic research has been applied to ethnic and racial groups in developed nations. As clinical trials continue to expand globally, it will be imperative that all stakeholders in the drug development enterprise apply these pharmacogenomic approaches to populations in underdeveloped and developing nations in an ethical manner, so that pharmacogenomic research during the drug development process minimizes risks and translates to benefit people and societies throughout the world.

21.2 PHARMACOGENETICS AND PHARMACOGENOMICS IN THE DRUG DEVELOPMENT PROCESS

Polymorphic expression of isoenzymes of the cytochrome P-450 (CYP) and other drug-metabolizing enzyme systems explain a significant amount of the variability of phenotypic expression of inter-individual responses to medicine [1,2]. The CYP2D6 enzyme, for example, of which there are over 100 alleles, is the primary catalytic enzyme in the oxidative metabolism for over 100 commonly prescribed medicines in the marketplace [1,2]. Expression of specific CYP2D6 alleles determines whether an individual is a "poor," "normal," "extensive," or "ultra-rapid" metabolizer of a particular drug, and theoretically provides highly predictive value about whether administration of a medicine in clinical practice will be safe and effective, and whether a subject in a clinical trial would be predicted to respond favorably to that drug.

In the field of Alzheimer's disease (AD), most of the globally marketed medicines for treatment of this disease, the cholinesterase inhibitors, have been studied in this regard because of their highly variable therapeutic effects and safety profiles [3–6]. Tacrine, donepezil, and galantamine are metabolized in the liver by CYP-related enzymes; rivastigmine is metabolized at the synapse and bypasses liver metabolism [3,7]. These medicines are partially and transiently effective in only about a third of patients, with adverse drug reactions and resultant poor compliance reported in more than 60% of patients [5,6]. The lack of robust clinical efficacy of cholinesterase inhibitors in patients with AD may be due to a mismatch between the mechanism of action of these drugs and pathogenesis of the disease, timing of treatment, interactions with other drugs, and pharmacokinetic and pharmacodynamic effects, as well as other individual genetic factors yet identified [6]. On the other hand, the safety issues are explained for the most part by the pharmacokinetic properties of these drugs [7]. For example, the influence of specific CYP2D6 alleles on the clinical response to donepezil has been evaluated in post-marketing trials, and provides evidence that extensive and ultra-rapid metabolizers of donepezil are less likely to have a significant cognitive benefit with this drug [8–12].

The genetic variation underlying phenotypic expression that has been observed in earlier post-marketing evaluations of drug responses in treated patients would be anticipated to be amplified when such assessments are performed in populations around the world. For example, the fact that nearly 10% of individuals of European ancestry cannot metabolize the pro-drug codeine due to absence of CYP2D6 alleles, whereas nearly all Saudi Arabians transform codeine into active morphine [13,14] illustrates a potential inherent limitation of the "one drug fits all" blockbuster approach to clinical drug development. Global clinical trials that include patients indiscriminately from various countries across continents simply based on phenotypic expression of disease state without regard to specific underlying genetic profiles have inherent "noise" in outcomes due to potential genetic variability across these ethnic and racial groups, which might obscure more meaningful underlying or safety measures [15].

As the genetic variability of ethnic and racial groups underlying common complex diseases and their pharmacokinetic attributes becomes better understood, the drive to implement a pharmacogenomic model of drug development studying homogeneous populations in clinical trials is developing momentum [16–20]. Thus, assessment of CYP polymorphism in early-phase human drug development programs could influence decisions regarding progression of a drug development program, and dictate stratification in later-phase study based on the ability of individuals to metabolize the experimental agent, or be the basis for exclusion of those who are ultra-rapid or poor metabolizers. Nevertheless, it has been argued that the stratification approach, with smaller sample sizes anticipated as numbers of sub-groups increases, might lead to spurious statistical interpretations [15]. In addition, the ethical dilemma of this pharmacogenetic stratification approach is that sub-populations might be excluded altogether in clinical trial programs based on genetic profiling [15], and these "orphan" sub-groups would be excluded by regulatory bodies from being formally approved for administration of the medicine because they were not studied during the drug development process. Further, pharmaceutical companies may decide strategically to defer pharmacogenomic assessments that might differentiate responders from non-responders prior to marketing, choosing rather to take the risk of studying heterogeneous populations across ethnic and racial groups to obtain regulatory approval for a medicine for the disease state as a whole, without regard to efficacy and safety of the medicine in genetically distinct sub-populations [21–23].

To date, there have been many examples of the application of pharmacogenomics *during* the drug development process. In the field of oncology, relevant genetic biomarkers and targets have been identified in the biopsied tumor tissue of living people using pharmacogenomic technologies. Medicines such as trastuzumab (Herceptin) to treat HER2-positive metastatic breast disease [24], imatinib (Gleevec) to treat KIT-positive metastatic gastrointestinal tumors [25], and cetuximab (Erbitux) to treat KRAS-mutation-negative colorectal cancer [26] were each developed through clinical programs that targeted individuals who demonstrated the relevant mutations to enrich clinical trials, requiring smaller numbers of individuals to demonstrate efficacy and safety. In another pharmacogenomic application, early-phase study of lapitinib (Tykerb; Tyverb), an ERBB1/ERBB2 kinase inhibitor which was subsequently approved for metastatic breast cancer, demonstrated that a sub-group of individuals who developed toxic adverse events (severe rash and diarrhea) in early-phase study were homozygous for the CYP2C19 allele [27], which would allow for exclusion of this genotype in subsequent clinical development trials of this drug. In clinical trials of patients with coronary artery disease, pravastatin have been shown to have a differential statin-lowering effect based on cholesteryl-ester transfer protein (CETP) carrier status [28]. Patients with schizophrenia who are homozygous for the 5-HT$_{2a}$ receptor C102 allele respond better in clinical trials to clozapine [29,30]. The efficacy of any of these medicines may not have been discovered if they had been studied without regard to underlying genotypic profile.

21.3 PHARMACOGENOMICS IN DRUG DEVELOPMENT FOR AD

The study of basic genomics in AD has certainly contributed to a better understanding of the complex nature of the underlying genetics of this common disease, in which over 200 genes may be contributory [2,31]. In addition to well-described genetic mutations of the APP, PS1 and PS2 genes [32–34], linkage studies in patients with late-onset AD (LOAD) have identified the E4 allele of apolipoprotein E (ApoE) as a highly associated genetic risk factor for development of this disease [35–37]. This association between ApoE and LOAD has been confirmed with genome-wide association studies [38], and remains the most consistently identified gene with the highest relative risk of any association gene identified in any common, late-onset disease [39]. Genome-wise association studies and gene expression studies have further highlighted the genetic complexity of LOAD by identifying additional novel gene variants that might also potentially contribute to disease phenotype based on the functions of the expressed proteins [2,38] (see also Chapter 20). Whereas gene expression of single mutations leads to familial forms of

AD, it is likely that in LOAD there is a complex convergence of expression of multiple genes, contemporaneously and/or sequentially, which initiate and contribute to the cascade of pathological events responsible for the LOAD phenotype, and which, with other genotypes, may delay or help prevent the disease. The genetic complexity of AD coupled with anticipated genetic heterogeneity of populations across the world, and as yet unidentified environmental factors that might also contribute to phenotypic expression in LOAD, makes the application of pharmacogenomics to identify appropriate therapeutic targets in the design of medicines that can be evaluated in relevant LOAD populations even more challenging.

To date several double-blind, placebo-controlled Phase II/III and post-marketing clinical trials have used an ApoE allele stratification strategy to assess the efficacy and safety of experimental medicines during drug development because of its consistent association with LOAD. ApoE carrier state has been shown to have an influence on the therapeutic response to cholinestersase inhibitor activity of Tacrine in post-marketing studies of patients with LOAD [39,40], though this finding has been questioned [41]. Phase II study of rosiglitazone, a peroxisome proliferator-activated receptor-gamma agonist, suggested that ApoE4-negative patients showed improvement in cognitive testing after 24 weeks of treatment [42]. However, a larger, double-blind, placebo-controlled Phase III study using ApoE4 stratification did not demonstrate efficacy in any subgroup [43]. A Phase II multiple ascending dose trial of bapineuzumab, a humanized monoclonal antibody directed against beta-amyloid, suggested improvements in cognitive endpoints in non-ApoE4 allele carriers [44]. However, a double-blind, placebo-controlled Phase III study did not identify improvements in any cognitive outcomes regardless of ApoE carrier status [45]. Within the design of a Phase II randomized trial of scyllo-inositol, which is thought to bind and prevent aggregation of amyloid, were pre-specified sub-group analyses based on ApoE 4 +/− carrier status, though these results have yet to be published [46].

A Phase III global double-blind, placebo-controlled trial is currently underway to evaluate the ability of pioglitazone, a perxoisome proliferator-activated receptor-gamma agonist, to delay the onset of mild cognitive impairment [47]. This study takes advantage of the close linkage of the ApoE allele with the TOMM40 gene, which codes one component of an outer mitochondrial membrane channel through which nuclear-encoded proteins enter mitochondria, and whose variable gene length is thought to predict delay of onset of mild cognitive impairment (MCI), the clinical precursor of LOAD. This approach will evaluate, for the first time, the combined effects of associated genes thought to have genetic bearing on AD, while studying otherwise normal individuals who will be stratified based on their predicted destiny to develop MCI due to expression of these particular alleles, which supports current thinking about the need to evaluate the utility of therapeutics prior to the phenotypic expression of this disease [17–20].

Additional medicinal clinical trials stratifying for ApoE4 carrier status for treatment of Alzheimer's dementia that are ongoing or have yet to be published include study of SB-742457, a 5HT6 antagonist (NCT00348192), pitavastatin (NCT00548145), and rivastigmine in MCI (NCT01602198) [48]. Randomized, controlled trials of pomegranate extract (NCT01571193), resveratrol, derived from plants and red grapes (NCT01504854), and fish oil supplementation in people with MCI (NCT00746005) are ongoing. ApoE carrier status is being studied for its influence to improve cognition with aerobic exercise in healthy adults (NCT0102791) and in African Americans with mild Alzheimer's dementia (NCT01021644) [48].

21.4 ETHICS RELATED TO PHARMACOGENOMICS IN GLOBAL CLINICAL TRIALS

Fundamental principles of informed consent, first addressed by the Nurenberg Code [49] after atrocities committed by Nazi scientists during World War II, and subsequently enumerated upon in the Declaration of Helsinki [50], the Belmont Report [51], the International Conference on Harmonization (ICH) guidelines [52], and the Council for International Organizations of Medical Sciences (CIOMS) [53], are the legal and moral linchpins upon which individuals who willingly volunteer to participate in clinical trials are protected. As outlined in the Belmont Report, individuals must be treated as autonomous agents, and afforded all of the information to deliberate independently about the risks and benefits of participation, while those people who are incapable of such self-determination must be protected during participation to the degree that risk is involved in the clinical trial (*respect for persons*). It is the obligation of all stakeholders (e.g., individual investigators, study sponsors, regulatory agencies, and society at large) to treat individuals in an ethical manner by respecting their decisions and protecting them from harm that might be unpredictably caused by the research enterprise (*beneficence*). Individuals must not be excluded from the benefits of the research, nor should burden be imposed upon them unduly; benefits should be distributed in a just manner (*justice*).

The recently published United States Presidential Commission for the "Privacy and Progress of Whole Genome Sequencing" [54] builds on the ethical principles of the seminal Belmont Report [51] and the more recent Presidential Commission's report, "New Directions: The Ethics of Synthetic Biology and Emerging Technologies" [55], to establish basic principles by which ethical genomic research should be conducted. Five fundamental ethical principles, derived from the ideal of respect for the individual, were established: 1) public beneficence; 2) responsible stewardship; 3) intellectual freedom and responsibility; 4) democratic deliberation; and 5) justice and fairness. Based on these tenets, the Commission made ethically important and practically useful recommendations about "what (ethically) ought to be done and what (legally) must be done" that would support the pursuit of public benefit anticipated from whole genome sequencing while minimizing the potential privacy risk to, and disadvantage of, the individual. These recommendations include:

1. implementation of strong privacy baseline protections for the individual, while promoting data access and sharing by clinicians, researchers and others with whom the individual chooses to share these data;
2. ethical responsibility and accountability in the public and private sectors for optimizing security of genomic data and access to genomic databases;
3. the development of consent processes that fully inform patients and research participants about the potential risks of genomic sequencing, and fully explain: what genomic testing is; how data are analyzed, stored and shared; what kinds of information will be provided to the individual; and how the individual might benefit from genomic discoveries in the future which were derived, in part, from those DNA samples;
4. ways to facilitate the progress in whole-genome sequencing so that the privacy of the individual is protected while potentially benefiting the public without imposing high barriers to data sharing; and
5. securing true public benefit, so that all segments of society, including minority racial and ethnic groups, are afforded opportunities to participate in this genomic enterprise, with the potential to benefit from the outcomes.

In practical terms, *informed consent* is the process by which an individual learns about the purpose of the research study, its duration, procedures involved, potential benefits and/or risks or discomforts, disclosure of alternative procedures or course of treatment that might be more advantageous to the participant, possible compensations including medical treatment, and how the confidentiality of medical records will be maintained. Being adequately informed, the subject signs a statement of voluntary participation with an option to discontinue participation at any time for any reason.

A fundamental concept of pharmacogenomic research in the drug development process, explicit in the President's Commission report [54], is the requirement that the principles of privacy and confidentiality be imbedded in the informed consent process related to the collection and storage of DNA/RNA samples that could ostensibly be used in future research endeavors. While genetic testing can be blinded relatively easily in a particular clinical trial so that confidentiality is adequately maintained through informed consent, the ethical concern is that during the long-term storage of tissue samples in biobanks for secondary, non-planned future use, the ongoing privacy and confidentiality of the individual donating tissue may not be adequately and appropriately enforced [56–58]. Intended or unintentionally inappropriate use of stored genotypic and/or phenotypic data by academic researchers, pharmaceutical companies, insurance companies, or government are perceived threats to privacy and confidentiality across the spectrum affecting individuals to society as a whole.

Theft of data through surreptitious access to electronic medical records or from mobile data storage devices is another potential concern. Re-identification might be attempted through linkage with available databases or by other means for the purpose of determining the owner's genotype or phenotype for future research endeavors or other untoward purposes [59–61]. Even though safeguards have been put in place in developed countries to de-identify, encrypt or delink personal information, there are still fears that the multiple locations at which tissue samples are collected and stored (in public, private and government-controlled databases and biobanks) may present serious challenges to maintaining anonymity and confidentiality [62,63]. In addition to potentially affecting the individual, such breach of privacy and confidentiality might also potentially affect family members, and inadvertently lead to discrimination or stigmatization against the individual, family members, ethnic or racial groups, and communities or populations to which that person is genetically identified, violating the *respect for persons* tenet.

With respect to giving consent for future, unforeseen pharmacogenomic research using personal biological tissue, reconciliation of the conflicting concerns for individual autonomy and confidentiality on the one hand, and the research and social interests of society in generating new health-related knowledge on the other, continues to be a matter of active ethical debate [64]. The most restrictive view is that research ethics and respect for persons dictate that informed consent be obtained from an individual for the use of all collected tissue samples for each current and yet unidentified future research study in which those specimens are studied [65]. This principle is codified into laws, regulations and guidelines of several organizational authorities (Council of Europe; Council of International Organizations of Medical Sciences; World Health Organization), consensus groups [66], and regulatory agencies of developed countries (e.g., Sweden, Switzerland, Italy, France) [67]. However, it is recognized that it may not be feasible logistically to obtain repeatedly renewed consent from the individual every time another research study involving previously collected tissue is undertaken well into the future [55,56].

Other less restrictive approaches, including "partially restricted consent" which allows use of specimens in current and *related* future research only, and "broad" ("open;" "blanket;" "generic") consent, which permits the use of tissue samples for *related* or *unrelated* future studies, are implemented by the United Nations Educational, Scientific and Cultural Organization and other developed countries (e.g., Australia, Germany, Estonia, Japan, Spain, United Kingdom, Iceland, Denmark, Norway) [56,59,65,67]. Implicit in this approach is the option for the individual to withdraw consent at some future date. However, as the value of the stored samples increases over time, and data are shared through collaborations and across countries, withdrawal of consent requiring removal of samples as well as data files, printed lists and questionnaires becomes impractical [68]. Therefore, the concept that individuals should not have the right to withdraw consent of use of previously collected samples in future research, only that they be assured adequate anonymity, has been advocated [63].

On the other hand, it has been argued that informed consent misrepresents the true nature of the relationship between the individual and the genomic research enterprise using biobanked specimens because it is impossible for the donor to make an informed choice about the risks and benefits of unspecified future research [69]. Nevertheless, it is universally agreed that the use of tissue or data in future research does require some type of formal oversight and authorization, regardless of the nature of the consent given by the individual, through rigorous review of each new research protocol by independent institutional review boards or ethics committees that represent the interests of the individual and are reflective of the society in which the research is being conducted [70,71]. In this regard, it is felt that ongoing transparent discussion by all stakeholders, including engagement of the community at large, is healthy and will assure that the autonomy of the individual in the clinical research process is balanced by the potential benefits to society [61,72–76] in consonance with the guidelines, regulations, and practices that have been established by these international organizations and countries.

The ethical issues of true voluntariness, coercion, exploitation, inadequate comprehension, and post-study benefit related to participation in clinical research are amplified in underdeveloped and developing countries where individuals are more likely to be poor, with limited access to healthcare, education and community or government resources [77–84]. *Voluntariness* refers to an individual's expression of free will to participate in research and is reflected by the formal process of informed consent. In developed countries, regulatory oversight dictates that the emphasis be placed on review between the investigator and participant of the informed consent document with signatures in place to establish voluntariness. It is recognized that in underdeveloped and developing countries where customs, practices and culture are uniquely defined and experienced, and where comprehension of a written document may be limited due to illiteracy and inadequate cross-cultural translation, or where signing a document may be dangerous in oppressive regimes, other ways of insuring understanding of the clinical trial process and obtaining voluntary consent may be required.

Further complicating the consent process, but requiring full attention, is the need in certain cultures to discuss the research process and protocol with local leaders, whether or not affiliated formally with government, for community approval for researchers to approach potential participants [78,85]. Involvement of the community in establishing recruitment procedures, disclosing information and obtaining consent in culturally and linguistically appropriate formats, implementing supplementary community and familial consent procedures where culturally appropriate, and ensuring the freedom to refuse or withdraw from the research study are guidelines that should provide protections for less advantaged individuals in the clinical trial process [80]. In certain countries or subpopulations, it might therefore be acceptable to provide detailed verbal consent about the research protocol that is both witnessed and verified, rather than requiring a participant's signature on a formal document [78].

When conducting pharmacogenomic research that involves collecting tissue samples for future unforeseen research, the ethical challenges regarding informed consent of individuals in developing or underdeveloped countries become much more complex [85]. What level and in what format informed consent for participation in pharmacogenomic research is obtained—influenced by the level of literacy and education, state of functioning of ethical review boards, and existence and level of local institutional regulatory and compliance policies—will require special attention by study sponsors if the autonomy, privacy and confidentiality of participants is to be achieved ethically. In the study of patients with AD, competency to make informed decisions about participation in a clinical trial must also be considered [86–90]. Indeed, some countries may still generally lack established local guidelines regarding the informed consent process. It must always be acknowledged that informed consent is considered an international human rights norm [83,85], and in situations where local laws, regulations, and guidelines are insufficient or lacking, sponsors must rely not only on internationally accepted guidelines and local rules of engagement, but should make public efforts to secure full engagement and support from local community representatives in the clinical trial process so that participants and local communities are fully enfranchised and do not feel exploited at some time in the future [91–93].

Whether to disclose the results of genetic research to the participant should be part of the informed consent discussion [85,94–98]. As with other ethical issues surrounding genetic research, societal and country practices and laws regarding this issue may not yet be firmly established in certain developing and underdeveloped regions of the world [94].

There are strong ethical and scientific arguments for and against sharing genomic data. Results of genomic research may not initially provide immediately useful information for prevention or treatment of disease in the participant, members of the family, or the community at large [93,95,97,98]. Knowledge of "premature" results may be misinterpreted and lead to unnecessary psychological, social, and economic stress upon the participant and family. There may be extensive financial, logistic, and time burdens dictated by the necessity to return study results to participants of genomic studies, which might significantly impede the drug development process [94,96]. It is argued that these concerns do not outweigh the respect for the research participant [99]. If study results are disseminated, the privacy of family members who do not wish to know their genetic predispositions must be addressed [95,100]. Withholding genetic study results may lead to the perception that study sponsors and investigators are exploiting participants and local communities in developing and underdeveloped countries whereas reasoned disclosure of study results provides reassurance to the participant and to the local community that there is a true partnership with other stakeholders in the research enterprise [85,93]. Thus, the hesitation by researchers and sponsors to disseminate genetic study results under all circumstances is contrasted with the ethical tenet of *respect for persons* which dictates that an individual should have the right to know personal and study results, or waive that right, as part of their initial agreement to participate [101].

The United States National Bioethics Advisory Commission of 1999 concluded that "disclosure of research results to subjects represents an exceptional circumstance," and only when research results have been scientifically confirmed and validated, have implications for the individual's health, and dictate an available course of action to provide treatment would it be reasonable to disclose genetic research results [102]. The CIOMS, the Council of Europe, UNESCO, and the World Health Organization (WHO) have more recently concluded that individuals must be informed of any findings that relate to their *particular health status*, as well as the individual's right not to know [103–107]. In its report "Genetic Databases: Assessing the Benefits and the Impact on Human and Patient Rights," the WHO stipulates that the research results must have been instrumental in identifying a clear clinical benefit to the identifiable individual, the disclosure of this information will avert or minimize harm to the individual, and there is no indication that the individual prefers not to know these results [107], which is the consensus of other international bodies including the European Medical Research Council and the 2002 Consortium on Pharmacogenetics [108,109].

Exploitation—the unfair distribution of the risks and benefits of research between sponsors and participants [82]—continues to be an ongoing ethical issue in the conduct of global clinical trials [78,80,81,83,85]. As greater amounts of clinical research are being carried out in countries with limited resources, there are ongoing concerns about the fair sharing of benefits derived from this enterprise. Historically, exploitation has been manifest by the recruitment of patients in developing or underdeveloped countries for the study of health conditions that are not locally prevalent. After completion of a clinical trial, participants might no longer have access to any experimental or previously approved interventions. In addition, if a study led to approval of a new medication, for economic reasons the sponsors might decide to limit marketing only to countries with high prevalence of the studied condition or to countries that could afford to pay for the medicine. It has been argued that it would be unethical to conduct a clinical trial in a developing or developed country if the intervention being studied would not be affordable or if the healthcare infrastructure could not support its proper distribution and use [78]. International conferences have codified this view, emphasizing that clinical research is justified in countries only where there is a reasonable likelihood the populations in which the research is carried out stand to benefit from the results of the research, and that at the end of a clinical trial, every participant should be afforded the opportunity to continue the best prophylactic, diagnostic, and therapeutic methods identified in the study [50,53].

Benefit sharing in pharmacogenomic research is a much more complex issue, as it can be anticipated that a significant amount of research using stored specimens will be conducted at some time in the future, related or unrelated to the condition that was originally studied [110,111]. Because most pharmacogenomic research is initiated by developed countries, and many developing and underdeveloped countries still lack the physical infrastructure to collect, store and process DNA samples, most tissue specimens are shipped to and evaluated in public and private biobanks in developed countries: so-called "South to North" collaborations [85]. Ultimate ownership of tissue samples, data and databases is still a matter of vigorous debate. There does not appear to be an ethical argument for an individual's ownership of donated DNA. The person's DNA derives value from the work on it performed by researchers supported by sponsors; thus, the rights of the scientists that have made the tissue valuable may exceed those of the donor [100]. Since tissue is ultimately controlled by "Northern" investigators, academic institutions and biobanks, future study might proceed, but without inclusion of researchers from "Southern" countries, who might still claim ownership rights and demand benefit from future research efforts of which they were not a part.

A further challenge is how to determine the relative contribution to a new discovery that occurs from future study based on the use of one's DNA sample collected decades previously. If there were to be financial dispensation, the practical challenge of locating anonymous individuals who donated tissue years previously would be daunting. As opposed to personal compensation, there is great support for the sharing of benefits through "payment" by sponsors from developed countries to the community, racial or ethnic group, or the country's society at large [62,85,110,111]. In addition to the health benefit of increased knowledge about the disease being studied, more direct benefit sharing might include free medical service or free medicine to individuals or populations participating in the research, even for some period after completion of study, and this should be delineated in the informed consent process [110]. Pre-arrangement for a portion of profits derived from the research to be donated to health sector organizations or to humanitarian or educational programs in the country where the research took place, and obtaining free access to treatments that were developed through biobanks, are other suggestions for benefit sharing [62,112].

In essence, then, as recommended by the Human Genome Organization Ethics Committee, all the details of the clinical trial should be addressed prior to beginning the research study—in collaboration with all stakeholders of developed, developing and underdeveloped countries, including research subjects, clinical investigators, lay representatives of the local communities, sponsors, ethics review boards, and regulatory bodies—to outline details of benefit sharing, informed consent, and sharing of research results, so that contributions and benefits are shared and the participants, local communities, and governments of developing and underdeveloped countries are considered as equal partners in the global clinical trial enterprise.

References

[1] Ingelman-Sundberg M. Pharmacogenetics of cytochrome P450 and its applications in drug therapy: the past, present and future. Trends Pharmacol Sci 2004;25(4):193–200.

[2] Cacabelos R. Pharmacogenomics and therapeutic prospects in dementia. Eur Arch Psychiatry Clin Neurosci 2008;258:28–47.

[3] Cacabelos R. Donepezil in Alzheimer's disease: from conventional trials to pharmacogenetics. Neuropsych Dis and Treat 2007;3:303–33.

[4] Jann MW, Shirley KL, Small GW. Clinical pharmacokinetics and pharmacodynamics of cholinesterase inhibitors. Clin Pharmacokinet 2002;41:719–39.

[5] Giacobini E. Cholinesterases in human brain: the effect of cholinesterase inhibitors in Alzheimer's disease and related disorders Giacobini E, Pepeo G, editors. The brain cholinergic system in health and disease. Oxon: Informa Healthcare; 2006. p. 235–64.

[6] Martorana A, Esposito Z, Koch G. Beyond the cholinergic hypothesis: do current drugs work in Alzheimer's disease? CNS Neurosci Ther 2010;16:235–45.

[7] Weinshilboum R. Inheritance and drug response. NEJM 2003;348:529–37.

[8] Varsaldi F, Miglio G, Scordo G, Dahl M-L, Villa LM, Biolcate A, et al. Impact of the CYP2D6 polymorphism on steady-state plasma concentrations and clinical outcome of donepezil in Alzheimer's disease. Eur J Clin Pharm 2006;62:721–6.

[9] Choi SH, Kim SY, Na HR, Kim B-K, Yang DW, Kwon JC, et al. Effect of ApoE Genotype on Response to Donepezil in Patients with Alzheimer's disease. Dement Geriatr Cogn Disord 2008;25:445–50.

[10] Pilotto A, Franceschi M, D'Onofrio G, Bizzarro DA, Mangialasche F, Cascavilla L, et al. Effect of a CYP2D6 polymorphism on the efficacy of donepezil in patients with Alzheimer disease. Neurology 2009;73:761–7.

[11] Chianella C, Gragnaniello D, Delser PM, Visentini MF, Setter E, Tola MR, et al. BCHE and CYP2D6 genetic variation in Alzheimer's disease patients treated with cholinesterase inhibitors. Eur J Clin Pharmacol 2011;67:1147–57.

[12] Seripa D, Bizzarro A, Pilotto A, D'Onofrio G, Vecchione G, Gallo AP, et al. Role of cytochrome P4502D6 functional polymorphisms in the efficacy of donepezil in patients with Alzheimer's disease. Pharmacogenet Genomics 2011;21:225–30.

[13] Bradford LD. CYP2D6 allele frequency in European Caucasians, Asians, Africans and their descendants. Pharmacogenomics 2002;3:229–43.

[14] McLellan RA, Oscarson M, Seidegard J, Evans DA, Ingelman-Sunderberg M. Frequent occurrence of CYP2D6 gene duplication in Saudi Arabians. Pharmacogenetics 1997;7:187–91.

[15] Issa AM. Ethical perspectives on pharmacogenomic profiling in the drug development process. Nat Rev Drug Disc 2002;1:200–308.

[16] Meyer UA, Zanger UM. Molecular mechanisms of genetic polymorphisms of drug metabolism. Ann Rev Pharmacol Toxicol 1997;37:269–96.

[17] Nebert DW, Menon AG. Pharmacogenomics, ethnicity and susceptibility genes. Pharmacogenomics J 2001;1:19–22.

[18] Xie HG, Kim RB, Wood AJ, Stein CM. Molecular basis of ethnic differences in drug deposition and response. Ann Rev Pharmacol Toxicol 2001;41:815–50.

[19] Tate SK, Goldstein DB. Will tomorrow's medicines work for everyone? Nat Gen 2004;36:534–42.

[20] Daar AS, Singer PA. Pharmacogenetics and geographical ancestry: implications for drug development and global health. Nat Rev Genet 2005;6:241–6.

[21] Sinha G. Drug companies accused of stalling tailored therapies. Nat Med 2006; 12:983.

[22] Smart A, Martin P, Parker M. Tailored medicine: whom will it fit? The ethics of patient and disease stratification. Bioethics 2004;18:322–42.

[23] Oliver C, Williams-Jones B, Godard B, Mikalson B, Ozhemir V. Personalized medicine, bioethics and social responsibilities: re-thinking the pharmaceutical industry to remedy inequalities in patient care and international health. Cur Pharmacogenomics Personalized Med 2008;6:108–20.

[24] Romond EH, Perez EA, Bryant J, Suman VJ, Geer Jr CE, Davidson NE, et al. Trastuzaumab plus adjuvant chemotherapy for operable HER2-positive breast cancer. NEJM 2005;353:1673–84.

[25] Heinrich MC, Corless CL, Demetri GD, Blanke CD, von Mehren M, Joensuu H, et al. Kinase mutations and imatinib response in patients with metastatic gastrointestinal stromal tumor. J Clin Onc 2003;21:4342–9.

[26] Lievre A, Bachet JB, LeCorre D, Boige V, Landi B, Emile JF, et al. KRAS mutation status is predictive of response to cetuximab therapy in colorectal cancer. Cancer Res 2006;66(8):3992–5.

[27] Zaks TZ, Akkari A, Briley L, Mosteler M, Stead AG, Koch KM, et al. Role of pharmacogenomic studies in early clinical development: Phase I studies with lapatinib. J Clin Onc 2006;24(185):3029.

[28] Kulvenhoven JA, Jukema JW, Zwinderman AH, de Knijff P, McPherson R, Bruschke AV, et al. NEJM 1998;338:86–93.

[29] Arranz M, Munro J, Owen MJ, Spurlock G, Sham PC, Zhao J, et al. Association between clozapine response and allelic variation in 5-HT$_{2a}$ receptor gene. Lancet 1995;346:281–2.

[30] Masellis M, Basile V, Meltzer HY, Lieberman JA, Sevy S, Macciardi FM, et al. Serotonin subtype 2 receptor genes and clinical response to clozapine in schizophrenic patients. Neuropsychopharmacol 1998;19:123–32.

[31] Selkoe DJ, Podlisny MB. Deciphering the genetic basis of Alzheimer's disease. Ann Rev Genomics Hum Genet 2002;3:67–99.

[32] Sherrington R, Rogaev EI, Liang Y, Rogaeva EA, Levesque G, Ikeda M, et al. Cloning of a gene bearing mis-sense mutations in early-onset familial Alzheimer's disease. Nature 1995;375:754–60.

[33] Levy-Lahad E, Wijsman EM, Nemens E, Anderson L, Goddard KA, Weber JL, et al. A familial Alzheimer's disease locus on chromosome 1. Science 1995;269:970–3.

[34] Goate Chartier-Harlin M, Mullan M, Brown J, Crawford F, Fidani L, et al. Segregation of a mis-sense mutation in the amyloid precursor protein gene with familial Alzheimer's disease. Nature 1991;349:704–6.

[35] Pericak-Vance MA, Bebout JL, Goskell PC, Yamaoka LH, et al. Linkage studies in familial Alzheimer's disease: evidence for chromosome 19 linkage. Am J Hum Genet 48:1034–50.

[36] Corder EH, Saunders AM, Strittmatter WJ, Schmechel DE, Gaskell PC, Small GW, et al. Gene dose of apoliprotein E type 4allele and the risk of Alzheimer's disease in late-onset families. Science 1993;261:921–3.

[37] Mahley RW, Weisgraber KH, Huang. Y. Apolipoprotein E4: a causative factor and therapeutic target in neuropathology, including Alzheimer's disease. PANS 2006;103(15):5644–51.

[38] Olgiati P, Politis AM, Papadimitriou GN, de Ronchi D, Serretti A. Genetics of late-onset alzheimer's disease: update from the Alzgene database and analysis of shared pathways. Int J Alz Dis 2011 doi:10.4061/2011/832379.

[39] Poirier J, Delisle M-C, Quirion R, Aubert I, Farlow M, Lahiri D, et al. Apolipoprotein E4 allele as a predictor of cholinergic deficits and treatment outcome in Alzheimer's disease. PNAS 1995;92:12260–4.

[40] Farlow M, Lahiri DK, Poirier J, Davignon J, Schneider L, Hui SL. Treatment outcome of tacrine therapy depends on apolipoprotein genotype and gender of the subjects with Alzheimer's disease. Neurology 1998;50:669–77.

[41] Rigaud AS, Traykov L, Caputo L, Guelfi MC, Latour F, Couderc R, et al. The apoliprotein E epsilon4 allele and the response to Tacrine therapy in Alzheimer's disease. Eur J Neurol 2000;7:255–8.

[42] Risner E, Saunders AM, Altman JFB, Ormandy GC, Craft S, Foley Efficacy of rosiglitazone in a genetically defined population with mild-to-moderate Alzheimer's disease. Pharmacogenomics J 2006;6:46–254.

[43] Gold M, Alderton C, Zvartau-Hind M, Egginton S, Saunders AM, Irizarry M, et al. Rosiglitazone monotherapy in mild-to-moderate Alzheimer's disease: results from a randomized, double-blind, placebo-controlled Phase III study. Dementia 2010;30:131–46.

[44] Salloway S, Sperling R, Gilman S, Fox NC, Blennow K, Raskind M, et al. A Phase 2 multiple ascending dose trial of bapineuzumab in mild to moderate Alzheimer disease. Neurology 2009;73:2061–70.

VIII. PHARMACOGENETICS AND PHARMACOGENOMICS CONSIDERATIONS

[45] Available from: <http://press.pfizer.com/press-release/pfizer-announces-co-primary-clinical-endpoints-not-met-second-phase-3-bapineuzumab-stu>; December, 2012.

[46] Salloway S, Sperling R, Keren R, Porsteinsson AP, van Dyck CH, Tariot PN, et al. Neurology 2011;77:1253–62.

[47] Crenshaw DG, Gottschalk WK, Lutz MW, Grossman I, Saunders AM, Burke JR, et al. Using genetics to enable studies on the prevention of Alzheimer's disease. Clin Pharm Ther 2012 doi:10.1038/clpt.2012.222.

[48] ClinicalTrials.gov, US National Institutes of Health. Available from: <http://clinical-trials.gov>.

[49] The Nurenberg Code. Available from: <http://www.hhs.gov/ohrp/archive/nur-code.html>.

[50] World Medical Association. Declaration of Helsinki: ethical principles for medical research involving human subjects. Available at: <http://www.wma/net/en/30publications/10policies/b3/index.html>.

[51] National Commission for the Protection of Human Subjects of Biomedical and Behavioral Research. The Belmont Report: Ethical Principles and Guidelines for the Protection of Human Subjects of Research. Washington, DC: Department of Health, Education and Welfare, DHEW Publications OS 78-0012. Available at: <http://www.hhs.gov/ohrp/humansubjects/guidance/belmont.html>.

[52] International Conference on Harmonization. Available from: <http://www.ich.org/fileadmin/Public_Web_Site/ICH_Products/Guidelines/Efficacy/E6_R1/Step4/E6_R1__Guideline.pdf>.

[53] Council for International Organizations of Medical Sciences (CIOMS). International ethical guidelines for biomedical research involving human subjects. Available at: <http://www.cioms.ch/publications/layout_guide2002.pdf>.

[54] Gutmann A, Wagner J. The Presidential Commission for the Study of Bioethical Issues: Privacy and Progress in Whole Genome Sequencing, October, 2012. Available from: <http://www.bioethics.gov/cms/node/764>.

[55] Gutmann A, Wagner J. The Presidential Commission for the Study of Bioethical Issues: New Directions: The Ethics of Synthetic Biology and Emerging Technologies, December, 2010. Available from: <http://bioethics.gov/cms/synthetic-biology-report>.

[56] Petrini C. "Broad" consent, exceptions to consent and the question of using biological samples for research purposes different from the initial collection purpose. Soc Sci Med 2010;70:217–20.

[57] Rodriguez E, Lolas F. The problem of informed consent content for genetic research using biospecimens stored in biobanks. Revista Bioethicos 2012;6(3):307–12.

[58] Rothstein MA. Expanding the ethical analysis of biobanks. J Law Med 2005;33(1):89–101.

[59] Lowrance WW, Collins FS. Identifiability in genomic research. Science 2007;317:600–2.

[60] McGuire AL, Gibbs RA. No longer de-identified. Science 2006;312:370–1.

[61] Lunshoff JE, Chadwick R, Vorhaus DB, Church GM. From genetic privacy to open consent. Nat Rev Genet 2008;9:406–11.

[62] Cambon-Thomsen A. The social and ethical issues of post-genomic human biobanks. Nat Rev Genet 2004;5:866–73.

[63] Lee SS-J. Ethical considerations for pharmacogenomics: privacy and confidentiality Altman RB, Flockhart ID, Goldstein DB, editors. Principles of pharmacogenetics and pharmacogenomics. London: Cambridge Press; 2012. p. 12–20.

[64] Lunshof JE, Chadwick R, Vorhaus DB, Church GM. From genetic privacy to open consent. Nat Rev Genet 2008;9:406–11.

[65] Shickle D. The consent problem within DNA biobanks. Stud Hist Philos Biol Biomed Res 2006;37:503–19.

[66] Caulfield T, McGuire AL, Cho M, Buchanan JA, Burgess MM, Danilczyk U, et al. Research ethics recommendations for whole-genome research: consensus statement. PLOS/Biol 2008;6(3):e73. doi:10.1371/journal.pbio 0060073.

[67] Salvaterra E, Lecchi L, Giovanelli S, Butte B, Bardella MT, Bertazzi PA, et al. Banking together: a unified model of informed consent for biobanking. EMBO Rep 2008;9:307–13.

[68] Mascalzoni D, Hicks A, Pramstaller P, Wjst M. Informed consent in the genomics era. PLOS Med 2008;5(9):e192.

[69] Rothstein MA. Expanding the ethical analysis of biobanks. J Law Med Ethics 2005;33:89–101.

[70] White MT, Gamm J. Informed consent for research on stored blood and tissue samples: a survey of institutional review board practices. Account Res 2002;9:1–16.

[71] Winickoff DE, Winickoff RN. The charitable trust as a model for genomic biobanks. NEJM 2003;349:1180–4.

[72] Hannig VL, Clayton EW, Edwards KM. Whose DNA is it anyway? Relationships between families and researchers. Am J Med Genet 1993;47:257–60.

[73] Kaye J. Genetic research on the UK population – do new principles need to be developed? Trends Mol Med 2001;7:528–30.

[74] Wendler D, Emanuel E. The debate over research on stored biological samples: what do sources think? Arch Intern Med 2002;162:1457–62.

[75] Edwards J. Taking "public understanding" seriously. New Genet Soc 2002;21:315–25.

[76] Chin R. Ethics and institutional review board capacity building Bairu M, Chin R, editors. Global clinical trials playbook: management and implementation when resources are limited: Elsevier; 2012. p. 175–97.

[77] Koski G, Nightingale SL. Research involving human subjects in developing countries. NEJM 2001;345:136–8.

[78] Shapiro HT, Meslin EM. Ethical issues in the design and conduct of clinical trials in developing countries. NEJM 2001;345:139–42.

[79] Brody BA. Ethical issues in clinical trials in developing countries. Statist Med 2002;21:2853–8.

[80] Emanuel EJ, Wendler D, Killen J, Grady C. What makes clinical research in developing countries ethical? The benchmarks of ethical research. JID 2004;189:930–7.

[81] Nundy S, Gulhati CM. A new colonialism? Conducting clinical trials in India. NEJM 2005;352:1633–6.

[82] Pace CA, Emanuel EJ. The ethics of research in developing countries: assessing voluntariness. Lancet 2005;365:11–12.

[83] Annas GJ. Globalized clinical trials and informed consent. NEJM 2009;360:2050–3.

[84] Altavilla A. Ethical standards for clinical trials conducted in third countries: the new strategy of the European Medicines Agency. Eur J Health Law 2011;18:65–75.

[85] Nyika A. Ethical and practical challenges surrounding genetic and genomic research in developing countries. Acta Trop 2009;112S:S21–31.

[86] Kim SYH, Appelbaum PS, Jeste DV, Olin JT. Proxy and surrogate consent in geriatric neuropsychiatric research: update and recommendation. Am J Psychiatry 2004;161:797–806.

[87] Kim SYH, Kim HM, McCallum C, Tariot PN. What do people at risk for Alzheimer's disease think about surrogate consent for research? Neurology 2005;65:1395–401.

[88] Noble Jr JH. Protecting people with decisional impairments and legal incapacity against biomedical research abuse. J Disabil Policy Studies 2008;18:230–44.

[89] Doody RS, Cole PE, Miller DS, Siemers E, Black R, Feldman H, et al. Global issues in drug development for Alzheimer's disease. Alzheim Dementia 2011;7:197–207.

[90] Bairu M. Bioethical considerations in global clinical trials Chin R, Bairu M, editors. Global clinical trials: effective implementation and management; 2011 p. 19–29.

VIII. PHARMACOGENETICS AND PHARMACOGENOMICS CONSIDERATIONS

[91] Weijer C, Emanuel EJ. Protecting communities in biomedical research. Science 2000;289:1142–4.

[92] Bhutta ZA. Ethics in international research: a perspective from the developing world. Bull WHO 2002;80:114–20.

[93] De Vries J, Bull SJ, Doumbo O, Ibrahim M, Mercereau-Puijalon O, Kwiatkowski D, et al. Ethical issues in human genomics research in developing countries. BMC Med Ethics 2011;12:5. <http://www.boimedcenter.com/1472-6939/12/5>.

[94] Beskow LM, Burke W, Merz JF, Barr PA, Terry S, Penchaszadeh VB, et al. Informed consent for population-based research involving genetics. JAMA 2001;286(18):2315–21.

[95] Knoppers BM, Joly Y, Simard J, Durocher F. The emergence of an ethical duty to disclose genetic research results: international perspectives. Eur J Hum Genet 2006;14:1170–8.

[96] Klitzman R. Questions, complexities, and limitations in disclosing individual genetic results. Am J Bioeth 2006;6(6):34–6.

[97] Murphy J, Scott J, Kaufman D, Geller G, LeRoy L, Hudson K. Public expectations for return of results from large-cohort genetic research. Am J Bioeth 2008;8(11):36–43.

[98] Lemke AA, Wolf WA, Hebert-Beirne J, Smith ME. Public and biobank participant attitudes toward genetic research participation and data sharing. Public Health Genomics 2010;13:368–77.

[99] Shalowitz DI, Miller FG. Disclosing individual results of clinical research: implications of respect for participants. JAMA 2005;294(6):737–40.

[100] Partridge AH, Burstein HJ, Gelman RS, Marcom PK, Winer EP. Do patients participating in clinical trials want to know study results? J Nat Canc Inst 2003;95(6):491–2.

[101] Fernandez CV, Weijer C. Obligations in offering to disclose genetic research results. Am J Bioeth 2006;6(6):44–6.

[102] National Bioethics Advisory Commission. Research involving human biological materials: ethical issues and policy guidance. Available from: <http://bioethics. georgetown.edu/nbac/pubs.html>; 1999.

[103] Council for International Organization of Medical Sciences (CIOMS): International ethical guidelines for biomedical research involving human subjects. Geneva: (2002). Available from: <http://www.cioms.ch/frame_guidelines_nov_2002.htm>.

[104] Council for International Organization of Medical Sciences (CIOMS): International guidelines for ethical review of epidemiological studies. Geneva: (1991). Available from: <http://www.cioms.ch/frame_1991_texts_of_guidelines.htm>.

[105] Council of Europe: Additional protocol to the convention on human rights and biomedicine concerning biomedical research. Strasbourg: 2004. Available from: <http:// www.assembly.coe.int/ASP/Doc/XrefATDetails_E.asp?FileID=17221>.

[106] UNESCO, International Bioethics Committee (IBE): International declaration on human genetic data. Paris, 2003. Available from: <http://portal.unesco.org/en/ ev.php-URL_ID=17720&URL_DO=DO_TOPIC&URL_SECTION=201.html>.

[107] World Health Organization (WHO): Genetic databases; assessing the benefits and the impact on human and patient rights. Geneva: 2003. Available from: <http://www. law.ed.ac.uk/ahrb/publications/online/whofinalreport.doc>.

[108] Medical Research Council (MRC): Human tissue and biological samples for use in research–operational and ethical guidelines. London, 2001. Available from: <http:// www.mrc.ac.uk/pdf-tissue_guide_fin.pdf>.

[109] Consortium on Pharmacogenetics: Ethical and regulatory issues in research and clinical practice. Minneapolis, 2002. Available from: <http://www.bioethics.umn.edu/ News/pharm_report.pdf>.

[110] Berg K. The ethics of benefit sharing. Clin Genet 2001;59:240–3.

[111] Ndebele P, Musesengwa R. Will developing countries benefit from their participation in genetics research? Malawi Med J 2008;20:67–9.

[112] HUGO Ethics Committee, Statement on benefit sharing. Available from: <http:// www.hugo-international.org/hugo/benefit.html>; 2000.

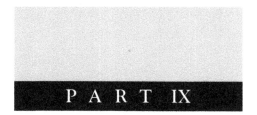

P A R T IX

HUMAN RESOURCES PLANNING

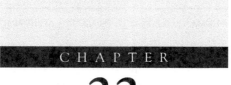

Long-Term Human Resources Planning for Alzheimer's Disease Trials

Nadina C. Jose[1], Lorne Cheeseman[2] and Stephanie Danandjaja[3]

[1]Anidan Inc, Singapore [2]Anidan Inc, Irvine, California, USA
[3]Sanofi, Singapore

Global aging is driving a marked increase in the prevalence of Alzheimer's disease (AD). A 2012 report, "Dementia: A Public Health Priority," [1] notes that "35.6 million people worldwide are living with dementia." It further estimates nearly 7.7 million new cases of dementia each year worldwide. That is nearly three times as many new cases as for HIV/AIDS (2.6 million per year) [2]. Assuming that incidence increases align with prevalence, by 2050 the annual increase could be 24.6 million new cases, with an average annual increase between 2010 and 2050 of 16.15 million. In addition to the 36 million people now living with dementia, we could have 646 million new cases during that 40-year period.

22.1 ADDRESSING THE URGENT NEED TO DEVELOP AD TREATMENTS

By 2050, the number of people who have lived with dementia over 40 years could reach 682 million. That number emphasizes the urgency of developing a cure or treatments that can delay the onset or progression of the disease. Pharmaceutical, biotech, and device companies are in various stages of developing new products that can help healthcare

M. Bairu & M.W. Weiner (Eds):
Global Clinical Trials for Alzheimer's Disease.
DOI: http://dx.doi.org/10.1016/B978-0-12-411464-7.00022-5

providers manage this rapidly growing public health priority. When planning global clinical trials, those companies have an obligation to create a solid infrastructure of clinical study teams that can navigate the variety of challenges presented by different countries and cultures.

A table in the "World Alzheimer Report" [3] shows the estimated prevalence of dementia regions with aging populations. Increased numbers of AD diagnoses are appearing in low and middle income countries of East and South Asia, Latin America, North Africa, and the Caribbean. Of the 1,188 AD studies found on ClinicalTrials.gov, 186 are being conducted in emerging nations: 112 in East Asia, 39 in South America, 9 in Southeast Asia, and 26 in Africa [4]. The numbers will continue to grow as more products enter development. Planning and implementing clinical trials in these regions must include planning for a sustainable workforce.

22.2 THE CHALLENGES OF EMERGING MARKETS

Creating a clinical research team involves recruitment, selection, hiring, training, and retaining the best possible team. Finding the right people for each position and building a competent team takes care in any setting. Each step in that process has unique challenges in each emerging market. A major emerging market is China, and clinical research organizations (CROs) can learn valuable lessons from clinical research professionals who have worked there.

22.2.1 Lessons Learned

Managing studies in large emerging countries like China and India can be time-consuming. Depending upon its type and scope, an AD study may require added resources in headquarters to ensure that there is enough qualified staff to support the local staff. Resource needs likewise increase with increases in the number of countries, because of each country's unique complexities and issues. Matters can grow even more complicated when the sponsor organization must deal with such country-specific items as clinical trial agreements, budgets, consent forms, investigational product import licenses, and translations. All of those factors have an impact on resourcing in terms of the time it takes to get them set up and completed—not to mention the time it takes for the documents to be reviewed and approved by the respective entities that handle them. Knowing in advance and having a full understanding of what is needed lessens the risk of delays and making the wrong choices.

22.3 HUMAN RESOURCES PLANNING FOR CLINICAL TRIALS IN CHINA

Conducting clinical trials in China is increasingly popular, but a multitude of human resource challenges arise when it comes to staffing trials there. Initial challenges during recruiting are followed by challenges in training the staff. All clinical trials teams need continuity through the trial, and retaining good staff presents unique challenges in China. Experience conducting clinical trials in China can teach important lessons that help improve the outcomes going forward.

Patient demographics and market potential make China an attractive region for conducting clinical trials. Although both of those attractions are valid, subtle and not so subtle forces in China can make it difficult to access its potential. While the availability of experienced staff is improving, it is not yet at the level found in regions such as North America and Europe. China's cultural approach to medical treatment includes the parallel use of traditional medicine alongside Western medicine. Consequently, diagnoses and standards of care may be quite different than in Western countries; and this is particularly the case for chronic central nervous system disorders such as AD.

Not only does considerable disparity exist between the level of medical care in the more developed and the less developed areas of the country, but it also exists between the treatment of poor patients and affluent patients within specific areas. The country's considerable nationalism leads to prejudiced decisions about the medicines that will and will not be available in hospital formularies. Although that prejudice is not a critical issue for clinical trials, it can cause a great many problems in the eventual marketing of a needed drug that may drive the placement of such a clinical trial in China. These forces form a backdrop that must be considered in any discussion about human resources for trials in China.

22.3.1 Recruiting Staff

Two demographic aspects are important to consider when recruiting staff in China. First, because of the large population, any open request for applications is likely to result in a large number of responses. That makes it necessary to plan for adequate resources to deal with the response and to have those resources in place. Second, because Chinese culture is driven by relationships between people, it is important to recognize that people are always more comfortable dealing with or working with someone they know. Although established relationship networks are important, it is possible to build new networks with the proper attention and time. Despite China being a developing country, it is critically important to maintain all sponsor organization standards for recruiting and staff quality. That is the reason for this focus on specific nuances of the process in China.

22.3.1.1 Dealing with High Rate of Responses

Most clinical trials conducted in China will have a coordinating or lead principal investigator (PI). The lead PI is an extremely important resource for the clinical trial or program being considered. This PI should be consulted early in the process for recommendations about key staff. Although the PI's recommendations may not always be suitable, it is important to give serious consideration to any candidates who meet the requirements for the roles to be filled. Likewise, it is important to consult staff members already part of the organization in China for their possible recommendations. It is, of course, necessary to take care to ensure that the people recommended will fit in with the larger study team and the culture of the sponsor organization.

22.3.1.2 Advantage of Response Rate

Along with the likelihood of a great many responses to job postings comes the opportunity for a high degree of selectivity. In China, most positions at the clinical research associate (CRA) level and higher can be filled with medical school graduates who have at least a couple of years' experience practicing in a hospital setting. Some might also have experience working with a multinational company. As a result of this initial experience, they should be fluent in spoken and written English. This competency should be thoroughly tested during the interview and should include talking with a native English speaker as part of the process. If this cannot be done in person, conducting such an interview by phone is also a good test, because once the project is running many interactions will take place by telephone. Furthermore, telephone sound quality may not be optimal, so it is important to ascertain that potential staff will be able to carry on a conversation under less than ideal conditions.

22.3.1.3 Initiative and Judgment Assessment

Time zone differences between China and North America or Europe mean that staff in China are often required to take the initiative in situations when no one at the sponsor organization is available. The sponsor organization needs to trust their far-flung staff's ability to handle those situations. That means it is important during the recruiting process to test or check applicants for initiative and judgment so you can be comfortable in these inevitable situations. Even when senior managers may be available in the same time zone, communication may not always be possible because international dialing on phones at hospitals or on mobile phones is still rare.

22.3.1.4 *Hiring Experienced vs. Entry-Level Candidates*

Depending on its long-term plans in China, a sponsor organization may find it preferable to recruit entry-level staff even when experienced CRAs are available. The quality of previous experience varies so widely that previous training may be useless and may even prove detrimental to further staff development. It could include learning bad habits that may be difficult to overcome. If the goal of a sponsor organization is to build a long-term CRO in China, then bringing on entry-level staff can be important. It requires an investment in training, but offers advantages in retaining staff.

22.3.1.5 *Hiring for the Long-Term*

To attract the best candidates, the hiring or sponsor organization needs to make itself attractive. The Chinese job market is hypercompetitive and compensation and benefits span a wide range of levels. Starting salaries are extremely low by Western standards, but rise quickly to levels similar to or even higher than those in Europe and North America. The importance of the speedy salary increases is that newly hired staff members expect to climb this ladder quickly. If they do not see an opportunity to do so they will go to competitors that offer better opportunities. It is not uncommon for entry-level staffers with less than a year with an organization to be offered double the salary by a competitor. Retaining staff in that environment is difficult but not impossible.

22.3.2 Retaining Staff Takes Commitment—on both Sides

22.3.2.1 *Organizational Commitment*

Potential employees in China are looking for many of the same opportunities as staff anywhere in the world. They seek

- to work for a reputable company, which in China means a well-known multinational company,
- an opportunity for high quality training to develop their skills,
- opportunities to grow and advance within the company, and
- international interaction with opportunities to travel outside of China on business.

Do not underestimate the considerable commitment to a staff; factor the costs and benefits of that commitment into any decision to establish and build a local presence. A potentially more affordable way to make international opportunities available to new employees is to station foreign experts in China or to bring them in as regular visitors. When recruiting key staff, it can be a definite advantage to emphasize the importance of the position by including a senior manager from the sponsor organization in the process.

22.3.2.2 *Employee Commitment*

An effective way to retain staff can be an employment contract that provides foreign assignments or training in exchange for the employee's commitment to stay with the company for a specified time period or be required to repay some of the travel and training expenses. Chinese staff members understand the value of foreign experience and the costs involved. They will generally accept a contractual agreement to be offered such opportunities. This can be an important tool not only for building local experience, but also for gaining the loyalty of key staff. With global organizations and projects, the cost and logistical challenges can make it tempting to omit Chinese staff from global meetings. Meeting those challenges, however, can pay off with retention of loyal staff members. It is important to weigh the costs of an individual project against the long-term benefits to the organization of staff development and retention.

Conducting clinical studies in China can cost less than performing them in North America or Europe. Still, during the strategic planning that precedes establishing a clinical trial organization in China, it is important to consider and plan for all the costs involved. Although recruiting and retaining staff in China can be a challenge, it is possible to build and maintain a high quality CRO there and to conduct high quality clinical trials. Case Study 22.1 shows how one organization accomplished team retention.

CASE STUDY 22.1 RETAINING A CLINICAL RESEARCH TEAM IN CHINA

A multinational company was running several projects in China. Within two years, three lead CRAs were promoted to clinician–study managers. For two years, a lead CRA with foreign experience was positioned full-time in China and worked alongside the clinician–study managers, company CRAs, and CRO-contracted CRAs. The lead CRA's assignment was to provide on-the-ground training and experience to the whole team and to facilitate interactions between the clinical teams in China and the US headquarters of the company. All three of the trainees were able to travel to the US to meet with colleagues on their respective projects, trips that included opportunities for training at US headquarters offices. One of them eventually transferred to the US headquarters, and all three remain with the company after more than 15 years.

22.3.3 Planning to Meet Staffing Challenges

Although staffing clinical trials teams in China presents a number of challenges, many strategies and tactics are available to meet those challenges. Some of them are outlined in Case Studies 22.2 and 22.3. The cost savings resulting from conducting trials in China and other emerging markets also provide resources to invest in the staff in ways that can increase retention and raise quality. Cultural and linguistic differences can make it easy to slip down to lower standards. So, no matter in what location the trials are conducted, remember the importance of adhering to global processes and standards.

22.3.4 Recruitment and Selection Lessons from China

With global standards in mind, managers rarely, if ever, underestimate the importance of training. Most know that comprehensive training is especially important in emerging markets, where new recruits generally have less applicable experience than is customary in North America or Europe. In such regions, it is critical to make thorough plans for delivering robust foundation-level training. Careful planning includes

CASE STUDY 22.2 REGIONAL TRAINER FOR A CRO

A CRO with operations in Asia had a trainer based in Singapore for the Asia Pacific region. At first, training was part of individual country budgets. That budgeting was seen to be unfair because it resulted in a disparity in the amount provided for training in different countries in the region. Another inequality resulted because the trainer was based in Singapore, and that office had a different cost basis for training. Local country managers in China worked with the regional headquarters for a central budget. Once the budget was managed by the regional training organization, that group became responsible for providing the same level of training to all the countries in its region. They struck a balance: Key staff traveled to Singapore for some training and the trainer traveled throughout the region to provide staff training at individual offices. That training approach resulted in opportunities for several staff members in the China office to advance to more senior positions that previously were unavailable to them. As a further benefit, the region could then offer additional services in China while also reducing staff changes—because employees saw opportunities for advancement in the organization.

CASE STUDY 22.3 TAG-TEAMING STRATEGY FOR A FAST-ENROLLING STUDY

The time to completion was critical for a study team in China conducting a large Phase III study. So they were concerned about the possible impact of changes to the study team. The study was to be fast-enrolling and conducted at only a relatively few sites, so the team decided to have two study managers and give the CRAs overlapping responsibilities for site monitoring. This ensured that each site had at least two CRAs assigned. Having two study managers meant better coverage for meetings with UK- and US-based headquarters, even when meetings took place outside of China's regular business hours. Some staff changes took place during the study, which also had several sick leave absences. Despite those setbacks, the redundancies outlined above were key to on-time completion of a study with an aggressive timeline.

consideration of language and cultural barriers. Otherwise, the result can be very different understandings of the training materials presented, particularly with the kind of remote self-training that has become common in our industry.

Language and culture are two factors often identified as risks when recruiting candidates who will best fit into an organization. Traditionally, sponsors will choose someone who originated from the country who just happened to be the perfect fit for the position, based on the person's qualifications and, more importantly, who is familiar with the culture and language. Sometimes, the choice of a team leader that is intuitively logical to corporate managers can backfire. Many managers have been surprised to learn that it's not always as effective to send a person to their country of origin. In some instances, there exist unrecognized stereotyping by the locals. Expectations of immediate engagement are only sometimes fulfilled. Similar issues can arise when corporate managers send a person to a region like Asia, where economic disparity is wide. Problems can arise when a team leader who has become an American or European citizen is assigned to the country where people of his or her ethnicity are generally blue-collar workers. When that leader exercises authority, local stereotyping can sabotage interactions.

22.4 RESULTS THROUGH TRAINING AND RETRAINING

Regular comprehensive training programs, followed up with retraining and assessment of trainees' comprehension, are important when working with staff in emerging markets. Training programs and their anticipated costs require careful planning. Because each person's learning style differs, it is important to combine different training methods to better reach each staff member. A strategic approach, for example, might include remote self-training, webinars, classroom training, specialized external training, and on-the-job training. That kind of coordinated planning not only develops staff competencies for conducting high quality clinical research but can also be a powerful retention tool (Case Study 22.1).

The same training provided to global staff must be available to staff members based in the emerging market—and with the same completion expectations. This may require such investments as creating IT training delivery options and even sending trainers to the far-flung site of the proposed new project. As much as possible, train staff everywhere in the world the same way.

When using in-person trainers, compare the cost of sending the staff to a central location against sending a trainer to the country where the trainees will be assigned. Balancing the costs for optimal efficiency and effectiveness differs with the level of training required in each specific situation (Case Study 22.2). Training programs require early planning. Travel plans, whether for trainers or trainees, involve passports and visas, and arrangements for transportation and lodging. Those logistics take time.

When staff members in an emerging country receive training similar to that of people elsewhere in the organization, it increases the likelihood that a company will enjoy greater staff retention. That has certainly been the case in China, where staff members appreciate such efforts at parity (see Case Study 22.1). That makes it important to budget for these expenses when planning a new project. Because training expense is likely to be a larger portion of the budget for a branch operation than for the global organization, it may be more difficult to maintain. The location of those funds in that organizational budget can make a crucial difference in ensuring carry-through for staff training.

22.4.1 Informal Training Opportunities

A great many excellent training opportunities can ensure that staff meet high standards of quality—*and* stay with your organization. Maximize interactions with colleagues from other countries by encouraging frequent contact, which can include individualized teleconferences. For example, some organizations found it highly desirable to send an international team to China to provide on-the-job training in the office and in the field. An organization with a dedicated training group can plan to spend time in an emerging market and provide both standardized group training and one-to-one work with individuals.

When a company's commitment to a region and the size of its programs justify it, placing long-term international staff there can provide extra value. It may not be easy to find someone for such an assignment; it requires a significant commitment from both the individual involved and the organization. Yet the company's return on investment—in quality of work and long-term staff loyalty—may far outweigh the initial cost and difficulty. By working alongside staff day by day, a person in that role can also create understanding across cultural and language barriers.

22.5 ENSURING CONTINUITY THROUGHOUT THE TRIAL

Staff change in any clinical trial is disruptive and can have a negative impact on quality. Because relationships are so important in business dealings in China, the impact of personnel changes can be even greater. To avoid as many of those problems as possible, try the retention steps described in Case Study 22.2. Additional steps, such as tag-teaming (Case Study 22.3) and ensuring that adequate handovers are in place can help to minimize disruption from inevitable changes (Figure 22.1). As with any study, it is important to ensure that up-to-date documentation is appropriately filed. Then, when a person leaves, the incoming staff member will have access to a complete, up-to-date picture of the study status. That kind of preparation is the best way to minimize disruption. Your organization's systems can make it more or less difficult to follow-up on study documentation status in an emerging market.

When a global trial master file (TMF) system is in place, it should include a follow-up plan for the status of documentation in any particular region, and a plan for keeping the documentation up to date. That means there must be a way to put metrics in place for filing monitoring reports, and a plan for regular TMF reviews for completeness. Any localized TMF should have a plan for regular reviews or even audits. Central study management should be provided with regular reports on the completeness of records. Electronic data capture (EDC) or clinical trial management systems (CTMS) can be helpful for centralizing data; but those systems need an oversight plan to ensure that data flow is timely and complete.

Once study sites start to enroll, in some areas—and particularly in China—the enrollment rate can be quite high. Thus it is feasible to have multiple staff working on a single study or at a single site. That introduces the possibility of tag-teaming or duplicating resources (Case Study 22.3). With that kind of staff redundancy, when a member leaves the organization at least one other is already familiar with the study and its

Risk Management Plan

RISK NUMBER Enter a unique number to be used as an identifier when implementing mitigation	RISK CATEGORY List focus areas	PROBABILITY The likelihood than an event will occur, described as: LOW <30% probability MEDIUM 31–64% probability HIGH >65% probability	IMPACT Identifies the impact of a positive or negative event on patient safety, data quality, timelines, ethics, study conduct, study product registration and launching; described as: LOW <30% negative or positive impact MEDIUM 31%–64% negative or positive impact HIGH > 65% negative or positive impact	RISK OWNER Accountable party responsible for monitoring, controlling, and updating the status of the risk throughout the project lifecycle. The person who generates risk mitigation and contingency strategies performs the cost–benefit analysis of proposed strategies, and determines which risks require mitigation and when to activate the contingency plan.	RISK MITIGATION Defines the specific action to take in order to prevent, minimize, or manage the risk while ensuring that patient safety is not compromised, and data quality is preserved, without jeopardizing either study product registration or launch.	COUNTRY LEVEL RISKS Please score: LOW 1 MEDIUM 3 HIGH 5	STUDY LEVEL RISKS Please score: LOW 1 MEDIUM 3 HIGH 5	COMMENTS
	Site Issues							
SUBTOTAL						0	0	
	Study Start-up							
SUBTOTAL						0	0	
	Recruitment/Retention							
SUBTOTAL						0	0	
	Monitoring							
SUBTOTAL						0	0	
	Study Management							
SUBTOTAL						0	0	
	Close Out							
SUBTOTAL						0	0	

Summary

Risk Categories	Country Level Risk	Study Level Risk
Site Issues	0	0
Study Start-Up	0	0
Recruitment / Retention	0	0
Monitoring	0	0
Study Management	0	0
Close Out	0	0

FIGURE 22.1 Sample risk management plan.

status. Although facilities may be relatively crowded at sites, particularly in China, usually no one objects to having more than one clinical monitor at the site.

Labor laws in China are very specific; they require that contract terms be in place and that the contract covers the specifics of notice periods, which are mandated at 30 days. Contracts can also stipulate repayment of training and travel expenses upon early termination, which may also be a deterrent to staff resignations. Additional aspects may be related to individual work dossiers in China. This differs significantly from most of the United States, where "at will" labor laws are common. Contractual requirements for certain notice periods can be used to reduce the effects of staff changes. Wherever you plan to set up a clinical trials organization, it is advisable to consult a human resources expert. An HR expert can provide information that can help to ensure that employment contracts comply with that country's labor laws.

22.6 DIFFERENT PLANS FOR DIFFERENT PLACES

Compliance with local laws is a necessity. Although it is not a legal obligation, it is a major training advantage to plan a training program that addresses cultural diversity. A good start for such a program is cultural immersion for the trainers.

An immersion curriculum should include illustrations and demonstrations of pertinent body language, facial expressions, and acceptable hand signals, words to use and words to avoid using. Because English is rarely the trainees' primary language, corporate staff needs, at minimum, a basic awareness of how to interpret the meaning when, for example, a local says *yes* or *no*. Do they understand their assent or refusal in the same way that the trainer does? When locals nod their heads in agreement, they may really be saying "maybe"—or even, "I'll go along with that for now so I won't displease you." Effective training requires thorough planning following the steps outlined in Table 22.1.

When English is not an employee's primary language, misunderstandings can easily occur. Team leaders and subordinates from different cultures may have entirely different attitudes toward communication difficulties. If an employee's culture defines *honor* as *saving face*, both the employee and the supervisor need a whole new skill set for verbal communication. When those skills are not yet developed, both parties could use the same dictionary or thesaurus. In that situation, written memos and instructions can be effective, though not foolproof.

Recognize that most developing countries are patriarchal societies. When corporate leadership is managed in a matrix environment rather than a hierarchical arrangement, local employees will find that alien to

TABLE 22.1   Some Steps to Ensure Effective Training

Research the country	Read about the country and inform yourself about its: demographics, terrain, business environment; school, banking, and political systems; food, holidays, and religion; local customs, traditions, and common spoken phrases. Interview people from the country to get current "real life" information.
Build relationships	Build a relationship with some local people. Be willing to experience them in their territory. Get to know their ways. Eat their food. Refrain from complaining about the weather or anything that appears illogical from your point of view.
Be open to learning	Be open to learning and to adapting. Couple that with developing the patience to let things run their course according to the pace of life in the country. Know when to push the agenda and when to take things more slowly, lest you delude yourself into thinking that you got through to local people, only to find out later that they were not truly engaged.
Give clear instructions	Use checklists and flow charts to provide accurate visual descriptions of what the instructions mean.
Delineate tasks simply	Delineate tasks simply. Identify responsibilities and accountabilities in an organized format that is easy to understand. One way is to use the RACI format.
Avoid colloquialisms	Avoid using "sayings," American or European proverbs or colloquialisms, any of which can cause misunderstandings and confusion.
Assign appropriate tasks	When you know that "saving face" can come first, assign tasks that you know local people can perform. Be realistic when planning which tasks to assign; it is better to ease newly hired staff into their roles rather than throwing them in to "sink or swim."

the management style they grew up with. Therefore, it is important to teach local teams how that unfamiliar system works. Otherwise, delays in engagement and subsequent performance are inevitable. A preferable alternative to failure is to avoid forcing a strange new system on a local team by creating, when possible, a hybrid environment.

22.7 ADAPTING AND APPLYING LESSONS TO OTHER MARKETS

Key elements to consider in building these clinical study teams are processes for recruiting, selecting, training, developing, and retaining these human resources. The same key elements have a profound impact on identifying investigative site teams to conduct trials in various regions. Scientific, ethical, business, economic, and cultural drivers are external factors that also influence human resource planning. Those

CASE STUDY 22.4 MONITORING TEAM SET-UP DIFFICULTIES IN INDIA

A regional head for Asia was assigned to set up monitoring teams in four countries: India, Singapore, Taiwan, and Korea. A feasibility checklist served as a guide for identifying the requirements for each country (Table 22.2). Next, to streamline the structure to be built in each country, a baseline risk management plan was developed (Figure 22.2). Together, Asia's regional head and the corporate manager developed a training plan and established a six-month timeline for setting up the monitoring teams. The timeline was based on information produced during study feasibility. Of the four countries, India was the country that had difficulty in meeting the timelines. A debriefing identified several issues at the root of India's delays.

Root Causes

Because of an inefficient process for reviewing candidates, it took three months for local human resources staff to shortlist the candidates for seven positions:

- One project manager
- Three senior contract research associates (CRAs) with at least two years of experience
- Two clinical project assistants (CPAs) with at least two years of experience, and
- One regulatory affairs manager.

In addition, the process was launched when several concurrent festivals were taking place, which meant people were not available for interviews.

Background checks and steps to validate applicants' resumes revealed that quite a number of applicants had falsified their credentials and training information.

Half of the shortlisted applicants failed when tested on their knowledge of the guidelines. Although they interviewed well, they could not describe the practical application of the guidelines. Because the scenarios presented were of the kind that forced thinking "outside of the box," the interviewer could tell that those applicants had memorized the information without really understanding its meaning. The regional head had failed to recognize that India's education system is very traditional and rote. Evidence of analytical thinking was rare among those applicants.

The ability of potential team members in India to be transparent was noted at an all-time low: just 30%. This indicates that they can answer honestly only when they perceive no possibility that they could lose face or appear to have limited knowledge.

State employment laws kept changing which confused everyone.

When the set-up of the monitoring team in India was finally completed, the next hurdle was ensuring the quality of the work. Quality was, and continues to be, a major factor to watch when conducting trials in India.

In 2012, most pharmaceutical and biotech companies reversed their view of India as a "go-to country." Although it still offers accessibility to large numbers of potential subjects and has a growing community of trained clinical trial sites, it is currently labeled as an "on-hold country." Among the reasons for that are political instability, poor intellectual property protection, an unreliable DCGI (India's version of FDA), and fraud. With no improvement in those situations on the near horizon, the chance that new studies will commence in India is severely limited.

TABLE 22.2 Going Global with AD Clinical Trials

Why Go Global?	Identify and Describe Key Business and Scientific Drivers For Global Trials

To evaluate potential clinical trial locations, a company needs answers to specific questions for each country under consideration.	What are the country's:
	 • AD prevalence rates?
	 • healthcare practice standards, including the medical community's general view of AD, its standard of care?
	
	 What is the availability and affordability of:
	 • trained clinical trial sites with trained staff?
	 • approved products for AD?
	 • adequate diagnostic facilities and specialty practitioners such as raters?
	
	 Important questions to ask about the environment, economics, politics and government, and culture of a potential clinical trial location include:
	     Is the country susceptible to regular natural disasters?
	     What is the political and economic environment?
	     How many holidays are observed each year?
	     What are the country's business practices?
	     What is the potential for currency fluctuations?
	     What is the predominant religion?
	     What language is spoken there?
	     What is the general public's attitude toward AD?
	     What is the quality of caregiver support?
	     What other cultural customs (gender roles, hierarchical structures), traditions, and/or sensitivities can affect work there?

RACI* Table for Study A

	Task	PM	Lead CRA	CRA	CPA	MM	CRO	Comments
	PRE-STUDY							
1	Proposal on study cost and resource allocation including outsourcing needs							
2	Feasibility activities							
3	Site communication and collection of feasibility information							
4	Site selection							
5	Protocol finalization							
6	Vendor selection / contracting (CRO, central lab, etc.)							
7	Set up CTIMS, IVRS, EDC, ePRO etc.							
	STUDY START-UP							
8	Country regulatory and health care authority handling							
9	Monitoring Plan							
10	Data Management Plan							
11	Risk Management Plan							
12	Clinical trial agreement preparation, negotiation, finalization with sites							
13	Vendor management and oversight plan							
14	Essential document preparation, EC/IRB coordination							
15	Documents translation							
16	CRF design, completion and creation of completion guidelines							
17	Investigational product management							
18	Supply management							
19	Study team training							
20	Organization/coordinate investigators meeting							
21	Site initiation visits							
	STUDY CONDUCT							
22	Project and Study Budget management							
23	Study monitoring							
24	Data tracking							
25	Safety monitoring							
26	Issues tracking, management and disposition							
27	Site management							
28	Trial master file management							
29	EC/IRB management							
30	Country regulatory, healthcare authority coordination							
31	Investigational product management							
32	Vendor Oversight Plan implementation and tracking							
	STUDY CLOSE-OUT							
33	Site Close-out activities							
34	Finalize study payments							
35	Trial master file management							
36	EC/IRB close-out letter							
37	Investigational product handling and disposition							
38	Data clean up, database lock							
39	Study files archiving							
40	Study team debriefing							

*RACI terminology

R: **Responsible** - persons who perform the task
A: **Accountable** - person(s) ultimately accountable for correct and thorough completion of the deliverable or task; person to whom R is accountable
C: **Consulted** - those whose opinions are sought
I: **Informed** - manager(s) kept up to date - often only upon completion of a task or deliverable

This living document will be used only for Study A. Its scope: Pre-study to Study Close-out. It can be amended as tasks are added or task ownership is revised.

Study Team
PM: **Project Manager**
Lead CRA: **Lead Clinical Research Associate**
CRA: **Clinical Research Associate**
CPA: **Clinical Project Assistant**
MM: **Medical Monitor**

FIGURE 22.2   Sample RACI.

influencing factors must also mesh with the regulatory-driven requirements to demonstrate effectiveness in different populations and regions where these myriad drugs, biologics, and devices will eventually be marketed. All are factors that further drive the trend toward globalization. Case Study 22.4 and Table 22.2 enumerate and describe steps to take that can minimize set-up complications.

Systems and solutions that leverage technology will likewise come into play to increase efficiency and manage overall operational risks. That is because, ultimately, the budget determines which systems and solutions can be used to meet the overarching goal of on-time completion of the clinical trials.

22.8 OPTIMIZING THE WORKFORCE

The pharmaceutical, biotech, and device industries need to be able to rely on the data's integrity coupled with their scientific validity in an ethically compliant, completed clinical trial wherever it was conducted. That means that creating certain benchmarks may vary because of differences in the socio-cultural, economic, and healthcare environments. When planning global clinical trials in various areas, researchers must also consider differences in the epidemiologic characteristics of AD between highly developed countries like the United States and Canada and developing countries with lower and middle income populations. In developing countries, such conditions as diabetes, heart disease, and infectious diseases are higher priorities than AD. Thus, the workforce required to support trials in so-called emerging regions will not be as robustly experienced and trained in conducting AD clinical trials.

In areas where there is a paucity of skilled and therapeutically experienced personnel, sponsors can opt to use local CROs or what some may call "boutique or niche CROs." This type of CRO is usually known for being "specialized" in a particular disease area. Criteria for outsourcing to a local CRO will have to be more stringent, with specific focus on three key areas: (1) depth of disease area experience of CRO staff and sites used; (2) level of training given to each CRO staff member and the sites they use; and (3) degree of quality control systems, including experience in implementing risk management plans. Table 22.3 lists some examples of local CROs.

One may argue that conducting and managing any clinical trial—regardless of phase, therapeutic area, and size—has International Conference on Harmonization-Good Clinical Practices (ICH-GCP) as its foundation. It is, nevertheless, the nature and specificity of the requirements and procedures, and the ability to provide statistically significant results, that sponsors need to have sites fulfill reliably and expertly.

TABLE 22.3 Local Contract Research Organizations in Asia

Gleneagles CRC Pte Ltd	www.gleneaglescrc.com Full service CRO and SMO with headquarters in Singapore, covering Asia and Australia
VCRO (Virginia Contract Research Organization Co. Ltd)	www.vcro.com.tw Taiwan-based, full serviced, covering Japan, China, Singapore, Hong Kong, Korea, and Southeast Asia
Prodia The CRO	www.prodiathecro.com First full service CRO in Indonesia, including central laboratory services
SiroClinPharm Pvt. Ltd	www.siroclinpharm.com Full service CRO with corporate headquarters in India and headquarters in Germany and the USA
Tigermed	www.tigermed.net Largest full serviced CRO in China based in Hangzou
LSK Global PS	www.lskglobal.com Korean full service CRO
Cognitech Clinical Research, Inc.	www.cognitechresearch.com Philippines-based full service CRO
CMIC Holdings	www.cmic-holdings.co.jp Full service Japanese CRO with Southeast Asian companies in Korea, China, Taiwan and Singapore

22.9 HUMAN RESOURCES PLANNING FOR CLINICAL STUDIES IN DEVELOPING COUNTRIES

Conducting clinical trials in developing countries generally means working with limited resources while trying to reach target enrollment and collect data of acceptable quality. Few people in those nations have the skills to run clinical trials that meet international standards, because trials are usually done in the same centers over and over, and the same teams repeatedly manage similar studies. In addition, few neuroscience studies have been done in developing countries. Sometimes that is because necessary diagnostic tests are too costly for the sites; sometimes because questionnaires have not been validated to the local conditions. These factors are compounded by the scarcity of study team members (on the investigator's or sponsor's side) experienced in any neurology-related studies.

To plan and form the right team for an AD study, it is important to consider several factors:

- the study volunteer's journey from diagnosis to maintenance,
- the relevant social and/or government support and management (if any),

- the cultural view of AD subjects that their families and countrymen hold, and
- specific requirements of the institutions that manage the study subjects.

22.9.1 Subject's Journey

In some countries, a neurologist or a psychiatrist (sometimes even an internist or geriatric medicine specialist) manages AD. They may coordinate with other specialists only when mental or neurological complications arise. By identifying who will first make the diagnosis and who will manage the subject later on, we can identify the correct study team member covering the right specialties and subject journey points. It may be necessary for the study investigators to be a team of psychiatrists, neurologists, and/or internists, with the managing specialist as the PI. Multispecialty teams like this may not yet be available in the institutions chosen as study sites. Consequently, the study will need a coordinator—not only to coordinate the investigators, but also to coordinate the nurses and social workers who support the subjects and help ensure that treatment is properly maintained and monitored.

22.9.2 Government Support

If AD is listed as one of the programs in the area where the study site is located, then healthcare professionals there are likely to be trained in the disease, and the institution will probably have an in-house process for diagnosing and managing AD. In this case, it is possible to select study team members who can adapt the institution's processes to accommodate the study protocol. The study coordinator should be able to help create an operating manual for subject management. In such cases, having government program support may also mean that the study team has more comprehensive management options available. That can be important when studying AD, or another disorder that benefits from multispecialty management. It might also simplify importing study products and supplying them to the sites.

If no AD program is available, then the investigator or coordinator should be someone with the authority to authorize conducting a study in the institution, even if no such program was previously available there. Sometimes that means the person must be able to convince the institution's management. In many instances, it means that the department head might have to be included as a study team member (or even a leader). In situations when referral or social supports are not readily available, other resources might be needed to support the subjects. Seeking potential undiagnosed subjects from general outpatient clinic

392 22. LONG-TERM HUMAN RESOURCES PLANNING FOR ALZHEIMER'S DISEASE TRIALS

records screening can require additional effort and resources, particularly when the protocol requires treatment-naïve subjects.

22.9.3 Cultural Acceptance

In most societies, AD is considered neither an embarrassment nor a taboo subject. Still, many people have no awareness of this neurological disorder and may think a friend or family member just has typical absent-mindedness. This can lead to denial about getting treatment—or even about seeking a diagnosis. Therefore, it is important that study team members can provide correct information and education to a potential subject and family members. An even more important qualification is the skill to communicate that information in a way that is suitable to the subject's cultural and social background. Skilled AD educators are still very rare, so the most suitable communicator might be a nurse or social worker rather than a physician.

Preparing the study team for optimal communication with subjects (and perhaps with related stakeholders) will require an investment in educational materials. Depending on the complexity of the study, the materials can be information that increases awareness, and facilitates monitoring of disease management and adverse events (e.g., through subject diaries, call centers), and instructions on how to respond to certain occurrences.

22.9.4 Institution Requirements

At sites where AD programs are available, the formal study team can be representatives of the program, and the whole system will be involved. Where there is no such program, however, the study team might have to involve all related function representatives to make the collaboration work practically and diplomatically. Bigger study teams require more sponsor support to coordinate the workflow and communication.

The situations above point to the possibility that a larger study team may be needed to compensate for the lack of structured programs led by skilled and experienced personnel in developing countries. In such a case, the sponsor's team will have more people to coordinate and more tasks to manage, which requires skillful project management. The extra human resource cost may not result in a higher cost per team, though, because individual wages are low in comparison with those for sites in developed countries.

This unique situation presents different challenges, however, because of frequent staff changes. When employees seeking career advancement and higher salaries leap from job to job, retraining becomes an

IX. HUMAN RESOURCES PLANNING

issue. Training must be offered more often, and that can make study progress choppy as key study people leave and are replaced. There are even times when a single person can be the life or death of a site, when there is really no suitable replacement person available in that area. In an area with such limited skilled personnel, it is critical to put in place a comprehensive risk management process. This process will ensure that emergency back-ups are available and comprehensive retraining can take place quickly. Sometimes the process can involve working with the institution to move in people from another department or speed up the hiring process. Similar arrangements are needed on the sponsor and CRO sides to make sure that study quality and operational controls do not falter while weathering the changes of its guardians.

Another unique challenge is the extra support needed for subjects and/or study sites. AD places a great burden on caregivers; the cost of caring for subjects may be huge, not just financially, but in the time needed for subject care. Many of those who enroll in the study are poor and may be referred to certain locales that provide "memory care," which are healthcare facilities far away from the study site. Some are even too poor to pay for the subject's and caregiver's transportation to the investigative site. In those cases, providing transport fees could be an important incentive for subjects to return regularly during the study. The same financial challenge can arise for laboratory tests and other tests considered routine in more developed countries and which are generally reimbursed by health insurance. In developing countries like Indonesia, subjects often must pay for testing out of their own pockets. To ensure that enough subjects enroll and stay through study completion and follow-up, a sponsor may need to pay in advance for testing. Reimbursement is unlikely to work because impoverished subjects are unlikely to have sufficient funds to wait for repayment.

Because magnetic resonance imaging (MRI) and positron emission tomography (PET) scans may be unavailable at the investigator's site, subjects may be referred to a centralized imaging laboratory, further increasing the cost of diagnosis. When a study requires biological marker or genetic testing, samples must be collected by suitable local laboratories, then sent to a central testing lab. Selecting a suitable lab requires considering not only the quality of its laboratory work, but also its handling of reagents, its sample distribution, and the quality of its travel and storage provisions. Where shipping samples out of a country requires government approval, the sponsor and/or site must have people who can navigate that process. Even then, the time needed for the government approval process may delay the study's start time.

To diagnose AD subjects, sponsors may have to pay for testing that excludes differential diagnoses. Even if such testing appears to be unrelated to the AD study, an incidental finding of dementia can reveal a potential subject. Without that diagnostic support, many subjects—and their physicians—may choose treatment based on empirical judgment. When investigators choose to maximize the use of limited resources works, it works to their advantage in identifying potential subjects.

Support for care outside of study treatment is another concern. The prognosis for AD can be affected by the quality of home care. Whether subjects have extended family support or the resources to provide adequate home care can affect the study outcome. Study teams may need to take action to neutralize significantly different levels of home care by providing social support, education for family members, and other appropriate steps.

References

[1] World Health Organization, Alzheimer's Disease International. Dementia: A Public Health Priority. [cited 2013 Jan 7]. Available from: <http://whqlibdoc.who.int/publications/2012/9789241564458_eng.pdf>.
[2] World Health Organization. Fast facts on HIV. [cited 2013 Jan 7]. Available from: <http://www.who.int/hiv/data/fast_facts/en/index.html>.
[3] Alzheimer's Disease International. World Alzheimer Report 2010: The Global Economic Impact of Dementia. Table 1, p. 15. [cited 2013 Jan 7]. Available from: <http://www.alz.co.uk/research/files/WorldAlzheimerReport2010.pdf>.
[4] ClinicalTrials.gov. [Internet] [cited January 2013]. Available from: <www.clinicaltrials.gov/ct2/results/map/click?map.x=762&map.y=62&term=Alzheimer's+Disease>.

Index

Note: Page numbers followed by "*f*", "*t*" and "*b*" refers to figures, tables and boxes respectively.

genetic/socio-demographic/socio-
economic, 5–7
lifestyle-related, 8–9
vascular, 7–8
total cases per country, prevalence of AD
vs., 161*t*–162*t*
Dementia Action Alliance (DAA), 27
Dementia India Report, 2010, 24–25
Dementia Management Law, 2012, 308
DIA. *See* Drug Information Association
(DIA)
Diabetes
as risk factor of dementia and AD, 7–8
DIAN study. *See* Dominantly Inherited
Alzheimer's Network (DIAN) study
Diet
and AD, 40–42
patients, and globalized trials, 68
Diffusion tensor imaging (DTI), 131–132,
139
acquisitions, 144–145
post-processing steps for, 145–146
measurements, multicenter variability of,
141–142
multicenter data, accuracy of, 146
Dimebon, 286
Disease-modifying drug (DMD)
clinical trials with, 163–168
active immunotherapy, 163–164
aim of, 169–170
Aβ anti-aggregants, 166
β-secretase, 166
χ-secretase, 165–166
passive immunotherapy, 164–165
global clinical trials of, 296–301, 298*t*–300*t*
DLB. *See* Lewy body dementia (DLB)
DNA (deoxyribonucleic acid)
variations, 330
Dominantly Inherited Alzheimer's
Network (DIAN) study, 12–13, 39, 89
Donepezil, 90
clinical development of, 291–295,
292*t*–294*t*
Drug Information Association (DIA), 209*b*
Drug Research Bylaws, 282
Drugs and Cosmetics Act 1940, 234–235
DTI. *See* Diffusion tensor imaging (DTI)

E
EADC. *See* European Alzheimer's Disease
Consortium (EADC)
Eastern Europe (EEu)
AD clinical trials in

conducting, countries in, 272–274
development and execution of,
emerging countries role in, 267–269,
267*f*, 268*f*
disease-modification treatment,
270–272
symptomatic therapy and, 270–272
overview, 263–264
prevalence of AD in, 264–267, 265*t*–266*t*
EC. *See* Ethics committee (EC)
Echo planar imaging (EPI) sequences,
141–142
EDPI. *See* European Dementia Prevention
Initiative (EDPI)
EDSD. *See* European DTI Study in
Dementia (EDSD)
Efficacy Working Party, EMA, 120
EMA. *See* European Medicines Agency
(EMA)
EMEA. *See* Evaluation of Medicinal
Products (EMEA)
Employee commitment, 380
ENCODE. *See* Encyclopedia of DNA
Elements Project (ENCODE)
Encyclopedia of DNA Elements Project
(ENCODE), 332
Enrollment, patient, 212–213
Ethical issues
global clinical trial and, 52–53
Ethics committee (EC), 280–281, 283–284
Ethnic difference
in drug development, 301–302
global clinical trials and, 54
European Alzheimer's Disease Consortium
(EADC), 147
European Dementia Prevention Initiative
(EDPI), 12
European DTI Study in Dementia (EDSD),
142
European Medicines Agency (EMA), 125,
259–261
Efficacy Working Party, 120
guidelines on dementia, 111
Qualification of Novel Methodologies for
Drug Development, 121–122
European Union (EU)
regulatory guidelines for AD, 120–122
and regulatory harmonization, 53
Evaluation of Medicinal Products (EMEA),
329–330
Exploitation, 366
Extrinsic differences, in international trials,
54

Positron emission tomography (PET), 131–132
  amyloid. *See* Amyloid PET
  goal of, 134
  quantitative imaging, requirement in, 137
  scanner, 137–138
Pravastatin, 81
Preclinical models, AD, 103–106
  vs. prodromal AD, 123–124
PreDIVA study. *See* Prevention of Dementia
    by Intensive Vascular care (PreDIVA)
    study
Presenilin-1 (PSEN1) gene, 12–13
Pre-study visit (PSV), 258
Pre-symptomatic treatment, AD, 12–13, 38–39
Prevalence, of AD, 3–4, 159–160
  in China, 247–248
  in Eastern Europe, 264–267, 265*t*–266*t*
  future projections, 14, 160*t*
Prevention, of AD
  defined, 34–35
  trials, 9–13, 37–40
Prevention of Dementia by Intensive
    Vascular care (PreDIVA) study, 11–12
Principal investigator (PI), 199
  role, and AD trials in China, 259–260
Privacy and Progress of Whole Genome
    Sequencing, 360–361
Prodromal AD. *See also* Mild cognitive
    impairment (MCI)
  preclinical AD *vs.*, 123–124
  treatment, 174–175
PROGRESS. *See* Perindopril Protection
    Against Recurrent Stroke Study
    (PROGRESS)
PROSPER (Prospective Study of Pravastatin
    in the Elderly at Risk) study, 81
PSEN1 gene. *See* Presenilin-1 (PSEN1) gene
PSF. *See* Point-spread function (PSF)
PSV. *See* Pre-study visit (PSV)
Psychometric assessments, 258–259
Pure placebo-controlled trial, 168–169
PVC. *See* Partial volume correction (PVC)
PVE. *See* Partial volume effect (PVE)
Pyritinole, 90–91

Q

Qualification of Novel Methodologies for
    Drug Development, EMA, 121–122
Quality of life (QoL), 64–66
Questionnaires
  implementation of, 303
  linguistic validation, 302–303

R

Randomized clinical trials (RCTs), 166
  for lewy body dementia, 285*b*
  Phase II/III, 285–287, 285*b*, 286*b*–287*b*
Randomized-Start Design, 91
Rater training, AD trials and, 170–171
RCTs. *See* Randomized clinical trials (RCTs)
Recruitment
  patient
    campaigns, 208–211
    caregivers and, 203–204
    cost of, 197–198
    as driver of globalization, 62
    educational material, 209*b*
    fighting fears with facts, 199–200
    market of, 197–199
    metrics to evaluate, 213*f*
    tactics, 206–208
    tips for, 207*b*
  staff, 377–379
    and commitment, 379–381
    demographic aspects, 377–378
    experienced *vs.* entry-level candidates,
      379
    response rates, 378
ReDeCAr. *See* Registry of Cognitive
    Pathologies in Argentina (ReDeCAr)
Registry of Cognitive Pathologies in
    Argentina (ReDeCAr), 223
Regulatory guidelines, for Alzheimer's
    disease, 111
  European, 120–122. *See also* European
    Medicines Agency (EMA)
  FDA, 122–124
Regulatory harmonization
  global clinical trials and, 53
Renal impairment, 108
Resource Utilization in Dementia (RUD),
    64–66
Retention, patient, 190–192
Risk/benefit ratio, 54
Risk factors, AD and dementia, 4–9, 6*t*
  genetic/socio-demographic/socio-
    economic, 5–7
  lifestyle-related, 8–9
  vascular, 7–8, 108
Risk factors, for vascular dementia, 108–109
Rivastigmine
  clinical development, difficulties with,
    295–296
Roche, 84–85
Rotterdam epidemiologic study, 80